WEIGHT LOSS
FOR LIFE

Lawrence J. Cheskin, MD, directed the Johns Hopkins Weight
Management Center for more than 30 years. He is currently an adjunct
professor at the Johns Hopkins School of Medicine and practices at
the Johns Hopkins Healthful Eating, Activity & Weight Program. He
is also professor and chair of the Department of Nutrition and Food
Studies at George Mason University's College of Health and Human
Services.

Kimberly A. Gudzune, MD, MPH, directs the Johns Hopkins
Healthful Eating, Activity & Weight Program, where she also practices as an obesity medicine specialist. She is an associate professor of
medicine at the Johns Hopkins School of Medicine with a research and
teaching portfolio focused on obesity prevention and treatment.

A Johns Hopkins Press Health Book

Weight Loss FOR LIFE

The **Proven Plan for Success**

WHY SCIENCE SAYS THAT DIETING IS NOT ENOUGH

Lawrence J. Cheskin, MD
& Kimberly A. Gudzune, MD, MPH

JOHNS HOPKINS UNIVERSITY PRESS
BALTIMORE

Note to the Reader: This book describes a personal approach to weight loss. It is not intended to take the place of your relationship with your health care provider or to substitute for medical treatment of obesity. If you are seriously overweight, are out of shape, are over the age of 40, or have a history of medical problems, we recommend that you seek the advice of a physician before beginning a weight loss program.

Drug dosage: The author and publisher have made reasonable efforts to determine that the selection of drugs discussed in this text conform to the practices of the general medical community. The medications described do not necessarily have specific approval by the US Food and Drug Administration for use in the diseases for which they are recommended. In view of ongoing research, changes in governmental regulation, and the constant flow of information relating to drug therapy and drug reactions, the reader is urged to check the package insert of each drug for any change in indications and dosage and for warnings and precautions. This is particularly important when the recommended agent is a new and/or infrequently used drug.

© 2021 Lawrence J. Cheskin
All rights reserved. Published 2021
Printed in the United States of America on acid-free paper
9 8 7 6 5 4 3 2 1

Johns Hopkins University Press
2715 North Charles Street
Baltimore, Maryland 21218-4363
www.press.jhu.edu

Library of Congress Cataloging-in-Publication Data

Names: Cheskin, Lawrence J., author. | Gudzune, Kimberly A., author.
Title: Weight loss for life : the proven plan for success / Lawrence J. Cheskin, MD, FACP, Kimberly
    Anne Gudzune, MD, MPH ; foreword by Jeanne M. Clark, MD, MPH.
Description: Baltimore : Johns Hopkins University Press, 2021. | Series: A Johns Hopkins Press health
    book | Includes bibliographical references and index.
Identifiers: LCCN 2020052635 | ISBN 9781421441948 (hardcover) | ISBN 9781421441955 (ebook)
Subjects: LCSH: Weight loss.
Classification: LCC RM222.2 .C4745 2021 |DDC 613.2/5—dc23
LC record available at https://lccn.loc.gov/2020052635

A catalog record for this book is available from the British Library.

Illustrations are by Jane Whitney.

Special discounts are available for bulk purchases of this book. For more information, please contact Special Sales at specialsales@.jh.edu.

To my wife, Lisa Davis, PhD, whose knowledge
of nutrition far exceeds my own
LJC

To the patients at the Johns Hopkins
Healthful Eating, Activity & Weight Program,
who have inspired this work and shared
their experiences to help others
KAG

Contents

Foreword

FOR THE PAST SEVERAL DECADES, Dr. Cheskin has been a leader in obesity medicine and research at Johns Hopkins and beyond. In *Weight Loss for Life*, Dr. Cheskin, Dr. Gudzune, and a team of experts have translated scientifically proven interventions into an approachable strategy that people can apply in their current lives. The text includes patient stories, distilled from decades of experiences with patients wishing to lose weight, to explain key behavioral processes that make the lessons described accessible and easy to understand. Everyone can take away important lessons from this book, both those attempting a lifestyle change for the first time and individuals who have been down this road before.

I have had the pleasure of knowing and working with Dr. Cheskin for more than 20 years. He is highly regarded for his commitment to science and clinical research. However, I most admire him for his dedication, compassion, and empathy with patients, which clearly resonates in this book. As the director of the Division of General Internal Medicine, I am overjoyed that Dr. Cheskin now practices at the Johns Hopkins Healthful Eating, Activity & Weight Program along with the program's founder and director, Dr. Kimberly Gudzune, coauthor of this book.

The approach to weight management covered here aligns well with the vision of our program. We focus on working with patients to make long-term lifestyle changes to prevent or ameliorate chronic disease and improve their overall health and well-being. We combine scientifically proven strategies with a compassionate and supportive approach to deliver high-quality care for each person.

The principles and strategies highlighted in this book echo the same priorities of the Johns Hopkins Healthful Eating, Activity & Weight Program. Our health care providers are at Johns Hopkins because they are dedicated to bringing patients the latest in care by pushing the boundaries of clinical innovation and biomedical research. By delivering personalized health insights rooted in the latest advancements in medicine, Dr. Cheskin, Dr. Gudzune, and the rest of our team help patients achieve a healthful lifestyle and weight.

I anticipate that the present volume will be an important resource for our patients as well as for the millions of individuals with overweight and obesity around the globe.

JEANNE M. CLARK, MD, MPH, FACP, FTOS
Director, Johns Hopkins Division of General Internal Medicine
Frederick L. Brancati Professor of Medicine and Epidemiology
Johns Hopkins University

Acknowledgments

IN A WORK LIKE THIS, there are many contributors and kinds of contributions. I would like to thank my son, Eric, for his devotion and understanding when the pressures of work and deadlines interfered with our time together; my parents, Al and Greta Cheskin, for instilling their belief that no goal is impossible, including writing a book that will help people lose weight; and my wife, Dr. Lisa Davis, for both her ideas and her steadfast support.

The inspiration for this book arose from the many thousands of people who came to the Johns Hopkins Weight Management Center to seek help and the current patients who receive care at the Johns Hopkins Healthful Eating, Activity & Weight Program. Through them I have learned much of what I write about in this book as well as about the value of persistence and commitment.

Credit for the success of the Johns Hopkins Weight Management Center was due mostly to the staff of the program helping people in need. The writing of this book was aided immeasurably by Linda Bunyard, MS, RD; Robin Frutchey, MS; Shavise Glascoe, MS; Corinne Roberto, RN, MSN; and Suzie Carmack, PhD, MFA, MEd, ERYT, NBC-HWC. Without them the nutritional, behavioral, exercise, and medical/surgical materials would have been only a shadow of what they now are.

There would not even be a shadow of a book, though, without the urging of my editor at Johns Hopkins University Press, Joe Rusko. I owe him a debt of gratitude for his sage advice while shepherding us ably (and persistently) through the writing. Also at the Press, my heartfelt thanks to Adelene Jane Medrano, who expertly handled the administrative phases of the editorial process; editorial director Greg Britton, whose encouragement, friendship, and wisdom about all things published are greatly appreciated; and press director Barbara Kline Pope, whose support of the technological features of this new revised work have made it an entirely different and far more highly evolved animal.

Without these individuals, there would have been no book. I am glad to have the chance to acknowledge their contributions and to express my thanks.

LARRY CHESKIN

About the Johns Hopkins Healthful Eating, Activity & Weight Program

THE PRINCIPLES DESCRIBED IN THIS BOOK capture the experience provided to our patients at the Johns Hopkins Healthful Eating, Activity & Weight Program. Our program focuses on working with patients to make long-term lifestyle changes to prevent chronic disease and improve their health. We combine scientifically proven strategies with a compassionate and supportive approach to deliver high-quality care for women and men.

We use a variety of evidence-based tools to help achieve these goals, including group and one-on-one behavioral counseling to promote a healthful diet and physical activity, meal replacements, psychological services including cognitive behavioral therapy, medication management, and eligibility for bariatric procedures including surgery and minimally invasive procedures. Our clinic is staffed by physicians board-certified by the American Board of Obesity Medicine, which recognizes their expertise in scientifically proven strategies to treat overweight and obesity. Program patients may work with other team members including psychologists, health coaches, and nutrition specialists. Our program works collaboratively with hepatologists (liver specialists focusing on fatty liver disease) and bariatric surgeons; these specialists work side-by-side with our obesity medicine physicians to deliver coordinated care to our patients.

Our health care providers are members of one of the world's leading academic medical centers, bringing the latest in care by pushing the boundaries of clinical innovation and biomedical research. By delivering personalized health insights rooted in the latest advancements in medicine, we help patients achieve a healthful lifestyle and weight. More information about the Johns Hopkins Healthful Eating, Activity & Weight Program is available at https://www.hopkinsmedicine.org/gim/clinical/lifestyle-weight.html.

WEIGHT LOSS
FOR LIFE

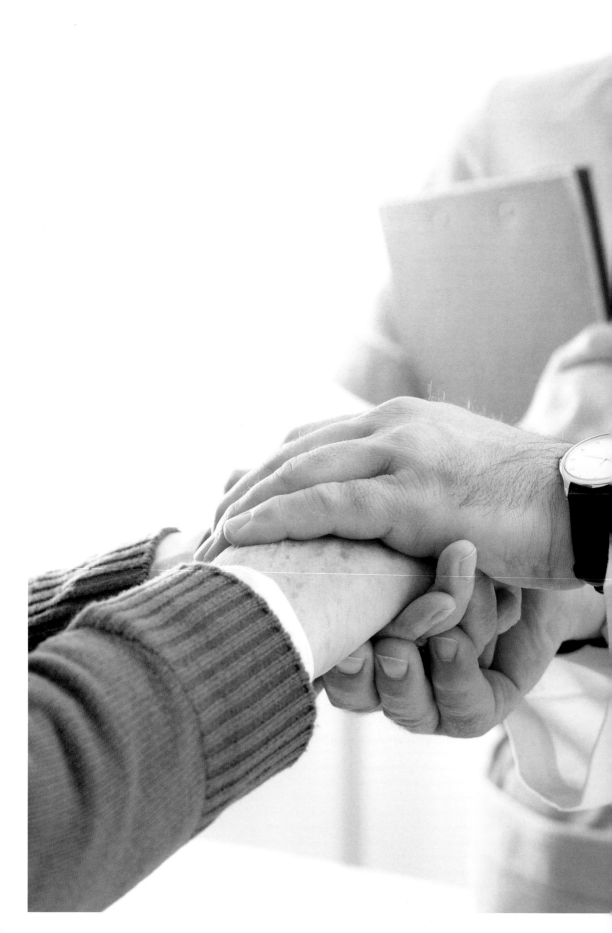

CHAPTER 1

We're Glad You're Here

IN THIS CHAPTER, WE WILL:

- **welcome you** as you begin your weight loss journey,

- **introduce you to** our *lifestyle* approach to weight loss and weight management, and

- **show you how** this approach will empower you to meet your weight loss goals.

IF YOU PICKED UP THIS BOOK, you are ready to lose weight for good. Congratulations on taking this step and welcome! We're glad you're here. As scientists representing the fields of medicine, nutrition, motivation, physical activity, stress management, and health promotion, we wrote this book to share our collective expertise with you. This is so that you can know, understand, and apply the science of long-term weight loss and weight management in your own life. You will be able to do this without getting caught up in the seemingly endless diets that are not based on established science and without feeling that you have to go it alone.

Whether this is the first time you have decided to lose weight or you have lost count of the number of diets or physical activity programs you have tried without success—or worse, losing weight only to gain it back—this book will give you the tools you need to manage your weight for good.

We understand that losing weight is challenging and that you may, like most people, lead a busy and stressful life. We have found in our research and our work with patients that successful and long-term weight management requires a holistic approach that acknowledges the realities of the world we live in. Although there are a (very) few lucky people with fast metabolisms who can lose weight easily and keep it off easily, most people (ourselves included) can't regularly consume high-calorie foods and live a high-stress, sedentary lifestyle while maintaining their optimal weight. These are real challenges, so please know that you are not alone. We wrote this book to give you the tools you need to take control of your health once and for all. In it, we will help you learn how to use a *lifestyle* approach that has already helped thousands of people lose weight and keep it off for good.

We'll walk you through the same step-by-step process that has helped our patients reach a healthy weight—and teach you how to adapt this approach for your weight loss needs in a way that will accommodate (and not ignore) your busy lifestyle. We'll also show you how to develop (or refine) your approach to stress management so that it is more strategic, because we know that this can make all the difference in your ability to keep the weight off. In this book you will learn how to:

1 **assess your needs** for weight loss and weight management,

2 **prepare yourself for challenges** of weight loss and long-term weight management,

3 **set attainable** weight loss and weight management goals that are truly right for you,

4 **develop** a *Personal Plan of Action* that is based on your unique history and future, and

5 **set yourself up for success** in the short term and the long term with:
   - a reliable support system,
   - a scientific approach to the process of change,
   - an accountability plan to keep you on track (even when it's hard), and
   - an emphasis on fun and flexibility so you can enjoy adapting your plan over time.

We are ready to support you every step of the way and to start you off on the path to success in the chapters that follow. But first, we need to ask you a very important question:

ARE YOU READY—REALLY READY—TO LOSE WEIGHT FOR GOOD?

If you find yourself hesitating, you're not alone and it's not your fault.

Beating the Odds

There is a highly publicized view that diets don't work and that you are better off either living with excess weight or, if you must lose weight, doing so at a rate not to exceed half a pound per week. The fact is that there are numerous examples of abuse and exploitation foisted on desperate people by the diet and fitness industries. Moreover, it is clear from various studies that the long-term success of most diet programs is poor. The available evidence is that for people who attend formal weight loss treatment programs, only 5% to 15% of those who lose weight will succeed in keeping most of it off five years down the road. For these people, nutrition programs (diets) and exercise programs work, but not for long. These statistics are discouraging when viewed in isolation, so it is helpful to put them in perspective. Let's see whether they can teach us something about how to become members of the "10% club"—those who lose weight and successfully manage it for the long term.

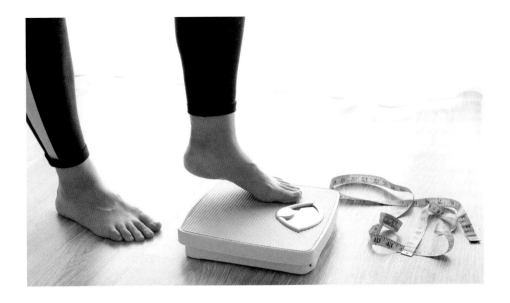

First, we invite you to come behind the scenes with us to look at a critical challenge that scientists like us face when we are studying and promoting weight loss. Here it is: most of the published research studies examining long-term weight loss report on the experience of a selected subset of people who try to lose weight. A close examination of these studies shows that they often recruit people who are referred by their doctors to university weight loss clinics. This means that the study population (the people trying to lose weight in the given study) often have other conditions or situations that make weight loss difficult (no matter how good the study's diet or fitness program may be). For example, the participants may have the medical diagnoses of severe obesity or depression, or they may be financially unstable. Since these studies often select groups with the most extreme situations, we must question the accuracy of the results. It can be difficult to know whether the diet or exercise regimen that is being examined in the study doesn't work; instead, it could be that the program is faulty or that some of the participants have conditions that make their weight loss efforts more difficult than people in the general population. This is one reason so many studies of weight loss programs do not show conclusive evidence of weight loss success.

The good news is that as we delve further into the science of weight loss, we do find that many people are a lot more successful at long-term weight loss than the public has been led to believe. The National Weight Control Registry is a large, voluntary, and ongoing research study of more than 10,000 people who have reported maintaining a weight loss of at least 50 pounds and keeping it off for at least a year. After ten years, nearly 87% reported maintaining a weight loss of at least 10% of their highest weight. This is important because we know that losing at least 5% to 10% of your highest weight can reduce your risk of heart disease and diabetes. So, if a person's weight is 300 pounds, a weight loss of 15 to 30 pounds would produce significant health benefits. These people are probably much more typical of individuals who have tried to lose weight than those people who participate in formal research studies. And the good news is, their success rate is much better.

And that is great news, because it means that this is a program that has great potential for you. Of course, you may be facing unique challenges in your weight loss program, such as stress, depression, or financial concerns. However, we'll address those challenges and offer tools to help you create a weight loss program that works for you. We look forward to sharing our approach to weight management, to support you in your success. As you'll discover, our approach is based on both the latest science of healthy living as well as the approach we have shared with thousands at our clinical programs for the past 30 years—and are currently sharing with patients at the Johns Hopkins Healthful Eating, Activity & Weight Program.

We know that your odds of success increase when you begin with the development of a Personal Plan of Action that is informed by your medical history but is also tailored precisely for your lifestyle and wellness needs—including your history of weight loss attempts, your personal motivations for losing weight, your daily dietary intake of water, your level of physical activity (including daily activity and weekly exercise), and your other lifestyle habits of strategic stress management, sleep, the responsible intake of alcohol, and the following of medical guidance (including pharmaceutical or behavioral prescriptions).

Overcoming Mindset Barriers

Although we know that this comprehensive approach to losing the weight for good holds great potential for anyone who has struggled to maintain their weight long term, we do find that there are two common mindset barriers that may prevent your success. We call them out now not to discourage you but in fact to encourage you. We hope that if you see yourself as having either or both of these mindset barriers, that you'll take the time you need to acknowledge them, address them, and, with our help, move past them.

The first most common mindset barrier to success that we see is a lack of personal commitment to weight loss and weight management because the person experiences what they see as unfair pressure to do so by friends, family, or society. They feel like others are trying to write their script for them, and they feel as though these other folks are shaming

BOX 1-1

Overcoming Mindset Barriers

Lose weight because YOU want to.

them into the journey of weight loss. Ironically, they can end up acting out against this pressure by either choosing not to lose weight or engaging in unhealthy behaviors.

If this sounds familiar to you, take a deep breath. Recognize that your friends and family care about you and want you to be healthy. However, this is not their journey. If you have this mindset barrier, the way to get past it (or remove it entirely) is to let go of the expectations of others and to get real with yourself about why losing weight is good for you—and no one else. You'll find some great reasons why you will want to commit to this journey later in this chapter and throughout the book, and you'll even get to design your journey yourself with your Personal Plan of Action.

The second most common mindset barrier to success that we see is almost the opposite problem. Instead of rebelling against other people's expectations of their weight loss, some people are choosing to lose weight because they are expecting the world to treat them better if they do. Interestingly, when people who hold this belief do lose weight, they are often surprised to find that the world does not necessarily treat them differently—which can in turn be demotivating. If this mindset barrier sounds familiar to you, acknowledge it and then recognize that you are in control only of yourself, not of other people's perceptions of you.

We recommend that you undertake your weight loss journey for no one else but you. Sure, there will be external pressures influencing your actions, and hopefully encouragement from loved ones, but we suggest that you place these motivations behind your commitment to yourself. If you remind yourself regularly of the reasons *you* wish to lose weight, you will enhance your resolve and your ability to stick to your program.

To help you get started with this perspective, we have included a "commitment" activity at the end of this chapter. We recommend you keep a weight loss journal. Start by taking some time to write in your journal the answers to these questions and save them so you can refer to the answers as inspiration throughout this journey.

Our Approach: Lifestyle Change and Obesity Medicine

This book introduces you to a scientifically based approach to a healthy lifestyle for weight loss and weight management. This idea that your lifestyle choices can have as much impact on the length and quality of your life as other medical protocols (such as pharmaceuticals or surgery) is a concept that we, as your author team, have known for years from the perspectives of our fields of public health and health care. It is also an idea that is now well recognized in both wellness promotion and health care fields.

In our fast-paced, modern world, chronic diseases caused by a lack of healthy lifestyle choices are rising steadily in developed countries. Moreover, these same countries are also seeing a rapid rise in "diseases of despair"—mental health challenges and illnesses caused by stressful, overworked, or overwhelmed lifestyles that are made worse by unhealthy lifestyle choices (mindsets and behaviors). It is not surprising that the number of people struggling with a higher-than-healthy weight and obesity is at an all-time high, with two in three American adults currently being overweight or obese.

To combat this rapid rise in both diseases of despair and chronic disease, there is thankfully a growing awareness of the need to promote the ways that the science of healthy lifestyles can be a form of medicine—and improve both the length and quality of people's lives. In fact, that is one of the reasons we wrote this book: to reflect the growing healthy lifestyles movement and the unique challenges of today's world. Another reason is that we know that the science of weight loss and

FIGURE 1-1

Global obesity rates

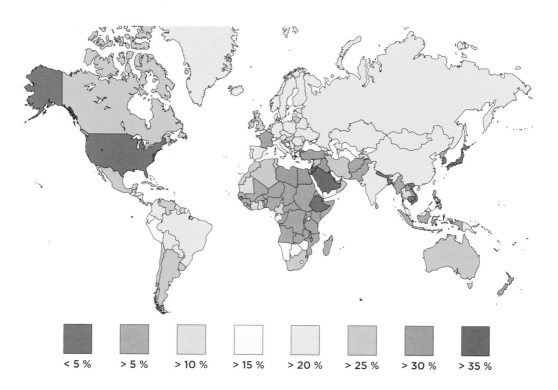

< 5 %   > 5 %   > 10 %   > 15 %   > 20 %   > 25 %   > 30 %   > 35 %

BOX 1-2

Meet the Team

As both a medical doctor and a professor of public health and nutrition, **Dr. Larry Cheskin, MD,** is a pioneer in the academic field and practice of obesity medicine. He was the founder of the Johns Hopkins Weight Management Center and currently practices at the Johns Hopkins Healthful Eating, Activity & Weight Program. This text will teach you the same approach Dr. Cheskin continues to share with patients at Johns Hopkins, along with additional recommendations in the fields of lifestyle change and obesity medicine contributed by the coauthors.

Dr. Kimberly Gudzune, MD, MPH, is an associate professor of medicine at Johns Hopkins School of Medicine and director of the Johns Hopkins Healthful Eating, Activity & Weight Program. She is also the director of the Obesity Medicine Fellowship in the Johns Hopkins School of Medicine and the clinical director of the Preventive Medicine Residency in the Johns Hopkins Bloomberg School of Public Health. In addition to being a practicing obesity medicine specialist, Dr. Gudzune has an active research portfolio focusing on obesity. Her research has won several awards in addition to being featured by major national and international news outlets.

Dr. Suzie Carmack, PhD, is an assistant professor of global and community health at George Mason University, where she trains future public health practitioners in their undergraduate and graduate (MPH) programs. As the award-winning and #1 best-selling author of *Well-Being Ultimatum* and *Genius Breaks*, she is globally recognized as a visionary in the field of well-being promotion and has helped hundreds of private and public sector organizations as a trusted adviser to their c-suite leadership. She currently conducts research exploring ways that tele-yoga interventions can reduce stress, burnout, and suicide prevalence in military, health care, and education contexts.

Robin A. Frutchey, MA, LCPC, received a master's degree in clinical psychology from Bowling Green State University, with a focus in behavioral medicine. She has obtained specialized training in the use of cognitive-behavioral, mindfulness, and motivational interviewing strategies to promote behavior change. For the past 20 years, she has been involved in research and clinical work aimed at disease prevention and management, as well as treatment of associated mental health conditions (for example, depression, anxiety, insomnia). She worked at the Johns Hopkins Weight Management Center for 11 years, focusing on individual and community-based weight management interventions. During that time, she also served as coordinator for the Global Obesity Prevention Center's Pilot Studies Core grant program for a number of years.

Linda Bunyard, MS, RD, LDN, earned her bachelor of science in human nutrition at the University of New Hampshire and her master of science in clinical nutrition at the University of Memphis. She completed her clinical internship at the University of Tennessee, Memphis Medical School. Her primary area of interest is nutrition counseling for weight management, behavior modification, and healthy nutrition. Linda has research experience in energy metabolism, weight loss, and reduction of cardiovascular risk factors, and her teaching experience includes Pepperdine University, LA County / USC School of Nursing, and Howard Community College. Linda is a registered dietitian with the Academy of Nutrition and Dietetics and licensed to practice in the state of Maryland.

Shavise Glascoe, MS, ACSM, EP-C, was the lead exercise physiologist at the Johns Hopkins Weight Management Center. Prior to her work at the Johns Hopkins Weight Management Center, she developed and implemented a number of health and fitness programs for community outreach nonprofit organizations, universities, public schools, and corporate offices throughout the country. She also has over five years of personal training experience, working with all age groups and experience levels. Her approach in training clients is to improve their quality of life and enable them to incorporate physical activity into their daily lives. Shavise holds a BA in exercise science from the University of Northern Iowa. Her passion for chronic disease prevention, weight management, and minority health led her to pursue an MS in health, physical activity, and chronic disease from the University of Pittsburgh. Shavise is a certified exercise physiologist through the American College of Sports Medicine.

Corinne Roberto, RN, DNP, is a graduate of the Johns Hopkins School of Nursing with a doctor of nursing practice in adult/gerontology primary care. She is an ANEW scholar and a recipient of the Johns Hopkins Nurses' Alumni Association Award for expertise in professional nursing practice and patient-centered health care delivery. Her doctoral project, "Weight Loss Maintenance Prevalence and Education to Improve Self-Efficacy for Physical Activity and Eating Behaviors," was completed at the Johns Hopkins Weight Management Center with mentorship by Dr. Larry Cheskin.

weight management has continued to evolve, and that it can be difficult for the public to know where to find accurate and timely health information that can help them lose and manage weight safely. And finally, we wanted to write this book, because we wanted more people like you to know how to use the same strategies and practices that we share with our patients—to make them available to those who would not otherwise be able to find or experience these solutions.

If you are now ready to apply the latest science of weight loss and weight management in your own life, you've come to the right place. This book will teach you how to do just that so you can "lose weight for life." You'll see that our entire approach is one that we use in our clinical practices and recommends the key lifestyle behaviors that have been shown to extend and improve both the quality and length of human life (box 1-3). We hope you are as pleased as we are to know that taking control of your health by committing to these behaviors will help you to not only lose and manage weight but also live a longer and happier life.

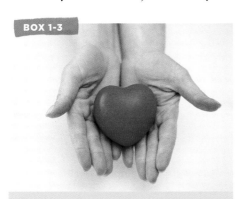

Six Ways to Take Control of Your Health

1 Increase physical activity (by means of daily activity and weekly exercise)

2 Follow a healthful eating pattern

3 Ensure adequate sleep and rest

4 Develop strategies for emotional wellness (a.k.a. stress management)

5 Use substances (for instance, prescription medicines) responsibly, limiting alcohol and avoiding tobacco use

6 Form and maintain healthy relationships

Our Strategy for Losing the Weight for Good: Meet Energy Balancing

Our approach recognizes that you are a busy person with multiple demands, and that you need a simple, straightforward, and strategic way to lose and manage weight. Therefore, we would like to share with you a strategy that one of our contributors (Dr. Carmack) created. The Energy Balancing Strategy (figure 1-2) is a way for you to rethink what is often called energy balance. As we will see later in this book in chapter 8, the concept of energy balance recognizes that, in order for us to maintain our weight, we must balance the energy we take in (that is, nutrition and water) with the energy we expend (through the physical activities of

FIGURE 1-2

Energy balancing strategy

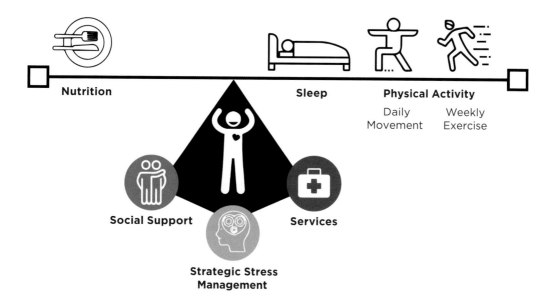

daily [functional] movement and weekly exercise). If we want to lose weight, we need to expend more energy than we take in; if we want to gain weight, we need to take in more energy than we expend.

With the Energy Balancing Strategy, you are encouraged to think of this energy balance not as a flat equation of numbers that stays relatively constant over time but instead as a dynamic "balancing act" that is constantly moving, changing, and evolving. This is why you'll notice that the strategy looks much like a seesaw at a child's playground—to reflect how the balance is never truly steady but instead is dynamically always in motion. You can interpret the balance as follows:

• **The seesaw goes "high left"** when your caloric intake is high, and when you get less than the recommended guidelines of sleep and physical activity. In any or all of these cases, you have a higher likelihood of gaining weight.

• **The seesaw goes "high right"** when your caloric intake is reduced relative to your physical activity, or when you follow the recommended guidelines for physical activity and sleep. In any or all of these cases, you have a higher likelihood of losing weight.

The seesaw approach is consistent with the well-known energy balance assumption that if you take in more calories than you expend, you'll gain weight, and if you take in fewer calories than you expend, you'll lose weight. However, our approach also recognizes the importance of other lifestyle factors: sleep, stress management, social support, and the use of health care or wellness provider services. Recent scientific studies have shown us that both a lack of sleep and experiencing high stress can cause unexpected weight gain and be a barrier to weight loss and weight management success.

Scientists are still trying to determine exactly why and how these two important healthy behaviors impact your ability to lose and manage weight, but two possibilities are emerging. Some recent research shows that lack of sleep and mismanaged stress can both slow down your metabolic system (that is, how well you process the energy you take in) and therefore your ability to lose and manage weight. Other research shows us that when you are not getting enough sleep or are not able to manage your stress well, your body begins craving sweets and storing fat more readily. Additional research shows us that when you are fatigued from lack of sleep or mismanaged stress, you feel more tired and are therefore more likely to skip your daily movement or weekly exercise. Whatever the reason, it's clear that getting adequate sleep and managing stress effectively will improve your weight loss efforts.

The Energy Balancing Strategy also depicts energy balance as being a challenge for each individual (as illustrated by the human that is attempting to balance their energy in and energy out). This element of the strategy is meant to convey the idea that we all are made up of different histories, genes, and biology, and we all may have different medical concerns. Some people have genetic compositions that make it easier for them to maintain a healthy weight easier than others. You may have heard that several hormones have been discovered that influence body weight and metabolism (leptin, *GLP-1*, as well as others). Some medications may either accelerate or decelerate our metabolism—and therefore disrupt our ability to get to and maintain a healthy weight. We also know that age and gender can influence weight loss and weight management ability as well. In short, we each have our own unique balance point (and tipping point) based on these many factors.

You may also notice that the Energy Balancing Strategy shows the fulcrum as sitting on three wheels that can move the fulcrum left or right—adjusting where the tipping point of energy balance resides. The left wheel is symbolic of social support that you can receive from friends or family members, which studies have shown is important for weight management program success. The center wheel is symbolic of your ability to strategically manage the stress that life throws your way—both "good" stress (getting a new job or starting a new relationship) and "bad" stress (finding out upsetting news or facing financial difficulties). The right wheel is symbolic of services that are needed to support you in your weight loss journey—from a wellness provider (such as a board-certified health coach) or a health care provider.

If you have the support of professionals on your weight management journey (as you do with this book), as well as the support of the people you care about (your family, your partner, your children, your friends, or your coworkers), you will have the help you need to stay committed to making your lifestyle healthier. You'll also feel better about the process since research shows us that social support predicts well-being. And, if you don't have the support of professionals who are trained in the science of obesity medicine or the support of people you care about, your fulcrum may go in the opposite (wrong) direction—making your energy balance that much harder to attain.

There is a lot more to weight loss than a simple "energy in and energy out" balance—it is a true balancing act of many factors. This is why so many people who are only focused on caloric consumption (energy in) and physical activity (energy out) are not always successful at losing weight in the short term or keeping it off in the long term. The good news is that you can learn to take control of many of these factors—and lose the weight for good. *And, that is exactly why we wrote this book.* We don't want you to feel alone in this process, trying to determine what recommendations are or aren't good for you. Instead, we will provide you with accurate and scientifically sound information in a way that makes it easy for you to apply in your busy life—and we will be here for you every step of the way through the step-by-step process included in this book. We'll also try to make the journey fun and easy for you by keeping the conversational tone you see in this chapter throughout the book.

In this book, we will share with you the benefits of our author team's experience, as well as practical tips that Drs. Cheskin and Gudzune share with their patients in their practice as physicians at the Johns Hopkins Healthful Eating, Activity & Weight Program. The book will help you to create your own customized plan, which we call your Personal Plan of Action. We will carefully and honestly describe methods that have helped thousands of other people lose weight, while at the same time offering some advice that can improve your health and psychological well-being. Please understand that cookie-cutter advice that is not individually tailored to match your needs is far less effective than what we can do together using your honest assessment of yourself and translating that into a Personal Plan of Action that will work for you.

Losing the Weight = Creating a Healthier and Happier Life

We also hope that you are as committed to your success as we are. That's because our work in the fields of health care, obesity medicine, and public health research has shown us that there are many advantages to losing weight—and keeping it off—that are not only good for you but also great for public health. For example, both medical and public health research has shown that being moderately to severely overweight and having an excess of body weight can compromise the quality of your life and take years off your life. We know that when you get to a healthy weight, you will

- decrease your risk of heart disease (the number one cause of mortality),
- lower your risk of cancer,
- lessen your risk of diabetes,
- decrease your risk of asthma,
- reduce the likelihood of snoring,

FIGURE 1-3

Benefits of maintaining a healthy weight

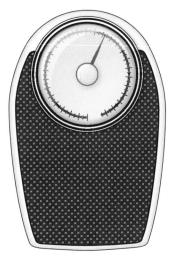

1 Decreased Risk of Disease People who maintain a healthy weight are less susceptible to disease. Obesity can lead to diabetes, cancer, and even asthma.

2 Better Heart Health Maintaining a healthy weight will keep your arteries clear of plaque buildup, lowering your risk of heart disease.

3 Better Sleep Excess body fat can interfere with both your airways and the body's chemical signaling to breathe. Maintaining a healthy weight improves lung function and quality of sleep.

4 Longer Life Every 33 lbs of excess weight increases the chance of death by about 30%. By this estimate, a healthy weight person will live 10 years longer than an obese person.

- reduce the pain of osteoarthritis,
- improve your ability to breathe and your lung function,
- improve your quality of sleep,
- increase the length of your life (by up to 10 years), and
- strengthen your immune system.

Why is it that a healthy weight can do so much good for the body, while unmanaged weight gain can cause so much harm? One reason is where your body stores extra fat. The way excess fatty tissue is *distributed* in the body is now believed to be at least as important as the *amount* of excess fat in determining a person's health risk. Are you an "apple" or a "pear" when it comes to body fat? Excess fat deposited around the middle (the apple figure) is much riskier in health terms than an equal amount of excess fat around the hips, thighs, or buttocks (the pear figure). In fact, excess abdominal fat, even when the body mass index (BMI) is normal, can increase health risks.

Being severely overweight is a risk factor for a host of medical problems, with the most common being high blood pressure, high cholesterol, heart disease, stroke, diabetes, and cancer. Another common medical problem, osteoarthritis, is not thought to be caused by obesity but is made worse when the joints are subjected to the strain of carrying around excess weight.

FIGURE 1-4

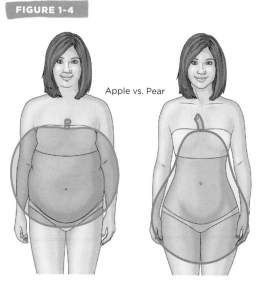

Apple vs. Pear

This image shows "apple"- and "pear"-shaped bodies. If your waist is greater than 35 inches for women or greater than 40 inches for men, you are more likely to be apple shaped. This means excess fat tends to be around your waist, rather than around your hips, thighs, and buttocks.

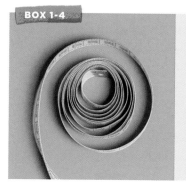

BOX 1-4

How to Correctly Measure Your Waist

The measuring tape should be snug against your skin but not pulled tightly. Measure just above your hip bones after breathing out.

FIGURE 1-5

Obesity and the risk of heart disease

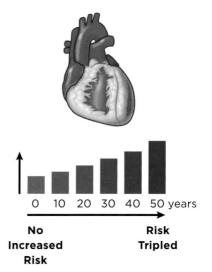

Risk of having heart damage:
25% increase for every 10 years staying obese

| 0 | 10 | 20 | 30 | 40 | 50 years |

No Increased Risk   **Risk Tripled**

BOX 1-5

A Note about BMI

Body mass index, or BMI, is an imperfect tool. For example, it doesn't take into account a person's body fat versus muscle content. Many Olympic athletes, for example, would have BMIs that would classify them as obese. BMI also does not consider waist-height ratio.

Body composition analysis provides a more accurate picture of body fat, muscle mass, and water weight. To use the most reliable body composition scales, look for one offered at your local gym, health club, or health care provider.

For some people, the medical advantages of losing weight are the most important, particularly if they have developed a worrisome health problem that is typically related to excess body weight. There is uncertainty, however, even among experts, about the health risks associated with being overweight by slight to moderate degrees. Overweight individuals have a 25% increased health risk, and "obese" or "severely obese" individuals are at increased risk of many diseases and conditions, as well as early death. BMI stands for body mass index, which is an estimate of body fat based on your height and weight. It allows us to estimate your health risks and is a good indicator of progress during weight loss and maintenance.

For many people who want to lose weight, though, medical concerns are not their only motivations. And even for those with medical conditions, the real payoff in reaching a healthy weight is just *feeling* better every day. Many people who have lost weight are pleased, for example, that their cholesterol is lower. But more tangible and infinitely more satisfying is the fact that, as 48-year-old Sofia said, "I can walk up a flight or two of stairs and not feel like collapsing. I don't get tired so easily anymore. I have so much more energy for doing the things I couldn't do before."

You will also likely find an increase in your self-esteem as you undertake a successful weight loss journey. You are likely to have more options when you go shopping for clothes, enjoy the increased energy, strength, and pride that comes with a more active lifestyle, take more pride in your appearance, and feel a tremendous sense of accomplishment that comes from having control over your body and body image.

TABLE 1-1

BMI interpretation, using World Health Organization criteria

BMI (kg/m²)	Interpretation
< 18.5	Underweight
18.5–24.9*	Normal Range
25–29.9	Overweight
>29.9	Obese

In Asian populations, the cutoff for overweight is 23 kg/m2.

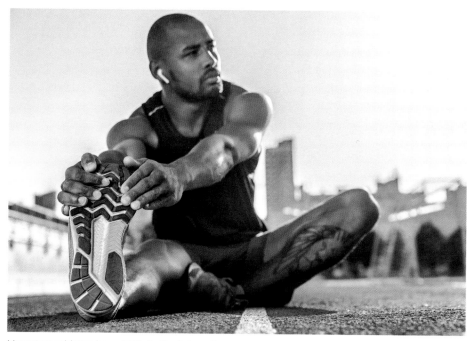

Many top athletes have BMIs in the "obese" range

- Height
- Weight
- BMI
- Blood sugar (A1C)
- Waist circumference
- Back pain (1–10 scale)
- Joint pain (1–10 scale)
- Mood (1–10 scale)
- Number of hours sitting per day
- Number of bouts of exercise per week
- Number of steps per day
- Number of minutes of cardio per week
- Number of strength training sessions per week
- Number of flexibility training sessions per week
- Number of hours of sleep per day
- Number of vegetable servings per day
- Number of sweets per day
- Other measures (as per your personal preference and your medical doctor's recommendation)

Medical Approval, Biometrics, and Key Behaviors

Before you begin any weight loss journey, it is important to gain approval from a medical professional. As part of this process, your medical provider may conduct several tests that can help you to track your current state of health and your progress over time as you implement your Personal Plan of Action.

Conclusion

Throughout this book, we will share both research and real-world advice with you—gleaned from the authors' combined knowledge in the areas of medicine, nutrition, motivation, physical activity, stress management, and health promotion, and from Drs. Cheskin and Gudzune's decades' long practice with thousands of patients at Johns Hopkins. We wrote this book to share our collective expertise with you so that you can know, understand, and apply the science of long-term weight loss in your own life without feeling like you have to go it alone. The book will provide you with practical step-by-step advice in making your own Personal Plan of Action—which you can tweak based on your own personal health history and lifestyle needs.

Congratulations on committing to the journey of losing the weight for good so that you can improve both the length and quality of your life. Again, we're glad you're here.

✏️ WEIGHT LOSS JOURNAL: Commitment Activity

Before you move on to the next chapter, take a moment to complete the commitment journal activity below so that you can document "why" you are committed to losing the weight for good. At this point, we also ask that you record your personal biometrics so you can track your "Day 1" status and track your progress over time. Many BMI calculators are available online; we typically refer our patients to the one on the National Institutes of Health website: https://www.nhlbi.nih.gov/health/educational/lose_wt/BMI/bmi-m.htm.

BOX 1-7

Date: _____

What does "losing the weight for good" really mean for you? _____
_____.

Why do you want to lose the weight for good—for you? _____
_____.

What dimensions of your life will be improved if you lose weight for good, and why?

☐ Physical   ☐ Financial
☐ Social   ☐ Mental
☐ Purpose/Career   ☐ Emotional
☐ Other

How can losing the weight for good help you in the roles you play in your life, and why?

☐ Worker   ☐ Friend
☐ Partner   ☐ Other
☐ Parent

Action Items

We will conclude most chapters of this text with a few calls to action, which will help you translate what you read into specific things you can do as part of your journey to live a healthier lifestyle and take control of your weight.

Weight Management Biometrics Baseline

The following questions will give you a baseline of where your health and weight are today, which you can then use to measure your success over time. We recommend that you seek a medical provider's help in collecting and documenting the data to respond to the questions. You should also seek the advice of a medical provider before starting any weight loss or weight management program, such as the one found in this book.

- What is your resting heart rate? _____

- What is your blood pressure? _____

- What is your cholesterol level? _____

- What is your weight in pounds? _____

- What is your height in inches? _____

- What is your waist circumference (at its narrowest)? _____

- What is your hip circumference (at its widest)? _____

- What is your neck circumference (at its narrowest)? _____

- With these measurements, use a free online tracker (we like the US Navy Calculator) to calculate your body fat percentage and record the number: _____

- Also with the measurements above, use a free online tracker (we like the National Institutes of Health Body Mass Index Calculator) to calculate your body mass index and record the number here: _____

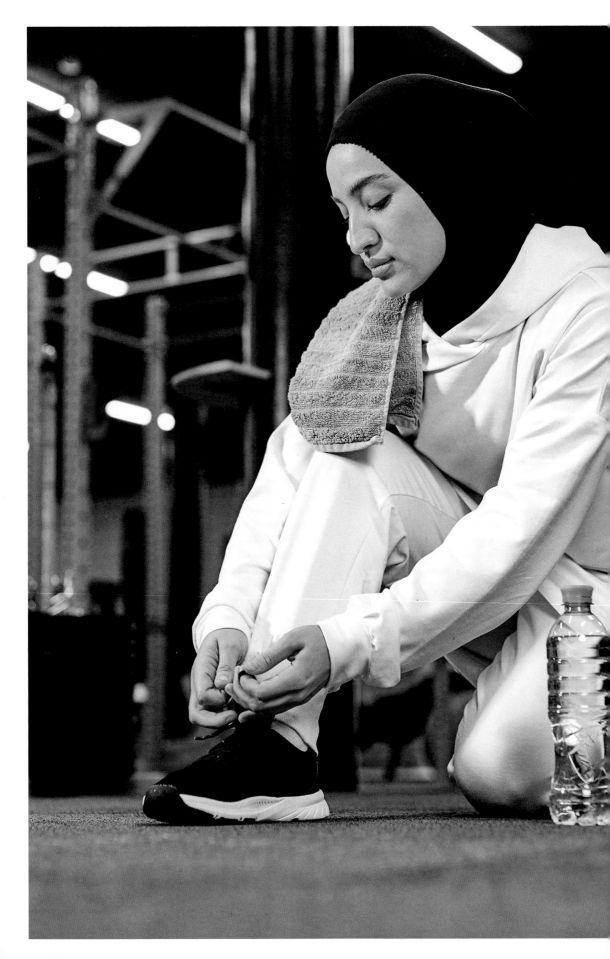

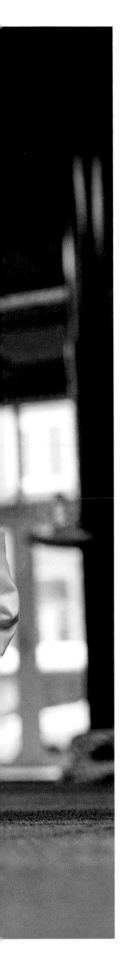

CHAPTER 2

Getting Ready

IN THIS CHAPTER, WE WILL:

- **help you assess your readiness** to begin a weight management program,

- **guide you to start** a weight loss journal,

- **describe** the behavior change process,

- **offer tips** for preparing for lasting change, and

- **give you the tools** to articulate your weight loss goals.

YOU ARE HERE BECAUSE YOU WANT TO LOSE WEIGHT for good. Again, congratulations. In this chapter, we'll explain how to prepare for the process of losing weight. Our research and our work with our patients have shown us that readiness is a key foundation for your future success.

What do we mean by readiness? Some people call it motivation, but it is more than that. Readiness can be understood as having two dimensions: 1) short term (commitment) and 2) long term (sustainability).

1 **Short-term commitment** is the urge, indeed the passion, to begin immediately.
2 **Long-term sustainability** is your conviction that permanent change is necessary and attainable.

The first is important in getting started in the process of losing weight; the second is critical for keeping it off for good.

Unfortunately, these two components of readiness can easily get out of sync. People most commonly have an abundance of short-term commitment but a shortage of long-term sustainability. We will see how to get these two factors more in tune with each other in this chapter and again in your Personal Plan of Action.

If change was easy, everyone would modify their lifestyle to improve their health. The reality is that most changes are messy and have some associated costs. It's important to weigh the pros and cons of change. You can ask yourself, "Is it going to be worth it for me to change?" "What will I have to give up to make this happen?" "What will I gain from making these changes?" Visualize yourself at your goal weight, and think about how you would like to see yourself at this weight. How would others see you?

It's also helpful to consider your values and how they are affected by weight. How important is your health to you? And how is it affected by weight? How important is your relationship with a romantic partner to you? And how is it affected by weight? How important is your family? How is your family affected by your weight? You get the idea. Many times, motivation and the desire to make a change come from the recognition that one's behavior is not in line with one's values. If, for example, you have young children who are very important to you, and you want to be able to play actively with your children and model healthy eating habits, you may be more motivated to start eating better if you recognize that the way you are currently eating is getting in the way of the things you value.

Your reasons for losing weight may be totally different from someone else's. You are not born motivated or unmotivated; your level of motivation depends on your readiness to change at any given time and will fluctuate. It depends on your reasons for wanting to make a change and your reasons for wanting things to stay the same.

Also keep in mind that what initially causes you to begin to lose weight may not be the same motivating factor that gets you to your goal. For example, you may be ready to lose weight now because you are worried about your recent lab results and because you're wearing the last pair of pants in your closet that still fit. However, after you've lost 30 pounds, you may be able to go off a cholesterol medication, and you may have a whole closet full of clothes that fit again. At this point, you may need to find something else to motivate you.

FIGURE 2-1

Weight loss motivation scale

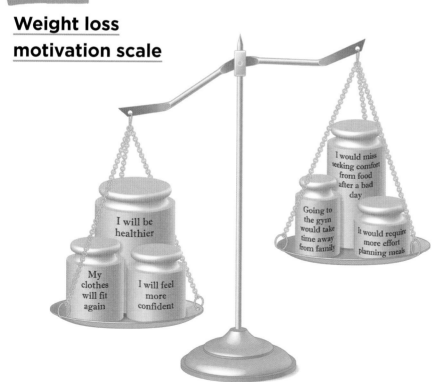

We find it helpful to picture motivation like the scales of justice (figure 2.1). On the one side, you will have your reasons for changing, and on the other side, you'll have your reasons for not changing. If the reasons for not changing outweigh the reasons for changing, you will be unmotivated to change. If the scales are balanced, you will likely feel stuck and ambivalent about changing. However, if the reasons for changing outweigh the reasons for not changing, you are likely motivated to change.

If you are feeling stuck or unmotivated, it can be helpful to look at the items on both sides of the equation. How can you make the advantages of changing (or pros of weight loss) more relevant and appealing? Is there anything you could do to address your cons of weight loss or reasons for not changing? For instance, if you are thinking that you don't want to attempt weight loss because you are worried about the effort required to plan calorie-controlled meals, you might try to use some premade meals or follow a simple meal plan. If you are concerned that going to the gym might cut down on the time you have to spend with your family, you might avoid the gym and purchase bikes for everyone in the family so that you can exercise together. Or perhaps you choose to go on family hikes rather than hitting the Stairmaster. Don't discount that your family and friends will likely be supportive of your efforts to live a healthier lifestyle. Addressing your barriers to change will likely help you feel more motivated.

 JOURNALING ACTIVITY: Am I *Really* Ready?

What would you say is the degree or intensity of your short-term readiness (desire to lose weight) and long-term readiness (commitment to taking the steps needed to lose weight)? Rate these on a scale from 1 to 10, 1 being not at all ready or committed, 5 being a moderate level of readiness or commitment, and 10 being the most ready or committed you can imagine yourself feeling.

In your journal, note the number that describes the strength of your short-term readiness and long-term readiness. Compare the two numbers you wrote down. It's not unusual for the first number to be larger than the second, because people are often more ready to commit in the short term than in the long term. This is especially true for people who've been disappointed with their long-term results when they have tried to lose weight in the past. If this is true for you, then this time around you'll want to make sure that the action stage (losing the weight) is rewarding (to help motivate you for the maintenance stage) as well as smoothly integrated with the maintenance stage (keeping the weight off). That way the maintenance stage is simply a natural extension of the action stage.

Look at your numbers again. If you rated your depth of commitment at 5 or lower, it is important to ask yourself what's holding you back. What specific doubts do you have, and where are they coming from? Any doubts or hesitation can limit your ability to succeed, so you'll want to identify them and address them before you can begin. For example, if you are concerned that your family won't want to shift to lower-calorie foods with you at mealtimes, consider ways you can stay focused on your goals while not causing conflict with your family. Perhaps you might consider making a batch of healthful foods to enjoy throughout the week, so you are not preparing multiple meals each evening. Or, if you are not a morning person, going to the gym before work is not sustainable. Consider other ways to get exercise in your day—perhaps a brisk walk during your lunch break. The bottom line is to be realistic about the doubts you have but be open-minded about ways to overcome them.

The Behavior Change Process

Research by Drs. James Prochaska and Carlo DiClemente has identified six stages in the behavior change process, which they call the transtheoretical model of behavioral change. These six stages cover the full path of any type of behavior (lifestyle) change, from before you even get on the path (precontemplation) all the way through the long-term path of success and into completion (where you ultimately forget there was a path at all). Take a look at these six stages of change, and see where you are so you'll know how close (or far) you are from long-lasting change.

Which Stage Are You In?

The person in the *precontemplation stage* is someone who is either unaware of the need for change or isn't yet thinking about making a change. In the case of weight management, the individual is either unaware of the need for change or is aware but doesn't wish to change anything in the near future. (Six months is often used to define the near future.)

The *contemplation stage* describes a person who is aware of a problem and wishes to do something about

BOX 2-2

Stages of Change

1 Precontemplation
2 Contemplation
3 Preparation
4 Action
5 Maintenance
6 Termination

it sometime in the next six months—but not right away. You may well be at this stage if you are reading this book. We sincerely hope that reading at least parts of this book will help you move to the next stage of change, the preparation stage.

The *preparation stage* describes a person who is aware of the problem, may have thought about taking action in the past, and has now decided to prepare for action during the next month (at most). This is the ideal stage to be in while starting to read this book. If you are at this stage, you will be ready to develop a plan and move directly to the action stage.

The *action stage* is self-explanatory. It describes a person who is acting on the change. We believe it is important to ground the actions of this stage within a strategic and customized Personal Plan of Action—and you will learn how to create such a plan for yourself later in this book. Such a plan is designed to support your individual needs so that you have a greater likelihood of success in carrying out the actions (behavior changes) needed to lose weight for good.

The *maintenance stage* describes a person who has ended an action stage and is now faced with the difficult task of transforming the temporary changes in behavior made in the action stage into long-term habits. This is undoubtedly the most important stage. It makes little sense to go to the effort to lose weight only to rapidly regain it.

The *termination stage* describes a person who no longer needs to make the change. However, this stage doesn't apply to all changes, including weight loss. We feel strongly that weight management is a part of an ongoing and active commitment to a healthy lifestyle. However, in time, maintaining healthy habits will become part of your everyday life, like breathing and sleeping.

 JOURNALING ACTIVITY:

What Stage Am I in for Long-Term Change?

Do you see yourself in one of the first five stages of the behavior change process? Take some time to journal about how you feel about being in this stage, and how you feel about progressing to the next stage.

Whether you are hopeful that you can progress to the next stage soon or feel nervous about the idea that you have to move to another stage at all, this exercise was designed to encourage you to acknowledge where you are on your own unique journey. We will circle back to this self-reflection later in your Personal Plan of Action and use it to inspire where we go next in your planning process.

BOX 2-3

I am currently in stage: _____

I feel _____ about being in this stage because: _____
_____.

I feel _____ about progressing to the next stage
(_____) because _____.

Before we do that, though, we have additional questions to share with you that will likely help you determine where you fall in terms of readiness to change. These are questions we ask of patients at the Johns Hopkins Healthful Eating, Activity & Weight Program. After you complete the questions, we will walk you through insights on what your responses can mean for your weight loss planning process.

Analysis: Preparing for a Lasting Change

The following questions may give you some quick ideas about what's inspiring you to lose weight—and what might be getting in your way. However, let's look closer at the significance of your various answers to these questions. We recommend that you read the discussions pertaining to your answers first and then read the other answers. Doing so will help you become better informed about the other answers and make it easier for you to recognize challenges in your own life should they crop up during or after you follow your Personal Plan.

1. WHAT IS YOUR WEIGHT HISTORY?

A. Childhood. About four out of five people who were heavy as children continue to have weight problems as adults. People in this category frequently have an inherited component to their weight problem. Obesity in childhood causes increases in the number of fat cells in the body. These cells can never be lost, only reduced in size. Because of this, some researchers believe that childhood onset obesity is a particularly difficult kind of weight condition to treat.

If you had a weight problem (overweight or obesity) as a child, it may indeed be more difficult for you to lose weight and keep it off from a physical perspective.

BOX 2-4

Readiness to Change Questionnaire

1 **What is your weight history?**
   a I've always been heavy, since childhood.
   b I've been heavy since my teens or twenties.
   c I've gained weight slowly over many years.
   d I've gained weight mostly in the past year or two.

2 **Are there specific factors that have contributed to your weight gain?**
   a Quitting cigarettes
   b Failure to return to prepregnancy weight after childbirth
   c Change in physical activity level (job change, retirement, illness)
   d Psychological concerns, such as depression, anxiety, ADHD, PTSD, or trauma
   e Change in appetite related to medications
   f None of the above

3 **Are you undergoing a lot of life changes or stresses at this time? Place a check mark next to the changes that are going on in your life now or that have taken place in the past year.**
   ___ marriage, divorce, separation, or breakup of a long-term relationship
   ___ death or dying of a loved one
   ___ job change, job loss, or promotion
   ___ beginning or end of school
   ___ personal serious illness or injury
   ___ change in residence
   ___ other major stresses

4 **What are your main reasons for wanting to lose weight? (Check as many or as few as you wish.)**
   ___ to improve my appearance
   ___ to improve my health or reduce my risk of medical problems
   ___ to improve my energy level and exercise tolerance
   ___ to avoid feeling embarrassed about my weight
   ___ to please someone important to me
   ___ to _____
   _____.
   (*Fill in the blank; list everything that comes to mind.*)

5 **Please rank, in order of importance from 1 to 5, whom you would like to lose weight for.**
   ___ spouse or significant other (or potential significant other)
   ___ family (children/parents/siblings)
   ___ friends
   ___ strangers/perceived societal pressures
   ___ myself, independent of others' wishes

6 **How much weight do you wish to lose?**
   a I wish to lose enough weight to get to a healthy body mass index (BMI).

b I wish to lose enough to get most of the way to a healthy BMI, but not that far.

c I wish to lose just enough to feel more comfortable or reduce my risk of medical problems, even if I am still moderately overweight.

7 **How many weight loss programs have you tried in the past?**

a I've never tried to lose weight before.

b I've tried to lose weight one to a few times before.

c I've tried to lose weight four or more times before.

8 **If you have previously tried to lose weight, what was the typical outcome in the short run?**

a I reached my goal.

b I got at least halfway to my goal.

c I got less than halfway to my goal.

9 **If you have previously dieted, what was the long-term outcome?**

a I kept off most of the weight for many years.

b I regained the weight after keeping most of it off for two or more years.

c I regained the weight after keeping most of it off for less than two years.

10 **Which statement describes how you believe you will behave while following a weight loss plan?**

a I will likely have a very hard time adhering to my plan.

b I will likely be spotty in adhering to my plan—some good days, some bad days.

c I will likely be consistently compliant with my plan.

d Other (describe): _____
_____
_____

11 **Which statement describes how you believe you will behave after the active weight loss phase has been completed?**

a I will likely go right back to old habits as soon as I've met my weight loss goal.

b I will likely start out with good habits, then slowly revert to the old habits.

c I will likely maintain the good new habits for a long time.

12 **What factors will play an important role in preventing you from successfully completing a weight loss program? (Check as many or as few as you wish.)**

__ lack of time

__ lack of physical resources (money, exercise equipment, etc.)

__ lack of motivation

__ lack of support from spouse, family, or others

__ major stressful event(s) intrude (change in job, residence, relationships, etc.)

__ need to lose weight becomes less important (for example, illness improves, special event like a wedding is over)

__ Other (describe): _____
_____
_____

And, from a mental (mindset) perspective, there may be additional concerns, too. We have seen many patients with a "there's no use in trying" mentality because they have always struggled with their weight.

We encourage you to restructure this thinking. To have the best chance of success, you must recognize the difficulties and consciously challenge your negative beliefs by replacing them with more accurate and helpful ways of thinking. While you may have struggled to lose weight in the past, there are likely things that you learned about yourself from each previous attempt. This book offers a completely new approach, and it offers new hope.

We also encourage you to rest assured that many people with childhood weight problems can and do overcome them. The National Weight Control Registry (discussed in chapter 1) is comprised largely of people who had struggled with weight since childhood and attempted many times to lose weight before achieving long-term success.

B. Teens and twenties. Like childhood onset overweight or obesity, the onset of weight problems in the teens or twenties is a common pattern. If you are still in this age group, take heart. Your eating patterns have not been entrenched for very long and are therefore more adaptable to change. In addition, you are likely to have a greater capacity for physical activity to help you maintain a lower weight once you reach it.

C. Extended adulthood years. Slow, subtle weight gain over a period of many years is so common that some recent weight tables adjust recommended weights for age. It is controversial whether weight gain with age in average amounts (typically a pound or less per year) is harmful to your health. Changes in body composition and decreased physical activity (in the face of undiminished food consumption) probably account for this gradual weight gain in most cases. Many men and some women tend to pack on these extra pounds around the abdomen. If this is the case for you, it is especially important to lose this abdominal fat because it is associated with a high risk of cardiovascular disease and diabetes (as discussed in chapter 1).

D. Recent. If you have gained a lot of weight only in the past couple years, you may be fortunate. This probably means that your heredity, food choices, or physical activity have protected you in the past from weight gain. Thus, a specific new factor is probably causing the relatively sudden change in weight. Specific factors are often easier to treat than the lifelong habits so often responsible for weight problems. Various specific factors are discussed next.

2. ARE THERE SPECIFIC FACTORS THAT
HAVE CONTRIBUTED TO YOUR WEIGHT GAIN?

A. Smoking. It is true that people who smoke weigh, on the average, a bit less than nonsmokers. The reasons for this are not entirely understood but may be related to one or more of the following: the slight appetite-suppressing effect of cigarettes, altered taste preferences in people who smoke, or an altered metabolism due to nicotine. In addition, it is common for people who smoke to increase their smoking when under stress; this behavior may help them avoid eating more when under stress. Commonly, people who smoke will gain weight when they quit smoking. The causes of this, too, are unclear but include reversal of the previously mentioned effects of smoking as well as a tendency to use food, especially mood-elevating foods such as sweets and chocolate, as a substitute for cigarettes after quitting.

For the typical smoker, quitting is accompanied by a gain of about 6 pounds, but the amount is highly variable. One patient of ours reported gaining 80 pounds in the two years after he quit smoking.

Many people choose not to quit smoking for fear that they will gain weight. Others go on a diet while attempting to quit in the hope of preventing weight gain. Our research suggests that dieting is associated with greater levels of smoking in heavy smokers. Thus, dieting at the same time may make it even harder to quit smoking. Since smoking is generally more dangerous than weighing a bit more, it is unwise to resume smoking in an effort to control weight.

If you are someone who has gained more weight than average after quitting smoking, there are specific strategies you can follow, and they do not include taking up smoking again. These strategies are described in detail in chapter 10.

B. Pregnancy. Just as the amount of weight gained during pregnancy is highly variable, so is the amount retained *after* pregnancy. Two years after pregnancy, the average woman weighs about 9 pounds more than she did prior to conception. This occurs with each pregnancy, of course. For women who have had several children or who had higher than average weight gain during a pregnancy, the numbers can add up to quite a few pounds. The causes are not well understood but may include hormonal influences (women who do not breastfeed, for example, may be more likely to gain than those who do) and changes in lifestyle after having a baby (including less regular exercise, snacking while prepping their child's food and clearing plates, or reduced quality and quantity of sleep).

There are specific things you can do to lose weight now, and to help prevent weight gain during future pregnancies. They include breastfeeding, if possible, and getting down to or near prepregnancy weight before becoming pregnant again. The role of physical activity is critical, as is understanding other baby-associated lifestyle changes.

C. Physical activity. If you believe that a recent decrease in your physical activity is a major factor in causing you to gain weight, take heart. This specific cause is not only treatable, but the treatment yields benefits beyond helping you lose weight. Chapter 7 contains information on how to design an exercise plan that will fit your specific circumstances and form an important part of your Personal Plan of Action.

The benefits of designing and carrying out a lifelong plan to increase physical activity include accelerating the pace of weight loss, making it much less likely that you will regain the weight you lose, and improving your cardiovascular fitness, stamina, and sense of well-being. As we will describe further in chapter 7, if you include a strength-training component in your Personal Plan, you will also build metabolically active muscle mass. This will enable you to eat a bit more than those who do only aerobic exercise and still not regain lost weight down the road.

D. Depression and anxiety. Depression and anxiety are common mental health concerns, especially in individuals struggling to manage their weight. The interaction between mood and eating is complex; we discuss it in more detail in chapter 5. We know for sure that there is a clear connection between mental health and body weight. The effect of excess weight on quality of life can trigger depression and anxiety; conversely, depression and anxiety can also cause problems with weight.

Depression can contribute to either weight gain or weight loss. People who are feeling chronically down may have trouble motivating themselves for any kind of change or activity, including weight loss. They may suffer from a lack of energy and

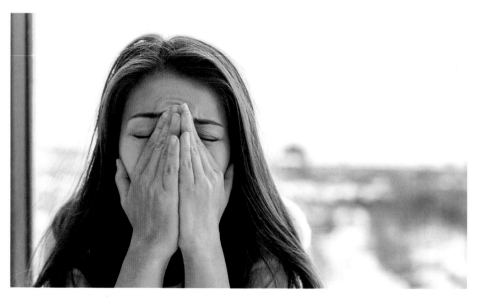

Mental health concerns, like depression and anxiety, are connected to weight management challenges

find it difficult to be physically active. Likewise, people who are feeling anxious may feel too overwhelmed by other worries and fears to focus on weight loss. Anxiety can negatively impact eating patterns (leading to skipped meals and binging) and food preferences (for example, anxiety can cause an increase in cortisol, a stress hormone, which can trigger cravings for high carbohydrate foods).

For people suffering from either depression or anxiety, their sleep may be disrupted, with some people sleeping more and others sleeping less. Sleeping too much or too little can contribute to weight gain because it interferes with your body's ability to perform the necessary regenerative processes that happen during sleep. Likewise, depression is often associated with changes in appetite, which can contribute to weight loss or gain. Both depression and anxiety can interfere with a person's confidence in their ability to successfully lose weight, and this lack of confidence (deemed "low self-efficacy") really dampens motivation. He or she might think, "Why even try if I don't believe I will be able to succeed?"

Many people who have experienced depression or anxiety have also gained weight because food provided comfort from their negative mood symptoms. The use of food for comfort in times of unhappiness is understandable; high fat and high sugar foods boost "feel good" brain chemicals, including serotonin and dopamine,

BOX 2-5

IF YOU THINK YOU HAVE symptoms of depression or anxiety, we encourage you to reach out to your physician to request diagnostic testing. If you have any thoughts of harm—for yourself or others—we urge you to seek medical attention (call 911) immediately. It is better to know for sure if there is a clinical diagnosis than to waste time (or risk harm) in guessing. If you are found to have either (or both) diagnosis/es, there are specific medications and psychotherapies available that can help you manage depression and anxiety symptoms. A detailed questionnaire for depression is included in chapter 5; however, this is only meant to support you in seeking out a medical diagnosis and is not meant to replace that process. Please note that some medications for depression and anxiety can impact your weight loss and management efforts; be sure to ask your doctor about this during the prescription process or your next medical appointment.

and also provide distraction. In the long run, though, eating for comfort is not helpful. It does little to relieve the source of the unhappiness, and it contributes to weight gain, which can lead to still more unhappiness and dissatisfaction. As hard as it may be, you *can* find other ways to comfort yourself when you are upset. If you find that you use food to console yourself, and that this has caused weight gain, you can incorporate the material on changing habits discussed in your Personal Plan of Action.

E. ADHD. Attention-deficit/hyperactivity disorder (ADHD) can cause problems with planning and organization, leading to poor food choices. ADHD is also associated with increased impulsivity, which can affect a person's ability to control their food intake. Usually, symptoms of ADHD will have been present since childhood; however, many adults are diagnosed with ADHD annually (both hyperactive and inattentive types).

F. Trauma. A trauma is a shocking and dangerous event that you see or that happens to you. During this type of event, you think that your life or others' lives are in danger. It is estimated that about 60% of men and 50% of women experience at least one trauma in their lives. Women are more likely to experience sexual assault and child sexual abuse, while men are more likely to experience accidents, physical assault, combat, disaster, or to witness death or injury. In individuals with a history of trauma, extra weight sometimes feels protective. Weight can be a way of shielding oneself from unwanted attention or intimacy.

If you have any of these contributors to weight gain or other concerns regarding a mental health condition not mentioned, they should be addressed by a physician or mental health professional. In many cases, you may want to wait to start a weight loss program until after you have taken the time to address the mental health concern. In other cases, you may be able to focus on weight loss while receiving treatment and support for your mental health condition.

G. Medication use. If weight gain has occurred after beginning a new medication, in many cases your physician will be able to substitute another that is less likely to affect your appetite or metabolic rate. Indeed, some medications can be stopped entirely, particularly when the medications are prescribed for a condition that often improves with weight loss, such as hypertension or diabetes. Medications that commonly contribute to weight gain include: steroids and progestins, including hormonal contraceptives; some medicines used to manage diabetes; some blood pressure medications; tricyclic antidepressants; phenothiazines (antipsychotics); and lithium.

H. Other. Even if none of these specific factors apply to you, you may be able to identify others that do. Identifying specific causes of weight gain is a useful exercise, because the causes often suggest their own solutions.

If you can't think of any reasons for your weight gain, you can still develop a Personal Plan that addresses your needs, but, as described in chapters 4 and 5, you may benefit from a period of *self-observation*. This often is the difference between just another diet that fails in the long run and making a permanent and satisfying change in your life.

3. ARE YOU UNDERGOING A LOT OF LIFE CHANGES OR STRESSES AT THIS TIME?

If you have checked off one or more recent, current, or imminent major life changes, we encourage you to assess how likely they are to interfere with your weight loss plans. For example, a recent serious illness or major life challenge (such as a divorce or death of a loved one) may impact your commitment to the long-term lifestyle changes that are needed for long-term weight loss. For some, this type of significant life event (stress) can be motivating, having a positive impact on their desire and ability to make the favorable lifestyle changes that need to be made in order to lose weight for good. On the other hand, experiencing such a difficulty can also seriously interfere with one's ability to concentrate on or commit to a Personal Plan of Action.

We encourage you to be completely honest with yourself regarding the likelihood of your stresses (life challenges) that might interfere with your Personal Plan of Action. While there is no "perfect time" to start a weight loss program, it is probably better to work on addressing any stressor that would prevent you from succeeding in your weight management goals first, so that you can more fully commit to your Personal Plan of Action.

If you didn't check off any of the items listed, this is the ideal time to begin the preparation and action stages of a weight management program. The fewer stresses and distractions you have, the easier it is to focus on the task of designing and carrying out your Personal Plan of Action.

4. WHAT ARE THE MAJOR REASONS YOU WISH TO LOSE WEIGHT?

There are many reasons why people choose to lose weight. The following are common reasons people want to lose weight. Consider your personal reasons, and say to yourself:

I want to lose weight . . .

☐ **to improve my appearance.** This is one of the most common reasons given. While appearance can be a strong motivator, it is best to have other motivators as well. This is because losing weight to improve appearance can easily turn into another form of losing weight—for others rather than for yourself. (We discussed how this is not generally a good idea in chapter 1.) If your self-image is tied directly to your weight, this is a prescription for unhappiness and disappointment. However, people who seek to lose weight in order to take better care of a body that they love and respect, perceived faults and all, will be more successful than those seeking to lose weight to alter a body of which they feel ashamed. Bottom line, be kind to yourself.

☐ **to improve my health and reduce my health risks.** This is certainly an important reason for wishing to lose weight. Unfortunately, it tends not to be motivating for many people because you usually can't see any immediate health benefits. For example, someone who is advised by his or her doctor to lose weight after suffering a life-threatening heart attack is likely to be highly motivated. This same person would not have been nearly as motivated if he or she had been given the same advice six months earlier (before the experience of the attack).

If you have medical concerns (hypertension, high cholesterol, diabetes, arthritis, etc.) that can be alleviated by weight loss, or if you are someone at increased risk for these problems because of your weight, you should be aware of the concept of immediacy. Because you may need to change your lifestyle for a while before seeing health effects such as lowered blood pressure or cholesterol, you may have some difficulty with motivation.

☐ **to improve my energy level and overall fitness.** Much of what was discussed earlier under health reasons to lose weight also applies to this category. Improving energy level and fitness can be a strong motivator, but one that is not easily sustained. Focusing on a *specific benefit* to be obtained tends to be much more motivating than something general like, "I want to feel better." For example, one young man we worked with came up with two specific reasons for losing weight that proved to be effective motivators for him. He said, "I have a one-and-a-half-year-old son who's now walking. I want to be able to get down on the ground and play with him." He felt very much left out of his son's life because of his weight. Second, his hobby had been repairing and renovating old automobiles, but he had given this up when he gained weight. His abdomen had grown to the point where he was getting stuck on the way out. He revealed, "I want to be able to fit under the cars to work on them."

Do you have specific things you used to do but are now unable to do because of increased weight and decreased fitness? Examples include sports, hobbies, forms of transportation (riding the bus, bicycling, and fast walking), and specific activities

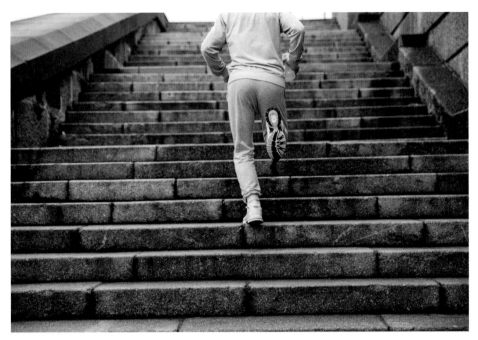

Choosing a specific weight loss benefit, such as being able to run up a flight of stairs, will help you stay motivated

(playing with children or grandchildren, running through the airport to catch a flight without risking collapse). Look for specifics instead of generalities, and you will find yourself more ready to change.

☐ **to avoid feeling embarrassed about my weight.** This reason is complex. It is similar to the already discussed "to improve my appearance." Because of our cultural peculiarities and pressures, it takes a high level of self-esteem or other defenses not to at times feel embarrassed when we stray from our culture's idea of an ideal body type. Although embarrassment is a powerful motivator, it is important that the source of the embarrassment be specifically identified and examined. Furthermore, it is important to differentiate between embarrassment and shame. Are you feeling embarrassed because you believe you overate or behaved in a way that caused you to gain weight? Or are you feeling shame, which is more about who you are as a person? Are you telling yourself that you are overweight because there is something wrong with you? To be clear, there is nothing wrong with you because you are overweight. It may be the case that you prioritized other things in your life over self-care, that your genes predisposed you to be heavier, or that you coped with life's challenges by eating. You may feel embarrassed about not doing something about the factors under your control, but remember that you are human. You are not alone, either; more Americans are overweight than not. Stating this reason for losing weight in more positive terms is a better way to motivate yourself for the long term. A more positive statement is: "I want to feel good about my energy level, fitness, and comfort in socializing. I want to feel proud of my efforts to take care of myself." Use specifics that apply to you when defining the benefits of weight loss.

☐ **to please someone important to me.** As noted in chapter 1, we encourage you to *beware* of this reason. You will improve your readiness for permanent change if you can find other reasons for losing weight than pleasing others. For example, it is common for people to decide to lose weight because of an upcoming event, like a wedding. This reason possesses many of the attributes that enhance readiness and motivation (it is important to you, is specific, and has immediacy). What it lacks, however, is long-term sustainability. What is likely to happen? Because of the pressure to lose weight by the wedding date, the caloric deprivation required will be extreme, perhaps with an intensive exercise regimen as well. There is unlikely to be an emphasis on permanently changing eating habits. Once the goal is achieved, or the wedding date arrives, the reason for losing weight departs with the guests, and old habits reemerge with a vengeance. Clearly, this is not a good way to enhance long-term readiness.

 JOURNALING ACTIVITY:

I Want to Lose Weight

As you consider why you want to lose weight—for you—we encourage you to first *make a list*. This should include medical as well as personal benefits of losing weight. Look at the list daily. You want to have these benefits at the forefront of your mind so that you can recall them anytime you need motivation to stick to your plan.

Second, *narrate the impact*. Carlos, a 55-year-old man we worked with, kept in his wallet a note his daughter had written on a paper napkin and slipped to him during a family dinner. It read, "Dad, I want you around for a long, long time. Please stop eating so much." He had suffered a heart attack three years previously, was seriously overweight, and had repeatedly been advised to lose weight by his physician. Previous half-hearted attempts to adhere to a diet had failed. The consequences

BOX 2-6

Example: My "Why Lose Weight?" List

1 To walk with my kids/grandkids to the park and back without needing to sit down and being left behind

2 To lower my blood pressure so I don't worry as much about having a stroke or heart attack

3 To go hiking or biking with my friends and not worry about holding them back

4 To feel proud of myself when I look in the mirror or at pictures of myself

5 To set a good example to my kids/grandkids so they will want to live healthier, longer lives

6 To sit comfortably in a chair or restaurant booth so I don't have to call ahead or be embarrassed if I don't fit

of failing health were insufficient to drive him toward definitive action until he realized, through his daughter's written message, that his declining health could rob him of the chance to see his daughter graduate college, get married, and so forth. He wanted to be there for those things. This shifted the balance sheet for him and helped him to stay the course when the barriers to successful change seemed insurmountable. He told me that he would take his daughter's message out of his wallet and read it whenever he felt his Personal Plan of Action was not working.

This process of narrating a story or letter in which you envision the true impact of your weight loss on those you care about can be a very powerful exercise in motivation. First, think about and write down all the benefits of weight loss in all of your dimensions of life. Then, rewrite this message as though it were a letter coming from someone important in your life. This exercise is meant to help you see and experience how losing the weight for good and getting healthier is not just about you—it makes a true impact on the people (and the world) around you.

5. FOR WHOM DO YOU WANT TO LOSE WEIGHT?

In this era of self-help, most people know that the "correct" answer to the above question is to rank "myself" as the number one person. Why is this desirable? Because losing weight for you means that you have explored and have come to understand the personal benefits of losing weight, *for you*. It's easier in the long run to lose weight when you do it because it would make *you* feel so much better physically and not

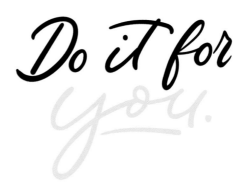

Do it for *you.*

You will have greater success if you want to lose weight for yourself rather than for others

because it makes your spouse feel so proud of himself or herself for having a svelte partner. When your primary motivation is to please others, as in this example, there is a high likelihood that the motivation will not sustain you in the long run, and may even foster feelings of resentment toward the person you are trying to please.

Wishing to please a spouse or significant other is a common reason for wanting to lose weight. For example, Zoe, a 30-year-old elementary school teacher, came to us for this reason. She had other reasons for wanting to lose weight, but her husband's disapproval was the strongest immediate motivator. It hurt her that her husband, David, admitted that he found her less attractive because of the weight she had gained (about 30 pounds) over the prior two years. The truth, though, was that there were other problems in the relationship as well. Interestingly, Zoe, like other people in her position, stated initially that she wished to lose weight primarily for herself and not for others. However, deep down, this was not the truth. She wanted to lose weight to end her husband's negative comments about her appearance and lack of self-care. She tried to make positive changes but was unable to stick to her diet and exercise plan. She dropped out of the program within a month.

While other factors played a role in her lack of success, Zoe's difficulty with weight loss stemmed from larger problems—an unhappy marriage, for one. The lesson to be learned here is that Zoe, like most people, was not likely to succeed in losing weight if she was doing it to please her spouse. The message her husband was sending her was a destructive one—in effect, he was saying, "My attraction and love for you is based on superficial rather than innate qualities you possess." Zoe might have done better if her marital problems had been addressed first, or if they had been addressed along with her weight problems.

Thus, it is important once again to examine your own motivations. Are you *really* doing this for you? You are much better off emphasizing the personal benefits you will reap through weight loss than by being a martyr and doing it for someone else.

You will greatly enhance your readiness for permanent change if you are able to do so. You are going to develop a Personal Plan for you, because *you* want to change.

It is also worth noting that if you come to the realization that you do *not* want to lose weight, that is okay, too. You may have other goals in your life that are more important to you at the moment, or you may have realized that you are happy at your current weight. You can still use the information in this book to improve your eating habits and level of physical fitness, if that is something that you choose to do.

6. HOW MUCH WEIGHT DO YOU WISH TO LOSE?

There is no right answer here, so let's look at the choices, and how your choice can impact both your readiness and the likelihood of achieving short- and long-term success.

☐ **Goal: Healthy BMI.** As discussed in chapter 1, body mass index (BMI) is a measure of one's body fat derived from a person's mass (weight) relative to their height. Aiming for a "normal weight" BMI may be reasonable in some cases but not in others. If you have always been in this range as an adult but tipped into the "overweight" or "obese" categories after a specific event like a pregnancy or quitting smoking, it is certainly possible for you to get into the normal BMI range again. If you have never been in this range, or last saw it on your sixteenth birthday, it is a virtual certainty that you

TABLE 2-1

BMI interpretation, using World Health Organization criteria

BMI (kg/m²)	Interpretation
< 18.5	Underweight
18.5–24.9*	Normal Range
25–29.9	Overweight
>29.9	Obese

*In Asian populations, the cutoff for overweight is 23 kg/m2.

will not be able to achieve or sustain that goal weight. Nor do you need to. Health risks seem to be minimal with modest degrees of being overweight. Aiming for normal body weight if you have not been this weight as an adult can sometimes mean aiming for frustration. In addition, it is also not a good idea to aim for a weight lower than a normal BMI. Not only are you unlikely to sustain such a weight, but it may be unhealthy for you to do so.

☐ **Goal: Most of the way to a healthy BMI.** This goal may be a reasonable one, but that will depend on a realistic assessment of your personal weight history. Again, if you have never been anywhere near a normal BMI, an initial goal even two-thirds of the way there may be unreasonable. For instance, if for your height, a normal weight is 125 to 145 pounds, but your usual weight has been 220 pounds, you would be aiming for a weight of 160 pounds, a loss of 75 pounds, more than a quarter of your total starting body weight. While this is by no means impossible, it is a major task to attain and maintain such a goal weight.

On the other hand, if your ideal body weight is also 125 to 145 pounds, but your current weight is 160 pounds, and you've been in the 140-pound range in the past, it is quite reasonable to set a goal of two-thirds of the way to normal body weight. This would entail a loss of 20 pounds, to 140 pounds.

☐ **Goal: Enough to feel more comfortable and reduce health risks.**
This is a common goal for people who have been very overweight for most of their lives. It is the most attainable and sustainable kind of goal. In many cases it is not necessary to put an exact number on it, since you may not know what weight improves physical comfort and health until you reach it. For many people who are seriously overweight, a loss of even 10% of their body weight is likely to improve fitness levels and reduce health risks, like high blood pressure and diabetes. This means if your weight is 220 pounds, your goal weight would be 198 pounds ($220 \times 10\% = 22$). While such a goal may not put you near our cultural "ideals" for weight, it can have a dramatic impact on the quality of your life. Such a goal should not be disparaged, only admired.

There is a tendency to believe that setting goals that are difficult to achieve improves the ultimate outcome—this is called "reach for the stars" reasoning. While striving for the nearly impossible is part of our folklore, it rarely works well in the long term, and it can be a difficult and frustrating process that may end up working against you. In weight loss, reaching for the stars is almost certain to result in disappointment, and it reflects a lack of appreciation for the magnitude of the task. Unreasonable goals will make even successful weight loss seem like a failure. In other words, if you cannot set goals that are reasonable for your personal situation, you are not ready to begin your Personal Plan.

What, then, is a reasonable goal weight for you? With the previous discussion and the material in the chapters that follow, you can set an appropriate goal and have the best chance of attaining and sustaining it.

7. HOW MANY WEIGHT LOSS PROGRAMS HAVE YOU TRIED IN THE PAST?

☐ **None.** This is often a good thing. You will not have had the experience of losing weight, then gaining it back. You probably have fewer preconceived notions about weight management programs and the likely outcome of your efforts. In general, we find that people who are attempting weight management programs for the first time have a good chance of successfully completing their programs.

☐ **I've undertaken a weight loss program one to a few times before.** This means that you have some previous experience with attempting to lose weight, but it is not a frequent practice. In an age where a majority of adults have tried to lose weight at least once, you are clearly not alone. Most people try on their own, sometimes with the help of friends or books like this one, rather than through a formal program. Read the discussion of the next choice to see what can be learned from your previous weight loss attempts.

☐ **I've tried weight loss programs four or more times before.** Although this sounds like a lot of times, it may reassure you that repeated attempts to lose weight are common. In any given year in the United States, 45% to 47% of women and 25% to 30% of men have dieted or participated in a weight loss program. Even if you have been initially successful in your previous attempts, having to repeat these efforts can be discouraging.

To enhance your readiness for long-lasting changes this time, it is critical that you view the previous attempts as valuable experience for the successful plan you are about to begin. In fact, previous weight loss programs do offer lessons you can learn from. In this way, then, you have an advantage over people who have never tried to lose weight before. We urge you to use this advantage to the fullest.

For example, you may, in retrospect, have wanted to do things differently during or after a weight loss program. Perhaps you began a previous diet when you were unable to commit the needed time and energy to the process, and now you can. Perhaps you were trying to lose weight for the wrong reasons before, and now you know better. Perhaps you were doing it for someone else in the past, and you will do it for you this time. Perhaps you had no coherent strategy during and after a previous attempt, but this time, you will formulate a Personal Plan of Action to see you through.

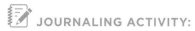 JOURNALING ACTIVITY:

My Past Weight Loss Attempts

Now you can see how to make previous weight loss efforts help your current effort. This is a practical use of your valuable past experience and will greatly enhance your readiness to change. We advise you to take full advantage of your personal dieting history—then you are much less likely to relive it.

BOX 2-7

Review the statements below. Think about your past attempts to lose weight and record your answers in your journal.

In the past, I _____ ,
but this time I will _____ .

Also in the past, I _____ ,
but this time I will _____ .

8. WHAT WAS THE TYPICAL SHORT-TERM OUTCOME OF PREVIOUS WEIGHT LOSS PROGRAMS?

☐ **I reached my goal weight.** Congratulations. You clearly have sufficient motivation to lose weight during the action phase. Since you have done it before, it's likely that you can do it again. This time, you will be following a plan that you will devise to meet your specific needs. You will be applying your considerable tenacity not just to a diet but to a comprehensive Personal Plan that addresses the habits causing you to gain or regain weight. This should be no more difficult for you than sticking with a traditional program, because you will have less deprivation on your Personal Plan. The emphasis will be on eating smart, making shrewd substitutions for the foods that get you into trouble, and recognizing and changing disadvantageous eating habits. The focus will not be on using sheer willpower to stick to a very restrictive diet plan. The fact that you have the proven ability to reach your short-term goals should make you feel quite confident about your ability to succeed with your own Personal Plan of Action.

☐ **I got at least halfway to my goal.** Congratulations again. Considering that most people seem to set their goals too aggressively, getting at least halfway there is usually quite an accomplishment. Too often, we focus on the part not achieved, rather than the considerable amount that was achieved. This is obviously self-defeating. Be mindful to avoid falling into this trap as you prepare your Personal Plan. You will be setting reasonable goals, with a plan geared to your specific needs, with a minimum of deprivation. That you were able in the past to get at least halfway to your goal without a Personal Plan is good evidence that you can do even better with one.

☐ **I got less than halfway to my goal.** Discouraging, isn't it? Perhaps you don't believe you can do much better this time. Your frustrations are understandable. However, don't let past experiences define you. Try looking at it this way. You can learn quite a lot from past experience. The methods you've used in the past may not have been the right ones for you. Read the third option under question 7 above and fill in the blanks if you have not already done so. If you set reasonable goals, develop well-thought-out reasons for losing weight, carefully devise your own Personal Plan, and talk positively to yourself about your ability to change, you will do remarkably well, regardless of your previous history.

9. WHAT WAS THE TYPICAL LONG-TERM OUTCOME OF PREVIOUS WEIGHT LOSS PROGRAMS?

☐ **I kept off most of the weight for many years.** You are to be commended. You are in a select minority. If you have now regained, it is likely that some specific factor is involved in your regain. If you have not regained but are still heavier than you'd like to be, you may wish to lose more weight. In either case, it is likely that you will again prove successful in managing your weight. Take advantage of the guidance available in these chapters, and begin with confidence.

☐ **I regained the weight after keeping most of it off for two or more years.** This, too, is an accomplishment to be proud of. Considering how common yo-yo dieting is, maintaining a majority of the weight lost during a diet for two or more years afterward is excellent. To do this, you had to succeed in continuing some form of diet or exercise-related behavior change for at least two years. It will be unhelpful if you focus on the fact that you eventually regained. Instead, take justifiable pride in the fact that you were able to sustain real behavior change for a prolonged period of time. If you could do that in the past, you can surely do it again now. And now you will have the advantage of past experience and an individualized program that will help you to address those specific areas that are causing problems for you now.

☐ **I regained the weight after keeping most of it off for less than two years.** Although you may feel discouraged, there is valuable information to be gathered here, too. Above all, don't get down on yourself for weight regain. View the past as objectively as you can. There can be many reasons why someone regains weight, and you can benefit from examining several different categories. These include your motivators for weight loss (see questions 4 and 5), the stresses and other circumstances that you lived through in the post–weight loss period (question 3), whether your weight goals were reasonable for you (question 6), whether you focused on changing your long-term eating habits or just taking off pounds, and any specific causes of weight gain that may have appeared in the post–weight loss period.

The bottom line is that you can learn more from mistakes than from success. Do it differently this time, and past mistakes become irrelevant. You will have a better long-term outcome this time if you learn from your past and incorporate this hard-earned wisdom into your Personal Plan.

10. HOW WILL YOU BEHAVE WHILE FOLLOWING A WEIGHT LOSS PLAN?

☐ **I will likely have a very hard time adhering to my plan.** If you believe this to be true, there are at least two things to be aware of. First, your belief that things will not go well is undoubtedly arising from your past experience in attempting to lose weight. As you are now aware, a bad past experience can be quite useful—*you can learn from it.* Second, your belief that you will be unable to adhere to a weight loss plan can have a tendency to make it harder to alter that dire prediction. It becomes a self-fulfilling prophecy—if you believe you will fail, you will fail. This is not the desired outcome, and such negative beliefs, no matter how compelling, must be countered. To counter them you must engage in positive self-talk and positive action.

Analyze why you believe you will experience difficulty. What did you do in the past that may have sabotaged your ability to stick with your plans? Was the diet you tried too limiting, entailing too much deprivation? Was the timing of the attempt wrong because of concurrent stresses? Were your goals unreasonable or not focused on behavior changes? Did you lack a good support system? Were you not convinced of the need to change at that time? Did you beat yourself up for small slips that then turned into big lapses because you were feeling demoralized? All of your answers are important, because all of these conditions can be changed this time to help you through. All that's required is a carefully thought out Personal Plan and your positive beliefs and actions.

☐ **I will likely be spotty in adhering to my plan.** Read the discussion to the first response option, as it applies equally well to this situation. Try to figure out what leads to your belief that your behavior will not be consistent. With what you have learned from past experience, you can set up your current goals, timing, motivators, support systems, and specific aspects of your diet and physical activity program so that you will be able to adhere consistently to your Personal Plan during the action phase.

☐ **I will likely be consistently compliant with my plan.** Congratulations. You either have had good success in complying with past programs or have taken to heart the advice to think positively. There is only one potential downside to consistent compliance during the action phase of a weight loss plan. Some people have little trouble with the initial adherence to a regimen but are prone to "all-or-nothing" behavior. To oversimplify, they are either being really compliant with a strict diet or really out of control with their eating, with no intermediate mode of behavior. If you think you are prone to "all-or-nothing" behavior, there are some things you can build into your Personal Plan that will help you to strike a healthy balance. These are discussed in chapter 5.

For the purpose of increasing readiness, the ability to adhere to a diet, even if only for a while, is valuable. The results you will see when you adhere to your Personal Plan will be very gratifying. They will help you to continue on your path to completion and beyond.

11. HOW WILL YOU BEHAVE AFTER THE ACTIVE WEIGHT LOSS PHASE HAS BEEN COMPLETED?

☐ **I will likely go right back to old habits.** Assuming that you are responding this way based on your past experience, one of the most important things you can do is examine your past behavior so you can learn from it. Were you dieting just for a specific occasion like a family wedding? Did you fall victim to all-or-nothing thinking? Were you not convinced of the need for long-lasting changes in your behavior? You can feel more confident this time, because before you begin you will have a Personal Plan of Action that includes ways to make the changes last.

☐ **I will likely start out with good habits then slowly revert to the old habits.** This is a common pattern. As discussed previously, readiness has a tendency to fade with time. You need a new set of skills to maintain behavior changes beyond the action stage. These include repetition, making your environment work for you, keeping track of your behavior, and using flexible responses. All of these tools can be learned and are discussed in further detail throughout this book. You will also incorporate many of them into your Personal Plan of Action.

☐ **I will likely maintain the good new habits for a long time.** Congratulations. That is the most important thing to be accomplished through your Personal Plan. Feeling confident that you will be able to maintain positive behavior changes indefinitely will help you to do so.

12. WHAT FACTORS WILL PLAY AN IMPORTANT ROLE IN PREVENTING YOU FROM SUCCESSFULLY COMPLETING A WEIGHT LOSS PROGRAM?

☐ **Lack of time.** To increase your readiness for change, it is important that you be realistic about how much time and energy you are willing and able to commit to this endeavor. If you decide to proceed, you will be better prepared if you make a specific time commitment on a regular, scheduled basis. For example, a typical patient at the Johns Hopkins Healthful Eating, Activity & Weight Program is asked to schedule about one hour per day for meal planning and preparation, a half hour per day for exercise, and one to two hours per

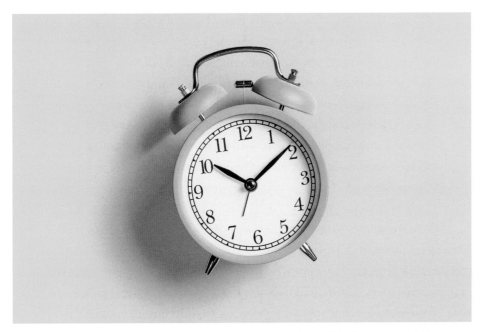

Be realistic about how much time and energy you can commit to achieving your weight loss goals

week for "school"—attending a group class, participating in online learning, or seeing the physician, health coach, dietitian, or psychologist. A similar schedule will apply to you and your Personal Plan. You will need time to plan meals so that you are not subject to the enticement of fast food, schedule a time for regular physical activity, and do your "schoolwork" at home. Your schoolwork will consist of recording your activities and progress in your Personal Plan.

☐ **Many people believe that they won't have the time to follow a weight loss plan properly.** If your life is busy, it can feel overwhelming to add more to your plate; however, the changes we are talking about likely take up less time than you think. To increase your readiness, you should remind yourself how important losing weight is for you. Refer often to your list of reasons. Spend a day or two tracking everything you do during a typical day and take inventory of how you are spending your time. Through a little creative time management, it is likely that you will be able to continue most or all of your previous activities and still devote enough time to your Personal Plan.

☐ **Lack of physical resources.** Lack of physical resources—namely, the funds to purchase exercise equipment, personal counseling, classes, and the like—is not necessarily an impediment to weight loss. In fact, there is some evidence that people are often more successful in keeping weight off long term on their own than through formal programs. Most formal weight loss programs treat everyone very much the same and fail to take into account the crucial differences between Marcella, Tamika, and Lucas, for example, each of whom needs to lose the same 40 pounds. Formal programs sometimes do not provide support during the all-important maintenance stage. Thus, it is quite feasible for you, with no more physical resources than this guide and your own commitment and planning, to achieve the goals you set in your Personal Plan.

Conversely, studies have shown that investing a significant amount of your physical resources in this endeavor to lose weight and keep it off can be a potent motivator. When people are given financial incentives to adhere to a program (for example, refund of a substantial deposit), they tend to do better. Having a financial and physical investment in your Personal Plan can make it more likely that you will follow through on it. The financial cost of devising and carrying out your Personal Plan can be nothing, or quite considerable. While it is sometimes helpful to have an "investment" in your plan, the lack of one does not mean you cannot carry out your plan successfully. Therefore, lack of physical or financial resources need not affect your readiness and commitment to change.

☐ **Lack of motivation.** This is the most commonly cited impediment to sustained change. In the past, you may have tried to begin a diet before adequately preparing, or you may have lost motivation midway through a diet. Perhaps your motivation began to suffer when your results were not as good as you had hoped, when you began to experience diet fatigue (for example, boredom with the meal plan, gym routine), or the wedding or other special event had passed. This time can be different. You have already examined and will continue to reevaluate your good reasons for embarking on this course of action. You will devise a plan that takes into account your specific needs as an individual. You will have reasonable goals, a strong support system, and the flexibility to adjust your plan to changing circumstances. In short, lack of motivation is not an ingredient in your Personal Plan. You will be well prepared this time. You will be ready.

☐ **Lack of support from family or significant others.** This, too, can be complex. Your best chance for success lies in "doing it for you" as your primary reason for embarking on a weight loss plan. Bearing in mind the benefits you will obtain from successfully losing weight and keeping it off will help you stay motivated. Sometimes, though, spouses or others, for reasons they may not even understand, will behave in an unsupportive or even a destructive manner. They may be jealous of your resolve or success. They may feel threatened. They may simply be unaware that their behavior is making it harder for you to adhere to your Personal Plan.

There is less of a chance that this problem will derail your plans this time around. Your motivations and coping skills will be stronger. You will probably build a "buddy system" of support into your Personal Plan. If you have decided to do this plan *for you*, pleasing others is not the point. While you cannot always control the behavior of others, you can control your own response to others' behaviors. Because you will be aware of the unsupportive behaviors of other people, you will be able to choose how to respond. You may decide that the behavior is irrelevant and choose to ignore it or to separate yourself physically from it. For example, you may choose to eat at a different time or in a different place when coworkers order in fast food for lunch and offer you some. Or, in the same situation, you may instead decide to address the unsupportive behavior directly. You can thank them for including you but ask that they not make such offers because it makes it harder for you to adhere to your diet.

When the unsupportive person is a spouse or someone else who is very close to you, you may decide to explore what's behind this behavior. Perhaps the other person is unaware of the behavior or the effect it has on you, in which case you'll need to talk to them about it. You can strengthen your coping skills by letting him or her know exactly what you would like him or her to do to be supportive. You may need to do this repeatedly. Whether the unsupportive person responds positively or not, you can stay on track (see chapter 5 for a more complete discussion of how to handle the would-be saboteur). You can rely on yourself and the Personal Plan you have devised for support.

If you have a supportive family member, you are in the best position to achieve your weight loss goals. Take Dr. Cheskin's patient Aaron, who worked as an architect. Even though Aaron's wife didn't appear on Aaron's balance sheet, she did all the cooking, and this was one reason Aaron had trouble losing weight. If Aaron's wife had been actively included in his Personal Plan, his chances of success would have been greatly improved. In fact, he and his wife could find that learning to cook together in new, healthier ways is a great hobby they both can share. Cooking, shopping, and even eating can become positive experiences, and the couple's time together could become one of the positive outcomes from Aaron's weight loss.

While it can be helpful to get the unqualified support of others, always remember that, by far, your most important booster is you.

☐ **Major stressful events intrude.** When stressful events occur, many people tend to abandon "optional" weight loss activities and fall back on tried-and-true coping mechanisms like eating. These old habits are tried, but they are not usually true. That is, *they don't work*, at least not in the long run. Although major stresses are indeed disruptive, eating does nothing to help a person deal with them. With luck, a major stress will not intrude anytime during or shortly after the action stage of your Personal Plan. If one does, though, you will be prepared. Your plan will include ways to deal appropriately with stress, without resorting to excess eating. Knowing that you have learned other ways to deal with major (and minor) stresses can make you less fearful of this form of intrusion into your plans.

☐ **Need to lose weight becomes less important.** This is a near-universal phenomenon. Your weight loss can lose priority at two different times. First, it can occur early in the action stage, before you have come close to your goal. Second, it can occur late in the action stage or during maintenance, when you have nearly reached your goal.

When it strikes early in the action stage, the cause is often lack of strong personal reasons for wanting to lose weight. This need not happen to you because you have examined your reasons and understand how to formulate them so they emphasize the benefits to you in losing weight. They are specific, they have immediacy, and they are important and can sustain your motivation. Your Personal Plan will include reminders of why you are committed to losing weight, which you can refer to when you think you are forgetting their importance.

When it strikes late, you are near your goal or in maintenance. The cause is often a false sense of security. You have gotten through the worst of it, you may believe. You have already obtained most of the benefits of weight loss. The last bit seems less important. What we can say from experience is: Not really. This time you have a greater respect and appreciation for the difficulties of maintaining weight loss, and you have incorporated maintenance into your Personal Plan from Day 1. You will not let down your guard when you near your goal, nor when you achieve it. You are ready for long-term success.

Set Rules and Condition Your Environment

Now that you have analyzed your past experience and current thinking, you have completed the hardest part of the task of making the most of your state of readiness for change. What remains is to set some rules and condition your environment so that it is supportive of your goals. Now, set the conditions in your environment that will help you get started by addressing this final set of questions.

IS THE TIMING RIGHT?

Weight loss programs often fail, not because the desire is not there or something is wrong with the program itself but because it's not the right time. Consider whether you have the time and mental bandwidth to focus on making major changes. Mere desire is a poor substitute for planned readiness. Desire to change is a necessary prerequisite to lasting weight loss, but it is only one component of readiness—and surely the most fickle. On the one hand, it can be a mistake to try to wait for the perfect time to diet, but, on the other hand, there are times that are better than others.

DO I HAVE THE SUPPORT I NEED?

Before beginning a new diet and exercise regimen, it's wise to get your doctor's approval. An appointment with your doctor is also an opportunity to discuss medication changes, laboratory tests, and a sleep study, if needed. Health insurance may cover office visits for nutrition and physical activity counseling, so if you have it, use it.

Decide whether to tell family, friends, and coworkers. On the one hand, telling others makes you vulnerable. Others will become aware that your weight is something that you want to change, and you may feel added pressure to succeed.

On the other hand, telling others may help you feel more accountable, and thus help with motivation. It may also increase the amount of support available to you. It is important to be specific with friends and family about what you need.

BOX 2-8

First, the Rules:

1 Remember: you are doing this for you, not for others.

2 Keep your personal reasons for wanting to lose weight in the foreground—review your reasons for losing weight daily and update them as needed.

3 Make your goals reasonable and attainable.

4 Monitor your progress regularly.

5 Vow to analyze and learn from past and future mistakes.

It would not be going too far to sit down with loved ones and to give examples of what would help you versus what would be unhelpful to you. Loved ones often try to help by policing the food intake of the person attempting to lose weight. They may be intervening with the best intentions; however, their comments are likely to backfire. It is not uncommon for someone dieting to eat more after being told that they should not eat something.

Share your specific reasons for wanting to lose weight with your loved ones. It may be a bit of a sacrifice for your significant other to agree not to bring ice cream into the house, for example, or to drink wine without you. But he or she is more likely to be on board with your decision if you've explained the effect your weight or your eating habits have been having on your life. Your spouse may think you look great and not understand that you get out of breath now when going up the stairs, or feel self-conscious in a sleeveless dress.

Family and friends tend to be most supportive when you sound satisfied with the choices you are making. If you go to a restaurant and appear disappointed to be ordering a salad, your dining companions will be more likely to urge you to order "what you really want." They internalize your feelings of deprivation and aim to alleviate your discomfort. If you remind yourself of your reasons for wanting to lose weight, you are more likely to truly want to make the healthier choice. If you sound excited and empowered about your meal choice, friends and family will likely be supportive. You might share enthusiastically, "I'm so excited to try this winter salad, it sounds fantastic" or "I'm challenging myself to eat only fresh

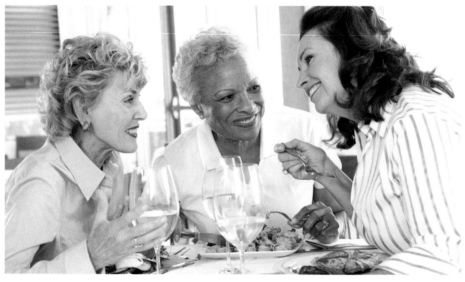

Decide for yourself whether telling friends about your weight loss plans will be helpful to you

vegetables and baked instead of fried foods." You may even notice others ordering healthful options after you.

If you do not feel comfortable sharing your plans with your friends or family but recognize that you would benefit from having support, you may wish to seek out an online weight loss support group, in-person support group (for example, Overeaters Anonymous, Taking Pounds Off Sensibly [TOPS], Weight Watchers), or professional counseling.

AM I PREPARED?

We recommend setting a start date, two or three weeks out. Use the intervening time to make sure you have done everything in your power to set yourself up for success. You want to reduce temptation whenever possible. This may mean clearing out your kitchen of items that don't fit with your meal plan, or particular foods that you frequently overeat (for example, ice cream, chips, cookies). This may require some discussion with your partner/spouse, roommate(s), or children. I have had some families come up with creative solutions when one person wants to keep something in the house that is problematic for another. One patient asked her husband to keep his jar of peanut butter in the spider-ridden basement that she was afraid to enter. Another patient, a single mother, had a separate drawer for her teenage daughter's snacks.

The "out of sight, out of mind" mantra really does have some truth to it. So, remove tempting foods from the house, keep them out of sight, or make them more difficult to access. Not only does making something hard to access make it less likely that you will want to expend the effort to go get it, it also cuts down on mindless, impulsive eating. If you have to climb up on a chair to reach the cupboard where the chips are kept (we love the cupboard over the top of the refrigerator for this purpose), you have a lot more time to second-guess the decision before eating the chips versus if they are on the counter. You may even forget that they are up there.

If you are someone who enjoys watching cooking shows and perusing foodie websites or books, think about whether this is likely to be problematic for you. Even the television, in and of itself, can be a trigger due to classical conditioning. If you are used to snacking in front of the television, just like Pavlov's dog, who salivated at the sound of a bell that had been paired with his dinner, you may find that without conscious consideration, you suddenly want to have a snack. Television commercials and pop-up ads can then provide added temptations. We often hear from patients that it is not until they start a weight loss program that they realize how many commercials for pizza and snacks they are exposed to.

Eating away from home can also present a challenge, and you should consider your social calendar and the level of temptation it presents. If possible, see if you can socialize with friends in ways other than going to bars or restaurants. Consider asking friends to join you for a walk, participate in a 5K, or go to a movie, concert, sporting event, art show, or theater performance. Be honest with yourself, and weigh the pros and cons of accepting invitations that would realistically put you in situations where it would be difficult to make healthful decisions. On the other hand, take care to avoid isolating yourself. Often when people overhaul their diets and begin eating healthier, they feel like they get less pleasure from their food. Over time, their palate will change, and they will figure out what healthful foods they enjoy. However, in the beginning, it can be tough. It is thus very important to try to find alternate sources of pleasure. Perhaps you used to look forward to picking up take-out on the way home from work. Instead, plan to eat a healthful dinner at home and then meet friends at a local park to go for a walk.

There are several other healthful practices you can adopt as you prepare to start a weight loss program. Each of these practices will be further described throughout this book.

REGULAR WEIGH-INS

First, we recommend that you weigh yourself regularly, at least once a week. Many patients find it helpful to weigh themselves daily, as it helps them better understand their body's responses. They learn how certain foods affect their weight, possibly due to water retention, and hopefully learn not to get upset or discouraged by minor fluctuations. It also helps them to more quickly identify and correct trends in the wrong direction. One may benefit from daily weighing by overcoming any fears of seeing the numbers on the scale.

TRACK YOUR SUCCESS

Additionally, we recommend finding a way to track your progress. Decide whether you will track progress solely via the scale or if you will also use other measures of success such as body measurements. Body measurements, such as waist circumference, are more time-consuming, but they may give you a better picture of your progress. Often when patients are strength training while dieting, they will put on muscle and lose fat at the same time. While fat and muscle weigh the same, one pound of muscle takes up less space than one pound of fat. Therefore, when you replace fat with muscle, your measurements are likely to go down (however, keep in mind that you will not necessarily lose fat in the same area where you put on muscle).

Track Your Physical Activity: Daily Movement and Weekly Exercise

In addition to measuring changes in weight and body composition, we suggest you track your daily physical activity. An activity tracker, such as a Fitbit, may be helpful in this regard. You could also track how long it takes you to run a certain distance, how much weight you can lift doing different exercises, and so forth. You may also want to measure how much sleep you are getting, how much time you spend practicing relaxation exercises, and so on. We often encourage patients to track both physiological (for example, body measurements, scale weight) and behavioral (for example, minutes spent exercising, percentage of time healthy meals were consumed) measures of progress, as sometimes the scale just doesn't reflect the progress that has been made. Many patients also find it helpful to write down the "wins" they had during the day—the times they were faced with temptation and stayed the course. Aim to recognize your success however you can, as this will help you stay confident and motivated.

Track Your Food Intake: Quality and Quantity

We also recommend logging your daily food intake for at least one week. Logging is tedious, indeed, but it is an effective tool for raising your awareness about your choices and your portions. It is a great way to increase your focus, be more accountable to yourself, and better understand your eating patterns and triggers for overeating. There are many ways to log your intake: written logs, phone apps (for example, Lose It, MyFitnessPal), and even taking photos of everything you eat. Use whatever is easiest and most intuitive for you.

SCHEDULE YOUR SUCCESS

We also recommend spending some time before you begin your weight loss plan working on structuring a plan for your meals, snacks, and physical activity.

People frequently ask whether it's better to eat according to their level of hunger or according to a schedule. Our answer is a little complicated and may sound a bit counterintuitive, but we generally recommend that people start by structuring their eating as much as possible, eating according to the clock at first. For many patients, we recommend scheduling three small meals and two to three snacks per day, eating approximately every two to three hours. Many patients that we have worked with come to us with irregular eating patterns. One common pattern is to overeat at night, resulting in not feeling hungry in the early part of the day, then heading into the evening in a calorie deficit and perpetuating the cycle of overeating in the evening. Others will overeat a large meal and then attempt to balance things out by skipping later meals. Eating according to a schedule is a way to structure and normalize one's eating habits.

People also ask "what is the best time to exercise?" As you will learn in chapter 8, exercise is not enough for your physical activity plan; we also encourage you to embed more movement throughout your day. Scheduling mindful movement breaks is one way to ensure you are taking time for stress relief and getting more movement into your day. This involves scheduling time to move different parts of your body throughout your workday—for example, moving your arms and legs at 10 a.m., your core at 12 p.m. (before lunch), your hips at 2 p.m., and your arms at 4 p.m. In addition, it is important to schedule exercise three to five days per week, aiming for a total of 150 minutes of movement weekly.

SLOW DOWN . . . TO EAT AND MOVE MORE MINDFULLY

Mindfulness has recently become a buzzword for stress management, even though it is a concept that has been in existence for centuries. Being mindful means being aware of one's experiences in the present moment. We know that when you take time to be more mindful about what you are eating and when, and how you are moving (in daily movement and weekly exercise), you will be more likely to stick to your Personal Plan of Action and enjoy the journey along the way.

Mindful Eating

In a perfect world, we'd like people to accurately assess their hunger level and eat only when they are truly hungry. On a 0 to 10 hunger scale, with 0 being not at all hungry and 10 being famished, it's probably ideal to eat at a 5 to 7. Wait too long and low blood sugar may begin to cloud your judgment regarding your food choices and portions. Eat when you are not truly hungry and you are likely to take in more calories than you need. However, many patients have a hard time assessing when they are truly hungry. Work demands, stress, and distraction can keep someone who is actually hungry from recognizing their need to eat, whereas boredom, stress, sadness, and frustration can feel a lot like hunger. Additionally,

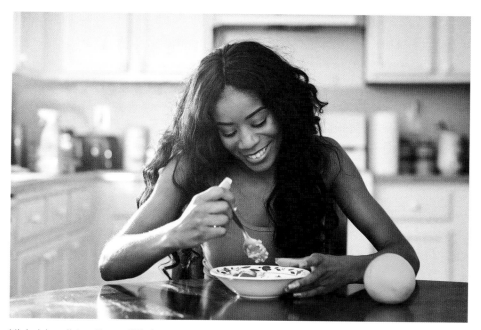
Minimizing distractions will help you enjoy your food and recognize your body's fullness cues

many hormones, such as cortisol, ghrelin, leptin, and estrogen, can have an impact on hunger levels. Therefore, we initially recommend that people eat according to a more rigid structure. Over time, it becomes easier to recognize if they are truly hungry or merely being triggered. At this point, they may transition from eating on a regular schedule to eating when they are feeling hungry.

That answers the question of when to eat, but what about *how* to eat? The answer is slowly and mindfully. Eat until you are no longer hungry. The goal is not to eat until you are full. For many, this is a huge adjustment in the beginning. If you find it hard to distinguish when you are no longer hungry, keep trying—you will quickly learn when to stop. You may also find it helpful to consider the marginal return you get from each bite. With your first bite, you get the most "bang for your buck"—that is the bite where your curiosity is satisfied, where you find out if it tastes as good as it looks, if it's new or familiar, and so on. You eat the first bite mindfully, paying attention to the flavor, texture, and aroma, but with each additional bite, you become habituated and your mind likely turns back to your conversation with your dining partner(s), and you may eat on autopilot.

If possible, establish one place in your home where you can sit down to eat meals. Avoid eating in the car, while working, while standing in the kitchen, or while walking. During all of these activities, your attention is at least somewhat divided. You are not able to give your meal your total focus, which results in the meal being less satisfying. In essence, if you are distracted, you have "missed" part of the meal, which leaves you wanting more later on.

It's also worth noting that the appearance of food plays a large role in our experience of eating. We recommend that our clients and patients use small plates, as this helps trick the brain into believing that portions are larger. A large body of research has shown that even when we believe we are compensating for large plates (by putting smaller portions on our plates), we are usually wrong. Larger plates lead to larger portions, even when we think we are compensating. Additionally, it's worth putting a little extra effort into the way you present the food that you eat. Plating the food attractively can increase satisfaction and satiety without adding calories. Again, these are important skills that can be practiced in the weeks leading up to the start of your diet.

Mindful Movement and Exercise

It is unfortunate that thousands of people hurt themselves in activities and exercise efforts every day, simply because they are not being mindful about how they are moving. It is not uncommon to see people watching television while they exercise on the treadmill, or to see people trying to multitask when they practice daily movement and activities. While this may feel like a great way to get more done in less time, multitasking can cause you to perform movements that are not right for your body.

In the movement field of kinesiology, it is often said that going "too far, too fast, too soon" is a great way to get injured. Unfortunately, many people have heard a different phrase: "no pain, no gain." This is actually not a recommendation based in science; in fact, you can hurt yourself if you push your body to the point of pain. We like to say that it is helpful to think of aiming between "easy and ouch" in your movement and exercise. If movement is too easy, you are less likely to be making progress over time. If movement is too "ouch," you may be pushing your body past its healthy limit—or worse, causing harm. So, challenge yourself but be mindful that you don't overdo it.

We also encourage you to be mindful about how you are moving, and to enjoy exploring movement as an expression and an experience. Explore how each movement your body makes is synchronized, with the muscles moving in concert, and how movement affects you mentally, as well as physically. Movement isn't just about our physical experience and strength; it also changes the way we think, feel, and interact. We know that movement is a great way to express ourselves, and recent studies have shown that our posture can influence how well we receive communication messages.

And finally, we encourage you to be more mindful about what you are telling yourself when you move and exercise. For example, you may think to yourself, "I am feeling really tight with this stretch" or "I am feeling out of shape on this walk." These thoughts are understandable; however, they can get demotivating over time. When you are mindful that you are saying these mean and unkind phrases to yourself, take a moment to "take them back" and turn them into a positive self-statement. For example, "I am feeling really tight today with this stretch" can become "I am getting more open as I stay in this stretch." Be mindful of what you tell yourself . . . because you are always right.

Believe That You Can

Henry Ford once said, "Whether you think you can, or you think you can't— you're right." We believe that you can lose weight for good, which is why we wrote this book. We recognize that it will be difficult, and we also know that you do difficult things every day. The boss gives you a terribly unpleasant task to do. There isn't anyone else who can do it, and so you do it. At home, at work, at school, in the community—there are endless difficult things to be done, and you do them. The trick with weight loss and maintenance is to convince yourself, with the help of the tools described in this chapter, that you *can* and *will* make the changes in your life that you desire to make, for the important and personal reasons *you* want to make them. You are already well on your way to the action stage, so take a moment to congratulate yourself for taking the time to learn more about your weight loss and management journey. Then, complete the action items in this chapter before moving on to chapter 3.

Action Items

If you haven't already, complete the weight loss journal activities from this chapter:

- Am I *Really* Ready?
- What Stage Am I in for Long-Term Change?
- I Want to Lose Weight
- My Past Weight Loss Attempts

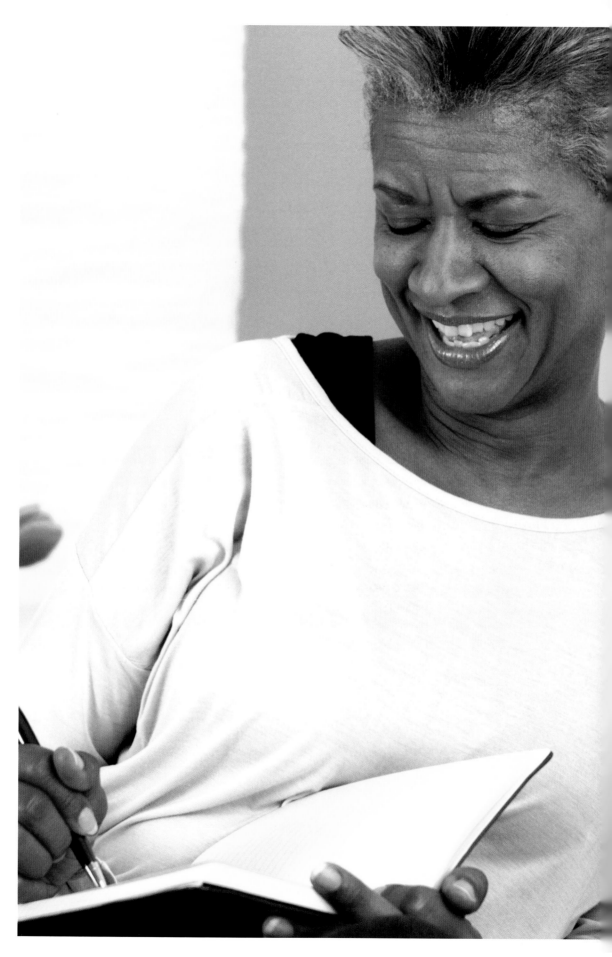

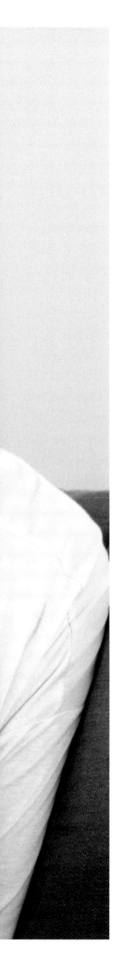

CHAPTER 3

Beginning Your Self-Assessment

IN THIS CHAPTER, WE WILL:

- **show** how modern American food culture promotes weight gain,

- **describe** a typical assessment process undertaken to develop an individualized weight loss plan, and

- **help you adapt** this process to conduct a personal self-assessment.

IMAGINE THE SETTING: a medium-sized conference room on the first floor of an office building. Around a conference table on this wintery Tuesday evening sit ten people, eight women and two men, who have gathered after work for a meeting. This is a diverse group brought together by one thing—they all suffer from obesity and are all serious about wanting to lose weight. The purpose of the meeting is to hear about an approach to help people lose weight and keep it off. Most of the people in this orientation meeting have tried to lose weight before, some many times, but none successfully in the long run.

The members of the group range in age from 20 to 68. They come from various walks of life—from a college student to an executive at a large corporation. They differ in income, race, and life experiences, and the factors that led them to become overweight are also quite varied. A few have been obese since childhood, but most did not gain weight excessively until their late teens or adult life. Some have been living almost exclusively on junk food, while others claim to eat a nutritious, varied diet full of fresh fruits, vegetables, and whole grains. Most are physically inactive, but one plays tennis regularly and another runs religiously three times each week.

The most interesting thing about this group is that its diversity is typical of people who want to lose weight. The 60-year-old restaurant owner who loves rich foods is clearly very different from the 35-year-old who has recently undergone a difficult divorce and gained weight in the process—even though both are women who find themselves to be 55 pounds over their "ideal" weight. However, this did not surprise us. Even if you selected ten equally overweight women of the same age, occupation, and race, all from the same town, you would likely find that each one of them gained weight for a different set of reasons.

A Different Approach: A Plan Tailored to *You*

At the Johns Hopkins Healthful Eating, Activity & Weight Program, our approach to weight management recognizes these individual differences and uses them to formulate the best plan for each person. Why is this individualization so important? Won't everyone lose weight if they just follow a strict diet? Does it really matter how the person became obese?

The fact is that, yes, everyone loses weight when they cut their intake of calories below their energy usage. Unfortunately, as many people have experienced firsthand, when a reduced-calorie diet ends, weight tends to be regained, sometimes with distressing rapidity. One thing that leads to regaining weight after a diet is that most diets don't address the *habits* that contributed to unwanted weight gain. The diet is often a short-term success—but a long-term failure—because it has provided little or no guidance about how to behave after the weight-losing phase has ended. This kind of guidance is crucial to long-term weight control. To be effective, a diet must be *individualized* to address the areas that caused problems for each individual person.

For example, it would make little sense to teach the 60-year-old restaurateur how to avoid eating to relieve emotional distress, as this is not one of her problem areas. Similarly, the 35-year-old divorcée already knows a lot about good nutrition and practices it—unless she is under emotional stress. Moreover, neither of them will be able to manage their weight in the long term by simply following the typical low-calorie diet. Both will likely lose some weight, but only temporarily.

We believe that an emphasis on individualizing one's approach is simply common sense: what works best is a low-calorie diet *combined with* an individualized, customized blueprint for change. You must place the long-term focus on altering the habits that caused the person to put on excess weight in the first place. To do this,

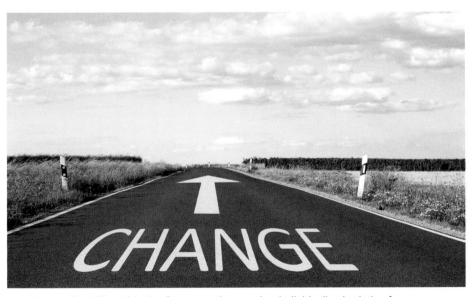

Your Personalized Plan of Action forms a path toward an individualized solution for lasting weight loss

a personalized assessment of each person's state of readiness is needed, as well as a review of his or her medical, dietary, behavioral, and physical activity profiles. The blueprint that results from this planning process is what we call a Personal Plan of Action: a plan designed by working from the specific needs of the individual.

Ideally, this assessment is done by a team of experts in the disciplines most relevant to the weight management process, and the various assessments add up to a comprehensive picture of the individual's current and past status. The different parts of the assessment overlap and interact with one another in various ways that can improve progress in weight loss. We have taken a similarly comprehensive approach in this book.

Our contributors include:

two physicians, to assess the person's medical status, develop a medical risk profile, and use advanced tools (including medications or procedures) when indicated;

a dietitian, to assess the person's current diet and offer suggestions for change;

a psychologist, to assess personal habits (the "why" of eating), enhance readiness for change, and encourage more mindful lifestyle choices;

a stress management and sitting disease (mindful movement) expert, to provide strategies for managing stress and incorporating daily movement as well as physical exercise; and

an exercise physiologist, to assess the person's current level of physical fitness and suggest improvements and ways to burn more calories (including daily activity and weekly exercise).

Obviously, not everyone has access to a team of experts. However, your author team includes experts in all the fields mentioned previously, and we've written this book to give you the tools you need to develop your own successful weight loss plan. Except for the medical evaluation, most people will be able to conduct a detailed self-assessment using this book alone. Nevertheless, some people will need professional help with some parts of the assessment. The information contained in this book will help you determine if *you* do. After the assessment, we will explain how you can use the information gained to formulate your own Personal Plan of Action.

If you have completed the questionnaires in the previous chapter and have thought about ways to enhance your readiness to change, you already know about developing a Personal Plan. You understand the importance of making lifestyle changes, and of acquiring the tools to make your changes a permanent part of your life. You are well beyond the contemplation stage and are actively preparing for change. Let's proceed with the rest of the assessment process—the medical, dietary, behavioral, and physical activity assessments.

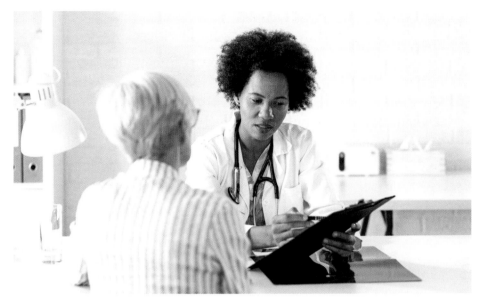

Unlike the other assessments, the medical assessment *must* be performed by a trained professional, such as a physician or other licensed medical provider

The Medical Assessment

Unlike the other assessments, the medical assessment *must* be performed by a trained professional—a physician or other licensed medical provider. In addition to assessing your overall health, the medical provider will concentrate on four areas while evaluating you before you begin a weight loss program:

- **an assessment** of the health consequences that being overweight has imposed, or is at risk of imposing, on your health;

- **whether your current medical treatment,** if any, is in conflict with the weight loss plan you are about to undertake;

- **a discussion of the pros and cons** of various weight loss techniques (rapid versus slower, diet versus exercise, etc.); and

- **a discussion of your hopes, fears, and aspirations.** A good medical provider will be able to address these issues in a forthright but empathetic way. (You may need to investigate several providers to find someone who can best meet your needs.)

Often this assessment can be performed by your primary care provider, although specialists in obesity medicine with expertise in this type of care also might be available in your area. Generally speaking, there are three parts to a medical assessment: (1) medical history, (2) physical examination, and (3) laboratory testing (when necessary).

Since a carefully collated medical history is often far more revealing than the physical examination, most medical providers start there. We begin the medical assessment of our weight loss patients with a medical history, using the insights revealed to help them develop a Personal Plan. Most primary care providers use a standardized format when recording a patient's history, generally following this order (though we will discuss them in a slightly different order):

- chief complaint (CC),

- history of present illness (HPI),

- past medical history (PMH),

- family history (FH),

- social history (SH), and

- review of systems (ROS).

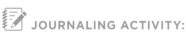 JOURNALING ACTIVITY:

Medical Exercise Assessment

As an exercise, let's imagine you are seeing us for a medical assessment. First, we are going to ask you some questions. Please note that *this is only an exercise*, and is not a substitute for an in-person evaluation by your health care provider. Before beginning any weight loss program, consult your medical provider in person for a history and physical, especially if you suspect or know that you have a medical problem, if you are age 60 or older, age 17 or younger, or if you are pregnant or breastfeeding. Now let's begin the medical history exercise.

Chief Complaint

What is your chief complaint? The chief complaint is traditionally logged in the medical record in the patient's own words, in quotes, like this:

CC: "I'm so unhappy with my weight; I have trouble even climbing a flight of stairs. . ."

You need to be specific, since, as you recall from chapter 2, the more specific, personal, and positive your goals are, the better your results will be.

What can you learn from your answer? The discussion of the various answers to question 4 (What are the major reasons you wish to lose weight?) in chapter 2 will provide some insight.

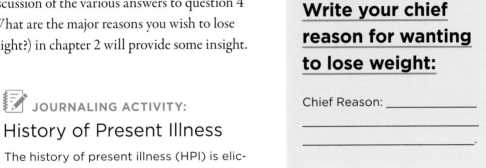

BOX 3-2

Write your chief reason for wanting to lose weight:

Chief Reason: _____

_____

_____.

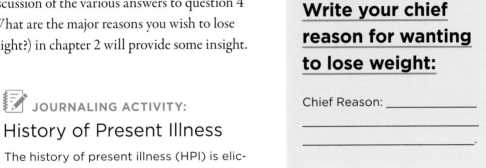 **JOURNALING ACTIVITY:**

History of Present Illness

The history of present illness (HPI) is elicited by asking the patient such open-ended questions as "When did you first notice the problem?," "What symptoms or consequences did it have?," "What happened next?," and "What do you think is contributing to the problem?"

The significance of your answers may be understood, at least in part, by revisiting your answers to questions 1, 2, and 3 in chapter 2, in which you considered your weight history, specific factors that contributed to weight gain, and any life changes or stressors you are experiencing. For the purpose of this medical self-assessment, we would like you to focus on the physical limitations being overweight may have caused, as well as the health, fitness, and quality-of-life improvements you stand to enjoy by losing weight.

REVIEW OF SYSTEMS

The review of systems is a systematic series of questions designed to uncover possible health problems that you may not be aware of. The following is an abbreviated version of the standard ROS; this version emphasizes causes of, or problems that result from, being overweight or obese.

If you experience any of the symptoms listed in the ROS, be sure to consult your physician. It is unlikely that having any of these symptoms will mean that you cannot or should not lose weight. Rather, they may provide additional insights and motivation you'll need for your weight loss plan.

Review of Systems

Do you suffer from any of these symptoms or illnesses, or have you suffered from them in the past?

General
Excessive fatigue? ___
Sleep disturbance? ___
Change in appetite? ___
Unexplained fever or chills? ___

Endocrine
Heat or cold intolerance? ___
Excessive thirst or urination? ___
Change in sex drive? ___
Excess hair growth? ___
Abnormal or absent periods? ___

Cardiopulmonary
High blood pressure? ___
Inherited heart condition? ___
Chest pains? ___
Shortness of breath
    with modest exertion? ___
    when lying flat? ___
Wheezing? ___
Chronic cough? ___

Leg pain while walking? ___
Ankle swelling? ___

Gastrointestinal
Frequent heartburn? ___
Change in bowel habits? ___
Bleeding? ___
Abdominal pains? ___
Nausea/vomiting? ___

Neurologic/psychological
Dizziness? ___
Numbness/tingling? ___
Blackouts? ___
Weakness? ___
Seizures? ___
Anxiety? ___
Depression? ___
Suicide thoughts/attempts? ___

In some cases, correctly diagnosing the cause of the symptom can lead to a treatment that makes it easier to lose weight. This was the case for Anna, a 37-year-old executive assistant who reported fatigue and cold intolerance on her ROS. Upon further evaluation, including blood tests, we learned that she was suffering from hypothyroidism (underactivity of the thyroid gland, which produces hormones that regulate our metabolism). Treatment of her hypothyroidism with a thyroid hormone medication made it much easier for Anna to lose weight.

In people like Anna, weight loss is easier or occurs automatically once their disease is treated. It is best not to expect this, however. Fewer than 1 in 100 people who are overweight or obese have gained weight because of an endocrine disorder.

A much more likely result of seeing a medical practitioner about any symptoms you checked off on your ROS is that you will learn that you have a specific medical problem. Many medical problems can be treated or even "cured" by losing weight and keeping it off. For example, Ahmad, a 56-year-old engineer, reported that he was getting progressively short of breath with physical exertion. This turned out to be the result of an early case of congestive heart failure with high blood pressure. In Ahmad's case, treatment of his high blood pressure and congestive heart failure with medications did not result in weight loss, because these problems were not a cause of his weight gain in the first place. The medications did, however, improve his shortness of breath and blood pressure. A silver lining of having this disturbing diagnosis, though, was Ahmad's enhanced state of readiness to commit once he learned about these medical conditions. He lost almost 50 pounds over a period of six months through a Personal Plan, which was geared to his specific problem areas, and he has kept the weight off.

Ahmad's motivation to continue to maintain his new, lower weight was boosted by the fact that weight loss made it possible for him to control his high blood pressure and mild heart condition *without* medications. The weight loss, in combination with a low-salt diet, enabled him to stop the medicines only a few months after they had been started.

Finally, Miriam, a 40-year-old retail sales associate with high-risk obesity, reported during her medical history that she often ate to settle her stomach. For the past four years, she had been experiencing abdominal pains in between meals and in the late evening. She had not seen a physician. It turned out that she had chronic ulcers, which were easily treated with a course of anti-ulcer medications. Eating to relieve her ulcer symptoms had not cured her ulcer. It had, however, contributed to her gaining 70 pounds in four years. The information that she had ulcers was very helpful to Miriam, who was able to keep her weight under control once she lost it with her Personal Plan. She no longer had the pain from her ulcers, so she didn't need to eat to try to feel better.

PAST MEDICAL HISTORY

Past medical history refers to medical, surgical, or psychiatric problems other than those described under the HPI. It includes past hospitalizations and other care, from birth to the present, as well as current medications used. These past and present problems may be relevant to the chief complaint; in addition, they serve as a reminder that the chief complaint has consequences beyond the obvious. For example, as discussed in chapter 1, heart disease, high blood pressure, type 2

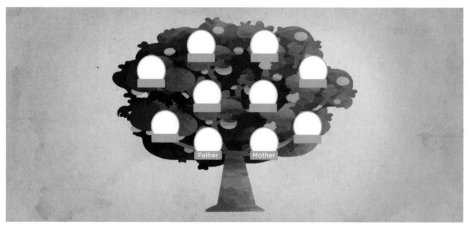

Family history is an important part of the medical assessment

diabetes, arthritis, gout, low back pain, and various other ailments are often the result of, or are made worse by, being overweight. If you have had any of these conditions or have symptoms of them, you should be under the care of a physician. Being aware that you have medical conditions or have had them in the past may give you another good reason to lose weight, as many health conditions improve, or may even be cured by, weight loss.

In your journal, note any medical conditions you've had, including past hospitalizations and medicines prescribed.

FAMILY HISTORY

Family history is important because genetics plays a definite role in determining whether you are likely to become overweight, and also whether you will suffer from various other illnesses. The most common illnesses and conditions with a strong inherited component include heart disease, diabetes, many forms of cancer, high blood pressure, and high choles-terol and triglycerides.

If any close relative has obesity or suffers from these conditions, you may be at increased risk yourself. Losing weight now can reduce your risk and increase your fitness as well.

SOCIAL HISTORY

Social history refers to your living arrangements, job, education, and various medically relevant habits such as whether you smoke and how much alcohol you consume. All of these things can have an impact on your weight and how you should approach weight loss. (See the discussion of questions 2, 3, and 12 in chapter 2.)

For example, if you are living alone, you may have an easier time making your home a temptation-free zone than if you are living with a spouse and children who seem to require vast quantities of non-diet-friendly foods to sustain them. A stressful job may have led you to use food to cope. Your previous education may or may not have taught you about the principles of good nutrition. Bearing children and quitting smoking could have made you more likely to gain weight. Finally, if you drink a significant amount of alcohol, it could be a potential dependency that is also contributing a lot of "empty" calories (see chapter 6 on designing your dietary plan).

Write down any of the features of your social history that will influence how you design your Personal Plan. It's important to remember to incorporate into your plan how you will deal with the following specific circumstances:

- living arrangements,

- job,

- education,

- smoking, and

- alcohol use.

As noted earlier, the medical history is followed by a physical exam and laboratory tests as needed to complete the medical assessment. A careful medical assessment can provide a great deal of useful information about your health and your future health risks. If you do have health problems, they will often be related to your weight in some way. Even if the problem is not one that tends to improve with weight loss, you will almost always benefit from finding out about the problem and getting needed medical treatment.

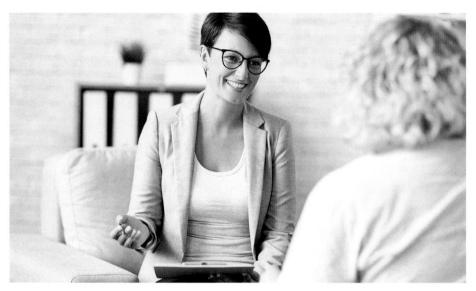

Use the questionnaires in this book or consult a counselor or psychologist to help you understand and manage your behaviors related to weight gain

The Behavioral Assessment

Behavioral assessments are often performed by a counselor or psychologist with expertise in behavior change. If a psychologist or similarly trained professional is not available to you, or if you do not wish to consult one, you can use the questionnaires provided in chapter 5 to guide your behavioral self-assessment. In general, the aims of the behavioral assessment are to:

- **assess your readiness** for change;

- **identify eating habits** and eating cues that influence your eating behavior;

- **assess your self-esteem,** explanatory style, and coping mechanisms;

- **diagnose eating disorders** like binge eating, bulimia, or anorexia;

- **identify and recommend treatment** for depression, anxiety, or any other problems; and

- **integrate** the behavioral assessment into your Personal Plan of Action.

The questionnaires in chapter 5 are designed to identify your mood, your attitudes toward eating, your coping style, your eating habits (like binge eating), and other information that will enable you to select an appropriate treatment effort. If you work with a counselor or psychologist, this information may be supplemented by an exploratory interview. This interview yields valuable information about the person's motivation for weight loss, past emotional traumas, the impact of the weight problem on his or her personal life, and current behaviors. We strongly urge you to consult a behavior change professional as you develop your Personal Plan. This specialist's insights and advice can be enormously helpful in developing a plan that is tailored to your specific needs.

The importance of this kind of assessment is clear in the case of Charlotte, a 41-year-old nurse's aide employed on an inpatient psychiatry ward who has been obese since her early teens. She came to us because of a hip problem, which would probably be improved with weight loss. She had never seriously tried to lose weight before. She related that her mother had been thin, and she had no recollection of her father, who was an alcoholic and left home when she was 2 years old. Her mother had remarried, and she had been raised by her mother and, from age 6, a stepfather whom she feared and disliked. At age 16, she left home and got a job. She later went back to school at night and became a nurse's aide. Although she had some friends, she had never been in an intimate relationship. Except for the recent hip problem, she was in good health. She had been prescribed an antidepressant once for depression but was no longer taking it because she felt she did not need it.

Charlotte's turned out to be a complex case, which is by no means typical of people trying to lose weight. Through a behavioral assessment, it was clear that Charlotte had a number of problems that would interfere with her ability to lose weight. She was still clinically depressed, for one. In addition, she revealed that she had been sexually abused by her stepfather, apparently with her mother's knowledge. It seemed likely that she had gained weight at least in part to fend off her stepfather's unwanted advances, since he was not attracted to people who had obesity. When she gained weight, the stepfather's sexual abuse stopped, but he became verbally and emotionally abusive toward her, causing her to leave home at a young age. Fortunately, the process of assessment helped Charlotte to deal with the aftermath of her troubled childhood. She lost only a modest amount of weight but felt much better about herself.

Although a good deal of information can be gleaned through a thoughtful process of self-assessment, there are a number of warning signs, discussed here and in chapter 5, of problems that are best handled by a qualified professional, such as a licensed counselor, clinical psychologist, or psychiatrist. We urge you to make an appointment with one of these specialists if you have a past history or current symptoms of any of the following:

- **depression:** chronic sleep disturbance, persistent feelings of hopelessness and helplessness, frequent crying, thoughts or plans of suicide;

- **eating disorders:** frequent binge eating, with or without purging by vomiting, laxatives, or water pills (diuretics); wish to lose weight when already below normal weight; prolonged fasting; distorted body image;

- **thought disorders:** recurring disturbing thoughts, hearing or seeing things that others do not, feeling that others are controlling you or plotting against you; and

- **anxiety or panic disorders:** intense chronic anxiety or fear, panic attacks.

If you have any of these symptoms, you will need additional help throughout your weight loss program, and you should seek it from a professional prior to beginning a weight loss program. Getting help for any of these problems may have the additional benefit of making it easier to manage your weight. Depression, for instance, will often sap a person's ability to sustain the kind of action required to design and carry out a good Personal Plan. Call your community hospital or a university center or your doctor or health insurance provider, if appropriate, and ask for the name of someone qualified to help you. To get the most appropriate reference, be sure to tell the person making the referral what you think your problem is—depression, eating disorder, thought disorder, or anxiety. Ask about the specialist's education (what degrees the person has and where they were earned) and how long the person has been in practice. If you're not satisfied, ask for additional names—or you may be offered the names of several specialists to choose from, even without asking.

The Dietary Assessment

Dietary assessments are often performed by a registered dietitian, and we recommend that you consult a professional dietitian. Nonetheless, with the information in this book, you can conduct an informative dietary self-assessment. The aims of this assessment are to:

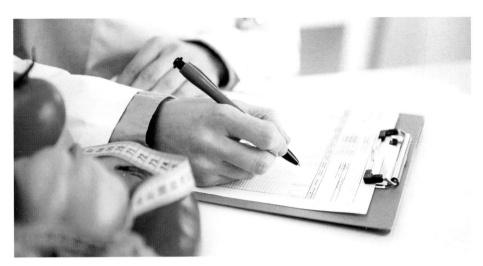

Though not a substitute for an assessment by a dietitian, this book will help you conduct a useful dietary self-assessment

- **define** your current weight category and weight history;

- **determine** your usual diet, including the percentage of your intake from fats, carbs, and protein, your food preferences, and your meal and snacking pattern;

- **create** an individualized weight-reducing diet; and

- **formulate** an individualized weight-maintenance diet.

Because the dietary assessment is so important, a highly detailed self-assessment is included in chapter 6, which will be of great assistance to you as you develop your Personal Plan of Action.

For our purposes here, though, please consider the following points right now. The dietary assessment will be useful to you only if you are completely objective and accurate about your usual diet, food preferences, and meal pattern. The individualized diet plan that you formulate in chapter 6 will only be as good as the information you provide. For whatever reason, a number of research studies have shown that overweight people are much more likely than lean people to underreport their actual food intake in surveys, diaries, and questionnaires. In most cases, we suspect this is unintentional and may reflect a lack of self-awareness of what and how much people are actually eating. To minimize the possibility of underreporting, you should do two things during your dietary assessment.

First, do not rely on recollections. We strongly encourage you to write down everything you eat and drink as soon as possible after you consume it. Set aside a week in which you know you will be following your usual eating patterns (not during holidays or vacations, for example). Make your food record from the day you start until the following week, not for the week just ended.

Second, we want you to resist the tendency to restrain or "improve" your eating during the period you will be recording your food intake. If, for instance, you sometimes grab lunch at the hotdog stand, it probably won't hurt you to do that for another few days while you are recording your usual eating patterns. To get the best idea of your diet, you should aim for recording a "bad" week rather than a "good" one.

Consider consulting a dietary professional if you find that you are having difficulty tracking your food intake.

As noted earlier, there is a good deal of overlap and interaction between the different parts of a comprehensive assessment. This is especially so with the dietary assessment and the behavioral assessment. In fact, it is somewhat arbitrary to distinguish the two. For example, what we eat at a meal is a result not only of our specific food choices but also of our habits, environmental cues, and our emotional state at the moment. As you probably are aware, a "good" diet does not guarantee good weight control. It is possible to gain weight on a genuinely low-fat diet if portion size is not controlled appropriately. Thus, it is important to perform not only a dietary self-assessment but a behavioral self-assessment, too.

The Exercise Assessment

The term *exercise* has negative connotations for many people, but really what we are talking about is not just exercise but movement—the full range of physical activity we engage in. It is rarely necessary to become an exercise "fanatic" in order to lose weight.

The aims of the exercise assessment are to:

- define your current and past levels of physical fitness and exercise tolerance,

- determine your usual patterns of physical activity and preferences for different kinds of exercise,

- measure your current resting energy expenditure via a test called "indirect calorimetry,"

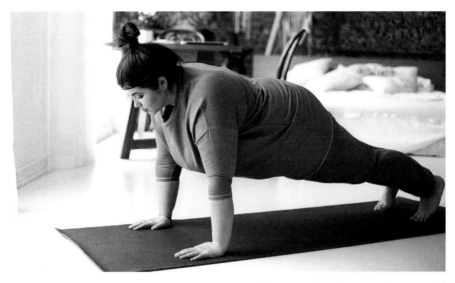

Though not a substitute for an assessment by a dietitian, this book will help you conduct a useful dietary self-assessment

- develop an individualized plan for gradually increasing physical activity, and

- set up physical activity monitoring for long-term maintenance.

Most of the details of the exercise self-assessment are provided in chapter 8. Some portions of the assessment, such as the indirect calorimetry test, you cannot do yourself. But you can do most of it. With the help of your honest answers to a series of questions, along with a willingness to try a variety of techniques to achieve your goals, you can make changes. Whether you are a "couch potato" or a "jock" or somewhere in between, finding enjoyable ways to increase your level of physical activity will make it considerably easier to achieve and maintain a lower weight.

When should you seek professional help to devise and carry out an exercise plan? First, when you have physical problems that make it difficult or unsafe for you to develop a traditional exercise plan. In that case, a consultation with your physician and an exercise physiologist, trainer, or physical therapist will make it possible for you to build an exercise component into your Personal Plan in a safe and effective way.

Second, if you experience difficulty in carrying out your exercise plan, an expert can guide you or even act as a personal trainer. This will help ensure that you follow through on a regular basis. Since such an approach is costly, we will describe a number of ways to improve your compliance with the exercise component of your Personal Plan—without having a personal trainer—in chapter 8.

Finally, if you experience any chest pain, light-headedness, severe shortness of breath, joint or muscle pain, or soreness as you carry out your exercise plan, you should stop doing your exercises and seek the advice of a physician and an exercise professional.

Comprehensive Assessment: The Synthesis

In many medical weight management programs, once all the assessments have been completed, a "synthesis meeting" occurs to review the recommendations from each professional who performed the individual assessments. This is done after the professionals have met and agreed on an approach. Feedback from the patient is important at this stage and may influence the plan that is ultimately adopted. The specifics of the weight loss plan are then discussed, and the plan begins.

In your case, the synthesis meeting will take place when you have completed the self-assessments and formulated the individual ingredients of your Personal Plan. At this point you will step back to make certain that all the components (medical, dietary, behavioral, and exercise) are consistent with one another, and that you can carry out the plan that you've put together.

Here are some broad considerations to keep in mind for your own synthesis meeting. When you have finished developing your Personal Plan of Action and are ready to assess it, ask yourself the following questions:

BOX 3-5

1 **Is it comprehensive?** To be comprehensive, your Personal Plan must address all the major areas that can influence your success on the Plan, including readiness, physical activity, and maintenance.

2 **Is it realistic?** To be realistic, your Personal Plan must incorporate reasonable goals to be achieved through specific actions. You must be capable of fitting these specific actions into your schedule, and you must be likely to carry them out. If there's anything in your plan that you do not believe you can or will do, you should strike it from your plan and put a more realistic approach in its place.

3 **Is it permanent?** To be permanent, your plan must incorporate a maintenance plan, enough flexibility to respond to changes in your life down the road, and techniques of self-monitoring that will enable you to detect major deviations from your overall plan before they get out of hand.

Now that you have been introduced to a medical weight management approach and have seen how you can adapt this approach to your own self-assessment, you are ready to continue. The next chapter describes the key ingredients of an effective Personal Plan and guides you in developing your own Personal Plan of Action.

Action Items

- Meet with your medical provider to discuss your plans to initiate a weight loss program.
- Working with your health care provider, complete the medical recommendations inventory located in the resources section of this book.
- In your weight loss journal, complete the medical assessment exercise described in this chapter.

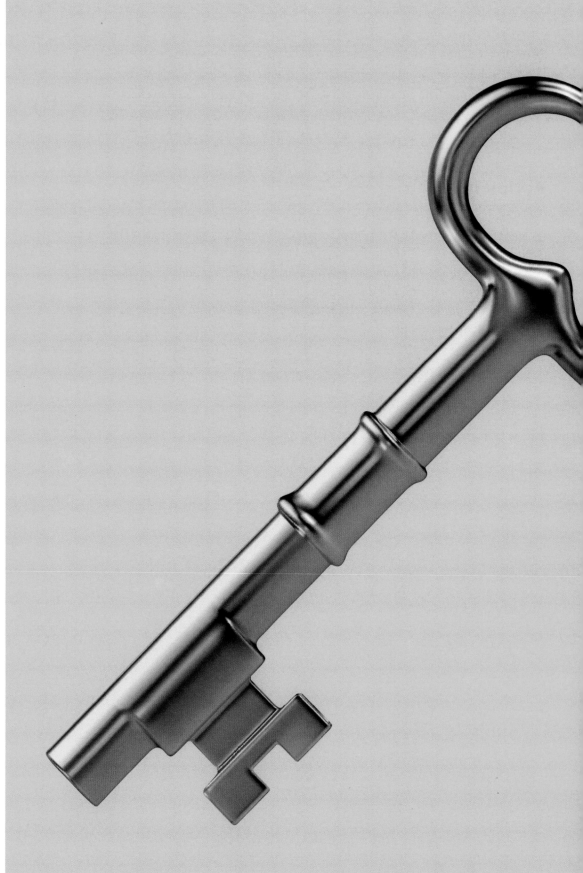

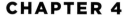

CHAPTER 4

Unlocking the Eight Keys to Your Successs

IN THIS CHAPTER, WE WILL:

- **identify** keys to help you develop a successful Personal Plan of Action.

SO FAR IN THIS BOOK, YOU HAVE LEARNED the holistic approach we will take in supporting you in losing the weight for good, which encourages you to become more mindful about food, physical activity, and stress management. You have also seen that this entire book is designed to help you develop your own unique Personal Plan of Action, which serves as a road map for the weight loss and weight management journey that is truly right for you.

In this chapter, we will share what we call the eight keys to your success. Think of these keys as principles to follow, and pull over and come back to, anytime you need support. Remember: this is your weight loss and weight management journey and no one else's.

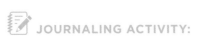 JOURNALING ACTIVITY:

Clear Away Distractions

Before you continue reading this chapter, make sure you have cleared away all distractions and have your weight loss journal open and ready. Formulating your Personal Plan of Action is crucial to your success and requires your undivided attention.

Key 1. Commit to the Journey (Not the Destination)

When you design your Personal Plan of Action, you will create your own road map to weight loss and weight management success, one that you will continue to travel and refine over time. When you commit to starting and sustaining this journey, it will be important that you shift your mindset from being all about the destination (weight loss) to being about the journey (committing to and enjoying the travel itself).

We take this approach because we have seen many patients focus on the destination instead of the journey. A destination approach is more like a diet—trying to take the fastest approach possible to get to a destination (weight loss). The patient takes shortcuts—short-term culinary sacrifices or sudden bursts of exercise and physical activity, resulting in swift yet transient weight loss. This approach may seem successful in the short term, but it doesn't usually work well in the long term. These shortcutters start to associate losing weight with pushing and punishing themselves, which can be hard (and not fun) to sustain over time. They end up living a lifestyle that only has two modes: "diet mode" and "between-diet mode." It is hard to maintain this back-and-forth, and all-or-nothing approach, which makes it easier for them to give up.

We don't want that to happen to you, which is why we have designed your Personal Plan of Action to be based on a journey metaphor. Much like you would enjoy planning for the ultimate vacation, we will take the time to enjoy planning, preparing, and packing for your losing the weight for good journey so that you enjoy the process of getting to weight loss and can continue the journey over time. This road map (your Personal Plan of Action) will be your "GPS" for how you are going to live for the rest of your life with respect to habits that affect your likelihood of gaining unwanted weight.

As you consider this long-term approach to lasting lifestyle change, you may be worried (as many patients are) about whether this approach will mean that you will never enjoy food again or will seek fulfillment primarily through training for marathons. Rest assured that the goal of your Personal Plan of Action is to make *gradual*, satisfying, and enjoyable changes in some of the ways you relate to food and physical activity—changes that you will choose and then want to make a part

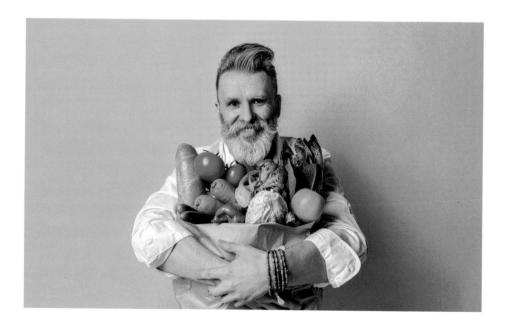

of your life for good. You will be justly proud of these changes and may even want to convert other people you care about to your new approach to life and health by sharing your inspiring story with others who want to create their own road map (plan) for weight loss and management success.

Key 2. Set Clear, Attainable, and Reasonable Goals

We achieve our goals most easily when they are clearly defined and, most importantly, when they are attainable. Accepting a realistic goal is critical to long-term success—and to your self-esteem. All too often we see people who have so thoroughly bought into the false idea that thinness equals happiness that they set goals based on a weight they passed on their sixteenth birthday. This is a guaranteed way to feel like a failure. Don't fall into the trap of setting as your goal an "ideal" body weight. "Ideal" weight is a misleading concept and should not be your target or your yardstick for measuring success. Your weight goals should be based on what's right for you, not on a perceived cultural standard.

At the Johns Hopkins Healthful Eating, Activity & Weight Progam, we have adopted a different concept, one that has gained widespread acceptance among weight loss professionals—"reasonable goal weight." If you have never been "thin," you will be fighting a losing battle with nature if you make it your goal to *be* thin.

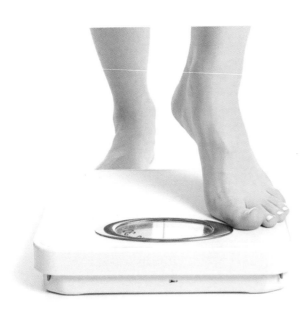

You will do much better if you aim for the following more reasonable goal: *the lowest healthy weight you have been able to maintain for one year or more since your early twenties.*

Some of our patients, like many readers, may still yearn to weigh less than their reasonable goal weight. Clinging to this dream hinders rather than helps progress, however. To help our patients let go of a frustratingly unattainable/unsustainable goal weight, we ask them to think about how much it would improve their lives just to get down to their reasonable goal weight, to

Aim for a goal weight that is reasonable for you

remember the benefits of losing even more moderate amounts of weight (see chapter 1), and to consider why so many people fail to achieve and maintain "ideal" weight. Extreme sacrifice can result in a brief achievement of the elusive goal of thinness, but the cost is enormous, and the achievement usually is only temporary. Some experts believe that unreasonable goals can lead to lowered self-esteem and possibly more serious eating disorders such as binge eating and bulimia. Don't set yourself up to be disappointed. Instead, take pride in what you can achieve. Your achievements can include healthful changes in your lifestyle, which are independent of just what registers on the scale. Your Personal Plan of Action and a willingness to learn will put your reasonable goal well within your reach.

For those who still want to take off those last pounds, we suggest the following: use your Personal Plan of Action to get to your reasonable goal weight, and then let yourself experience life at this weight for six months or so. This will allow you to get comfortable with your ability to maintain that weight. Then, if you wish, slowly reduce further. Under no circumstances do we recommend that people lose so much that they weigh less than their personal concept of an "ideal" body weight. We have had patients who say that they want to lose "just a few extra pounds" so when they "finish" dieting they can eat "whatever they want" and still be below their ideal weight. As you can imagine, this is a formula guaranteed to cause rapid weight regain and yo-yo dieting.

Key 3. Find a Reliable Support System

A strong support network will help keep you on track for the long haul. Having someone make lifestyle changes with you is the ideal situation as employing the buddy system has been shown to improve a person's chances of successful weight loss. Probably the best buddy is a good friend or relative who is enthusiastic, tenacious, and wishes to lose about the same amount of weight as you do. Your buddy need not fit this description to a tee, but you must be able to cooperate and support each other. Be careful if you choose a spouse or significant other as a buddy. In most cases, this arrangement is loaded with potential pitfalls. Spouses and significant others may think they are being helpful, but they bring their own emotional baggage to the table, and it often gets in the way. Even though significant others do not usually make good buddies, they can be helpful by not making it harder for you (for example, not eating chocolate ice cream while you are having a salad) and by being a nonjudgmental, one-person cheering squad.

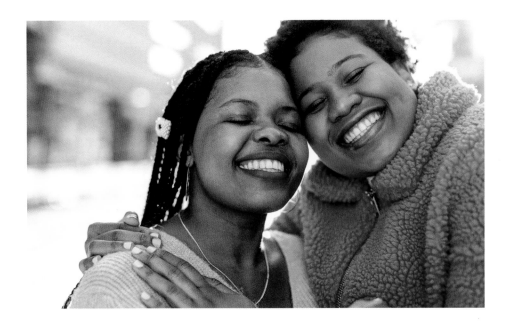

What should you and your buddy do once you have found each other? The idea is not that you will do exactly the same thing at the same time. Your Personal Plans do not have to be at all alike. What is important is that you let each other know the details of each other's plans and understand what kind of support you need from each other. One example of such support might be agreeing to talk with your buddy, by phone or text message, any time you have the urge to do something outside of your plan.

Checking in on a twice-weekly (or, better yet, daily) basis with your buddy is also a good idea, for two reasons. First, it makes you accountable for your actions to someone you like and trust, someone who can both praise your accomplishments and encourage you after your setbacks. Second, it sets up a competitive challenge for each of you, since neither of you will want to report that you did not do as well as your buddy did.

Of course, competition can be a double-edged sword—it tends to make you lose weight faster, but it may also undercut the supportive aspect of the buddy system if it becomes too intense. To avoid this problem, try to focus any competition not on the number of pounds lost each week, but on the changes in behavior (nonscale victories) that are critical to long-term success, such as your newfound appreciation of healthier foods. Agree with your buddy at the outset that you will not discuss the specific number of pounds either of you has lost, and then stick to that agreement. That way, your buddy and you can both "win" in this competitive event.

Key 4. Master Your Mindset: Be Nice to Yourself

No matter how good your plan is or how motivated you are initially, you will be unlikely to succeed in the long run unless you have faith in your ability to lose weight and you consciously remind yourself of the great reasons for doing so. Think of this process of being nicer to yourself in your self-talk as mastering your mindset.

How do you talk to yourself? Though it might seem strange at first, we recommend that you actually say encouraging words out loud—things like "I really did a good job of avoiding the donuts in the breakroom this morning." Always be upbeat and hopeful, and speak with authority tempered by humor. Expect setbacks, but never let them get in your way. And never get down on yourself if you slip up. Remember, what you are doing is not easy, and you are still the same good person you were before that unfortunate encounter with the Boston cream pie. Be as patient with yourself as you would be with an infant who has to fall about 200 times before she gets the hang of walking. You are the infant this time around. Will talking to yourself really work? The short answer is *yes*.

Most of us have had the experience of talking the wrong way to ourselves. Too much negative self-talk can have a devastating effect on one's sense of self. If we tell ourselves we are incompetent, out of control, socially inept, fat, or whatever too often, the danger is that we begin to accept those negative thoughts as truth. The result is a negative self-image and a lack of motivation—two states that can seriously impede your ability to make positive changes in your life. However,

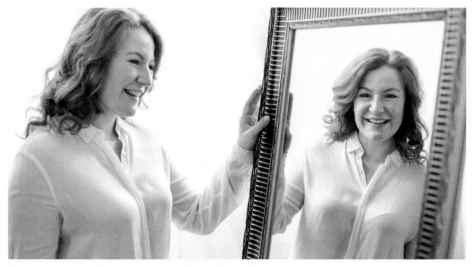

Encourage your weight loss efforts with positive self-talk

talking to yourself positively will have an equally strong influence, but one that will increase your self-confidence and motivation. You are strong and capable, and mistakes are merely opportunities for reflection and growth. First believe, then you will become.

We are not born with a high level of self-confidence. It is usually achieved through the effects of a stable and supportive upbringing and positive feedback in adulthood when we act in ways that show we believe in ourselves.

This attitude should not be construed as license to lose sight of reality and to unashamedly lie to yourself and the world. When you talk to yourself the right way, you can tell yourself the truth ("Yes, I slipped up pretty badly" as well as "I did a good job") and learn from your mistakes and your successes. Since you believe in yourself, there's no reason to hide the truth. When things go right, pat yourself on the back. When they don't, you will want to assess what went wrong and formulate a strategy to better handle such challenges going forward. If you understand what happened and why, then you will have the best chance of learning from experience.

An important distinction that many people aren't aware of is the difference between self-confidence and *self-efficacy*. There is a relationship between these two concepts, but they are different, and understanding the difference can help you make things happen more smoothly when it comes to successfully carrying through with your Personal Plan.

Self-efficacy is a narrower concept than self-confidence; it is specific to a task or situation. For example, if you have bicycled since you were a child and knew you were very good at it, even if you haven't biked for the entire year, you have confidence that you can get back on a bike in the spring and not worry about immediately falling off. In other words, you have high self-efficacy regarding your ability to ride a bike.

Therefore, in order to be successful at losing weight, you need not be a person who is highly self-confident overall. You simply need to gain positive experience

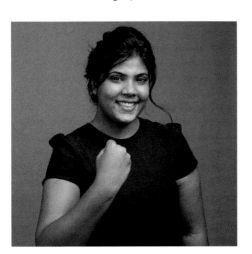

in losing weight to the point where you recognize that you are knowledgeable and skillful in doing the specific tasks that are part of your Personal Plan. You are then like the bike rider: you have high self-efficacy in yet another skill: losing weight.

Self-efficacy is often a subset of self-confidence, in that people who are highly self-confident are more prone to believe they can accomplish anything they set their minds to, while people with low self-confidence may be

BOX 4-1

Mindset Mastery Statements

1   I am kind to myself when I commit to my weight loss and weight management as a journey.

2   I am in control of my eating; I choose what I can say yes or no to.

3   Food cravings last only a few minutes. I can distract myself until the feeling passes.

4   I take a walk when I need to clear my mind, avoid eating, and relieve stress.

5   As a reward, I use praise, gifts, or quality time with friends instead of food or clothes.

6   I am doing great so far; I don't need to stray off the path that I have created.

7   I have the strength to say no to poor habits and yes to positive lifestyle changes.

8   I feel so much better when my clothes aren't tight.

9   It is my choice to eat healthy foods or unhealthy foods, and I choose wisely.

10   I deal with the things that are stressful to me (and I don't eat to solve them).

11   I avoid situations that encourage overeating or I prepare myself for them.

12   Social occasions are important to me because of the people who are there, not the food.

13   I eat to please myself, not someone else.

14   I eat in response to my body's needs, not my emotions.

15   I eat slowly and enjoy my food without distractions.

16   I respect my body and choose well-seasoned foods instead of unhealthy ones.

17   I eat only when I'm physically hungry, and I stop eating when I'm no longer hungry (rather than when I'm stuffed).

18   When I stray from my Personal Plan of Action, it is merely a temporary setback. I take stock of what I can learn from the experience and get right back to my routine.

19   I eat at least three meals a day, including breakfast. This helps me control urges and avoid eating in the evening.

20   I nourish my body and improve my health when I choose to eat fruits and vegetables daily.

21   My focus is on health, and I challenge myself to include plenty of fruits and vegetables in every meal.

unsure of themselves even when they may be well trained or experienced in accomplishing a specific task. For our purposes, it is self-efficacy, knowing you have the skills down pat, that will make you successful. Self-confidence in the absence of skill will not work. So let's focus on building your self-efficacy for weight loss and not worry about the squishier area of self-confidence.

To help you learn what to say to yourself in stressful food situations, read the mindset mastery statements aloud.

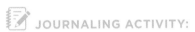

Mindset Mastery Statements

In addition to saying these statements out loud on a regular basis, you may also want to write some of them down in your journal so you have them when you need them (in moments of weakness with regard to your weight management challenges). We also encourage you to create mindset mastery statements that you find helpful. They can help strengthen your resolve. At the very least, they will entertain and distract you.

Key 5. Make Gradual Changes

One of the key ingredients in your Personal Plan of Action is a technique you will see illustrated repeatedly throughout this book. It is based on principles of behavior modification and recognizes how difficult it can be for us to change habits all at once. Applying the technique of *gradual change* to your Personal Plan of Action will make it more likely that you will permanently replace the old habits with the new.

For example, what do you do if you were brought up on whole milk, hate the taste of skim milk, but drink a lot of milk and wish to cut down on fat? Do you

    a hold your nose and swallow the skim milk,
    b limit your whole milk to one glass per week,
    c keep the whole milk and try to cut fat somewhere else, or
    d do none of the above?

The answer is *d*. None of the other solutions is very good. As we have seen, if you take solution *a*, it's likely that you'll either return to drinking whole milk or suffer with an unnecessary feeling of deprivation. Option *b* will also be seen as deprivation, and *c* constitutes a lost opportunity to cut down calories and fat in a relatively easy way.

Instead of choosing one of these unproductive ways of dealing with the situation, make the gradual change approach a part of your Personal Plan. Switch from whole milk to 2% fat milk. (By the way, this is a misleading figure, since even whole milk is only 4% fat by volume, but fully *55% of the total calories* in whole milk are from fat. See page 173 for information on how to read food labels and not be misled.) While it may taste somewhat less creamy than whole milk, 2% should be close enough to keep you from feeling deprived. Use 2% fat milk for a month or so, then switch to 1%. (For an even more gradual change, you can mix equal amounts of 1% and 2% as an intermediate step.) You will notice something interesting at this stage. The whole milk that you used to prefer will now taste too oily. Taste preferences are complex, and they are changeable. Foods you liked to eat as a child you no longer eat; foods you wouldn't even taste as a child you now rank among your favorites. You can use the changeability of taste to your advantage in fine-tuning your dietary choices now.

Ironically, the surest way to change is often the slowest, most gradual route. The same principles can be applied to other aspects of your Personal Plan, such as increasing physical activity and adding fiber to your diet. A side benefit of using the gradual change technique is that you can avoid the trap of endless sacrifice. Feeling that you are depriving yourself in order to lose weight sets you up for reverting to old habits, since no one wants to be deprived indefinitely. With gradual change there is little or no deprivation or suffering, only satisfaction, as the changes you've made become a part of the rest of your life, a part that you can be justifiably proud to have achieved.

Key 6. Make It Fun—and Enjoy Yourself

You can enjoy designing and carrying out your plan. This will be obvious once you realize that you don't have to put things in your Personal Plan of Action that you are going to hate. If, for example, you would rather be trapped alone in an elevator listening to the piped-in music for half an hour three times a week than spend the same amount of time jogging, we will help you find some other way to increase your level of physical activity.

Not only will you hate it if you do something you don't enjoy, but it will not work in the long run because it will never become part of your life. If you force yourself to do this unpleasant thing, you will resent having to do it, and you will drop the activity in short order.

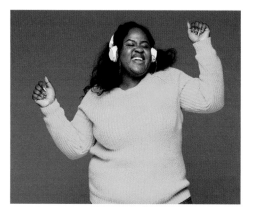

Again, the concept of talking to yourself properly is important here. Ask yourself if there was ever a time in your life when you liked to do a particular physical activity—a team sport, for example. Then ask yourself what it was about that activity that you really enjoyed. Many people recall the camaraderie of being on a team as being an important factor in their enjoyment of a particular sport. You may not be able to play a team sport regularly now, but you can recapture the joy of camaraderie by choosing an activity that fits your current lifestyle, such as exercising with a friend. Instead of telling yourself, "Exercise is boring," ask yourself, "What can I do to have fun?" It might be joking around with your neighbor while you play basketball, or seeing how many birds you can identify on a long walk. It doesn't matter, as long as it is something you can enjoy even a little bit.

And don't underestimate the personal satisfaction of learning more about yourself and making positive changes in your life. Most people spend their adult lives locked into patterns they acquired during childhood, never to change. We all know the saying, "You can't teach an old dog new tricks," but there's another popular saying that is preferable because it is much more positive: "You're never too old to learn."

The personal growth you can achieve through developing and completing your Personal Plan of Action is a wonderful reward. People often believe that if only they were thinner they would get the love and respect they deserve. The truth is, these things come with the self-confidence you achieve when you take control of your life.

If you think of yourself as someone who can't change, this is the time to practice talking to yourself the right way. For example, your Personal Plan of Action may require that you change the kinds of food you eat. If you are trying to cut down on carbs or fats, you will have a hard time if you wrinkle your nose and say to yourself, "Foods don't taste as good if they're not cooked in butter," or, after trying a sugar substitute, you frown and say, "Not as good as old-fashioned sugar." These statements are being made by the old dog in us, the part that doesn't want to succeed in making changes. Instead, try saying to yourself, "You know, fried and fatty foods are not as tasty as well-seasoned foods, because all you taste is the grease, not the food under it" or "I respect myself and I want to be healthy. Eating these foods will not help me achieve my goals. There are many other healthy, delicious foods out there for me." In addition to changing the way you talk to yourself, try new foods, new forms of physical activity, and new coping styles—they can all be enjoyable and empowering.

There are few greater sources of enjoyment and satisfaction than learning about and improving yourself. Remind yourself of this periodically, and take pride in your accomplishments. You will enjoy the process of change a lot more.

Key 7. Be Flexible

The final ingredient in your Personal Plan of Action is flexibility. Your plan is not etched in stone. Though the plan is capable of carrying you far into the future, it will only be useful as long as you build in flexibility, the capacity to change and adapt to new situations or changing needs. How do you build in flexibility? There are at least two ways. The first is to regularly reassess your needs and how your Personal Plan of Action is addressing them. The second is building in backup plans.

The plan that seemed perfectly adapted to your needs when you devised it may need adjusting as you carry it out. For instance, you get a new job with a new schedule and new stresses; you decide that you really don't like salads, which for a long time have been the major ingredient in your diet; or they close the local pool where you've been swimming for the season. If you have built enough flexibility into your original plan to absorb some changes, and if you are willing to adjust your plan, you'll be better able to deal with these kinds of situations.

How have some of our patients dealt with the need to change their plan? Bob changed jobs in the middle of implementing his Personal Plan of Action, and in his new job he had to attend business lunches virtually every weekday to entertain sales clients. Instead of being able to bring his carefully planned healthy lunches from home, he would be eating in restaurants. Since he had built flexibility into his plan, he was able to swap his lunch and dinner menus. He had his larger meal at lunch, allowing him to choose from a broader range of restaurant offerings, and he ate his healthier "lunch" at dinnertime. As a bonus, he discovered that he felt less hungry when he got home after a filling lunch and was less tempted to snack in the evening.

Marcella put together the diet for her Personal Plan of Action with a heavy emphasis on salads to provide fiber

Don't be afraid to change course as needed to meet your goals

and bulk. About a month into her plan, however, she told us that if she saw one more piece of lettuce, she was going to start wiggling her nose like a rabbit. Because there is more than one way to cut down on calories and improve the quality of food intake, she was able to make substitutions that worked for her. Now, instead of salads, she eats carrot sticks and broccoli florets as well as some crunchy snacks like pretzels. This increased her satisfaction with only a slight hike in total calories. In the past, Marcella might well have substituted potato chips or rich desserts.

Ximena loved to swim when she was a teenager and was excited about getting back into swimming as part of her Personal Plan. She joined her neighborhood outdoor pool and had a regular routine of lap swimming. She felt better and had more energy. Then the summer ended, and the pool was about to close for the season. What to do? Join a more expensive and less convenient indoor pool? Stop swimming and get off track with her weight loss goals? Ximena had built flexibility into her exercise plan by selecting backup exercises. Expanding on the theme of enjoyable childhood activities, she switched from swimming to ice skating and rollerblading. Since she was not going to do these things as frequently as she had been swimming, Ximena also began taking a brisk walk around her office complex at the end of her lunch hour each day.

Even if nothing seems to have changed in your life, you should periodically reassess your needs to avoid burnout. You need to step back from your plan and see which components are working for you and which are not. This will give you an ongoing reminder of which areas you need to work harder on, as well as positive feedback for the areas you are handling successfully.

How frequently should you reassess, and how is it done? Ideally, reassessment is an ongoing process, but it helps to set specific time intervals for a formal reassessment, such as one, three, six, and twelve months after beginning.

Key 8. Journal the Journey

In this chapter, you learned more about the key principles of a successful weight loss plan. Now you're ready to choose among the tools available in this book to develop a plan that's tailor-made for you, one that will help you create a path for losing weight safely and keeping it off. Your Personal Plan of Action will help you chart this path (road map) to success.

As you work your way through this book and create your plan, we also encourage you to "journal your journey." Take notes throughout the process, possibly journaling your journey in a personal diary or by sharing your story on social media. These notes can also be used as a quick reference guide for you whenever you need a refresher course, and they can also be motivating for others who are, or want to be, on a weight loss journey.

Documenting your progress in your personal weight loss journal will be very helpful in assessing your progress. For example, keeping an ongoing record of the date, circumstances, and outcome of each episode of emotional eating will enable you to see if the frequency of these events is decreasing, and whether you have been able to alter your response or at least change the kinds of food you eat when you are upset. Remember, for any given problem, you should not expect immediate or complete changes right away. Use your skill of positive self-talk and the technique of gradual change to keep yourself motivated and moving in the right direction. For many problem areas, extensive record keeping is not necessary. Write yourself notes to document your successes, as well as the areas requiring more work or a shift in strategy.

Action Items

- Develop your mindset mastery skills.
  - Review the mindset mastery statements in this chapter. Choose the ones that resonate most with you and write them in your journal.
  - Come up with a few personalized mindfulness statements of your own and add them to your Plan as well.
  - Try repeating your mindfulness statements each morning to start your day on the right track.
- Journal your journey. Start by tracking any problematic patterns in your weight loss journal.
  - Problematic eating patterns include instances of eating for reasons other than hunger (that is, emotional or stress-based eating), eating outside of designated meal times, or barriers you confronted that prevented you from making healthy food choices. Problematic movement patterns include sitting throughout the day (without taking time to stretch and move) or an irregular activity schedule.
  - When you document a problem, try to document a solution that may go with it, which could help you avoid the problem in the future.

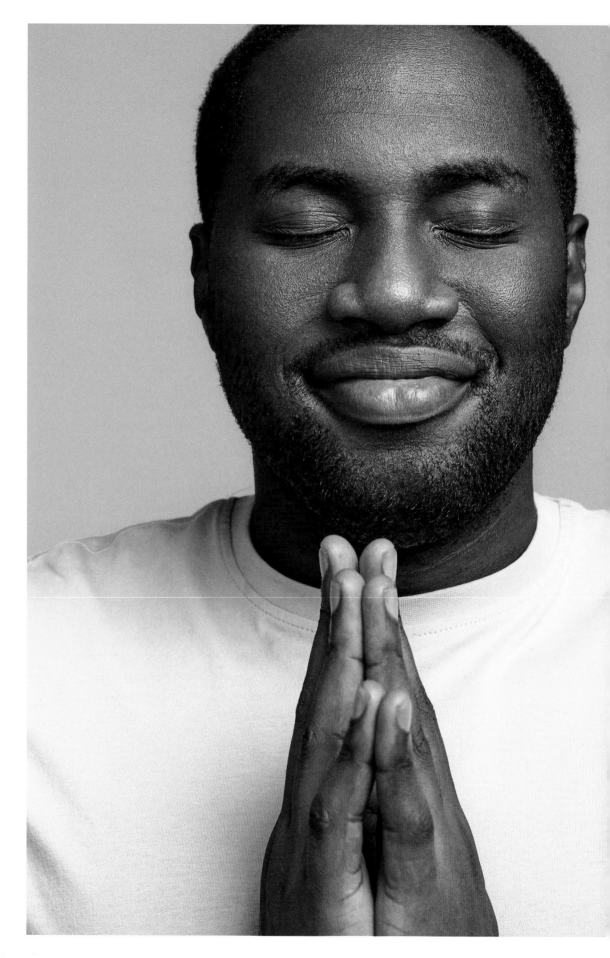

CHAPTER 5

Strategic Stress Management

IN THIS CHAPTER, WE WILL:

- **discuss the importance** of strategic stress management (the combination of stress reduction, rest, relaxation, and sleep behaviors that you need to optimize your weight loss and weight management efforts);

- **explore the difference** between "good" and "bad" stress, and how they both can impact your energy balance equation (and therefore your weight loss and weight management efforts);

- **introduce you to** the 5-Step Transformation Challenge to help you understand your current eating habits. As part of this assessment, you will look at:
  - patterns of problematic eating and how to respond;
  - different approaches to eating, addressing restraint, explanatory style, self-efficacy, and self-esteem;
  - binge eating disorders; and
  - the connection between depression and weight management; and

- **ask you to observe** your own behaviors related to eating and dealing with stress, to inform your Personal Plan of Action.

THROUGHOUT THIS BOOK, WE HAVE EMPHASIZED the ways that weight management is a true balancing act. You have learned that weight loss occurs when caloric expenditure exceeds caloric intake, and that weight management occurs when you can balance the calories in with calories out. You have also learned that this balance is not as simple as it might seem, because it is influenced by other factors such as your metabolic rate (which is impacted by your age, medical conditions, prescriptions, and behaviors such as sleep and stress management). This is why it can be difficult for each person to find the balance that they need to either lose or maintain their weight over time.

Although age, medical conditions, and prescription use are generally unchangeable, we have the ability to change eating, sleeping, and stress management practices to support weight loss and weight management efforts. That is why this chapter's focus is on what we call *strategic stress management*—the combination of self-observation, stress reduction, eating, relaxation, and sleep behaviors that you need to optimize your weight loss and weight management efforts.

Our work with patients as well as lifestyle research have shown us that inadequate stress management can easily derail weight loss and weight management efforts. That is because stress can compromise both sides of the energy balance equation: causing cravings for sweets and other unhealthy choices (including alcohol) on the food and drink intake side, and compromising physical activity performance on the expenditure side.

To support you in considering ways that you can get strategic about stress management as part of your weight loss and weight management efforts, we provide you with a series of self-assessments that we hope will serve as a mindfulness exercise. As you go through this chapter, we ask that you be mindful of your past and current behaviors and mindset patterns so that you can learn more about the ways that you are and aren't managing stress strategically.

We also hope that while you complete these assessments and use the results to inform your Personal Plan of Action, you will do so in a way that practices self-compassion (the ability to recognize challenges while having hope and optimism for being able to solve them). By taking the time you need to complete each action item that is included (and not rushing), you will discover more about yourself and your past patterns so that you can better identify (and eventually adjust) those that you find are no longer serving you and your weight loss or weight management goals.

A Few Words of Caution

Before we proceed further, we want to share three important cautions. First, we want to remind you that this assessment process is not meant to feel critical or judgmental—like a test that you feel you have to "pass." Instead, consider it a way to be honest with yourself about your prior mindset challenges so that you can identify those you would like to change moving forward. Second, as mentioned earlier, we ask you to be compassionate with yourself throughout this process. Try to let go of self-judgment and self-criticism with regard to prior patterns you do not like to see within yourself. Allow your desire to lose the weight for good inspire you to transform any discomfort you might have about past choices into pride that you are now committing to a whole new relationship—with yourself. Just as you would build a new relationship with another person slowly over time, with trust and honesty, consider this self-assessment an opportunity to begin the same process—with you.

And finally, please remember that not all stress is bad. Some stress is actually good—stress that we welcome or even seek to find! Stress can mean excitement or motivation. Getting a new job, asking someone out on a first date, getting married—these are just a few examples of "good stress," which must also be managed strategically to support your weight loss and weight management efforts. By doing so, you'll be able to improve your performance in the great opportunities that life asks of you (good stress) *and* be ready for the tough stuff that life throws at you (bad stress).

"Why Do We Eat?"

Although "We eat when we're hungry" is the most obvious answer, once you start paying attention to your eating habits, you will likely find that you eat for a number of reasons other than hunger. You might discover specific triggers that tend to drive your choice of *what and how much to eat.*

In this book, our approach to weight loss draws on several fields of science and medicine, including behavioral science—the study of human habits, culture, and social interactions. In this chapter, you will identify *your* "whys"—reasons for

BOX 5-1

The Four As of Stress Management

Stress Management Strategy #1: Avoid Unnecessary Stress

Not all stress can be avoided, and it's not healthy to avoid a situation that needs to be addressed. You may be surprised, however, by the number of stressors in your life that you can eliminate.

Learn how to say no. Know your limits and stick to them. Whether in your personal or professional life, refuse to accept added responsibilities when you're close to reaching them. Taking on more than you can handle is a surefire recipe for stress.

Avoid people who stress you out. If someone consistently causes stress in your life and you can't turn the relationship around, limit the amount of time you spend with that person or end the relationship entirely.

Take control of your environment. If the evening news makes you anxious, turn the TV off. If traffic's got you tense, take a longer but less traveled route. If going to the market is an unpleasant chore, do your grocery shopping online.

Avoid hot-button topics. If you get upset over religion or politics, cross them off your conversation list. If you repeatedly argue about the same subject with the same people, stop bringing it up or excuse yourself when it's the topic of discussion.

Pare down your to-do list. Analyze your schedule, responsibilities, and daily tasks. If you've got too much on your plate, distinguish between the "shoulds" and the "musts." Drop tasks that aren't truly necessary to the bottom of the list or eliminate them entirely.

Stress Management Strategy #2: Alter the Situation

If you can't avoid a stressful situation, try to alter it. Figure out what you can do to change things so the problem doesn't present itself in the future. Often, this involves changing the way you communicate and operate in your daily life.

Express your feelings instead of bottling them up. If something or someone is bothering you, communicate your concerns in an open and respectful way. If you don't voice your feelings, resentment will build and the situation will likely remain the same.

Be willing to compromise. When you ask someone to change their behavior, be willing to do the same. If you both are willing to bend at least a little, you'll have a good chance of finding a happy middle ground.

Be more assertive. Don't take a back seat in your own life. Deal with problems head-on, doing your best to anticipate and prevent them. If you've got an exam to study for and your chatty roommate just got home, say up front that you only have five minutes to talk.

Manage your time better. Poor time management can cause a lot of stress. When you're stretched too thin and running behind, it's hard to stay calm and focused. But if you plan ahead and make sure you don't overextend yourself, you can alter the amount of stress you're under.

Stress Management Strategy #3: Adapt to the Stressor

If you can't change the stressor, change yourself. You can adapt to stressful situations and regain your sense of control by changing your expectations and attitude.

Reframe problems. Try to view stressful situations from a more positive perspective. Rather than fuming about a traffic jam, look at it as an opportunity to pause and regroup, listen to your favorite radio station, or enjoy some alone time.

Look at the big picture. Take perspective of the stressful situation. Ask yourself how important it will be in the long run. Will it matter in a month? A year? Is it really worth getting upset over? If the answer is no, focus your time and energy elsewhere.

Adjust your standards. Perfectionism is a major source of avoidable stress. Stop setting yourself up for failure by demanding perfection. Set reasonable standards for yourself and others, and learn to be okay with "good enough."

Focus on the positive. When stress is getting you down, take a moment to reflect on all the things you appreciate in your life, including your own positive qualities and gifts. This simple strategy can help you keep things in perspective.

Stress Management Strategy #4: Accept the Things You Can't Change

Some sources of stress are unavoidable. You can't prevent or change stressors such as the death of a loved one, a serious illness, or a national recession. In such cases, the best way to cope with stress is to accept things as they are. Acceptance may be difficult, but in the long run, it's easier than railing against a situation you can't change.

Don't try to control the uncontrollable. Many things in life are beyond our control—particularly the behavior of other people. Rather than stressing out over them, focus on the things you can control, such as the way you choose to react to problems.

Look for the upside. As the saying goes, "What doesn't kill us makes us stronger." When facing major challenges, try to look at them as opportunities for personal growth. If your own poor choices contributed to a stressful situation, reflect on them and learn from your mistakes.

Share your feelings. Talk to a trusted friend or make an appointment with a therapist. Expressing what you're going through can be very cathartic, even if there's nothing you can do to alter the stressful situation.

Learn to forgive. Accept the fact that we live in an imperfect world, and that people make mistakes. Let go of anger and resentment. Free yourself from negative energy by forgiving and moving on.

Reprinted with permission from Helpguide.org © 2001–2010. All rights reserved. For more articles in this series, visit www.Helpguide.org.

eating that may or may not be due to hunger, which can interfere with your body's natural ability to maintain a stable and reasonable weight. It's important to learn how to label your triggers and understand their role in your eating behavior. This awareness will allow you to figure out how to avoid your triggers when possible, and to respond to them differently when they cannot be avoided. In this chapter, we will explore a variety of triggers for overeating. Read this chapter slowly, and spend at least a week paying close attention to your triggers and building strategies to incorporate them into your Personal Plan of Action.

Losing weight for life, as we emphasize in this book, involves more than merely going on a diet. Understanding your reasons for eating is probably even more important for weight maintenance than for weight loss. In the short term, people can often power through temptation and avoid overeating because their level of motivation is so high when they are just getting started. However, to succeed long term, triggers must be identified and managed.

Take our patient Alison as a case in point. Alison had gained 10 pounds over the course of six months because she had started coping with a stressful job by unwinding each evening after work with a glass of wine and some snacks. She told herself, "I deserve a little wine after everything I put up with today. I am so frazzled, nothing else is going to help me relax." However, as she slowly but steadily put on weight, her pants began to get to the point where she could barely button them. At her yearly physical, her doctor commented on the weight gain. This was enough to compel Alison to act. She swore off wine and extra snacks completely for two months. When she had a bad day at work and thought about having a glass of wine, she remembered her pants not fitting and she was able to forgo it. However,

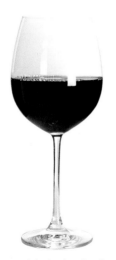

Be careful of using food and drink to manage stress

she never found anything else to manage the stress at work, so she just suffered through. When she lost the 10 pounds she had hoped to lose, she returned to having a glass or two of wine after work. She told herself, "I know this caused me to gain weight before, but I'm only going to have a drink tonight. I'm not going to do it every night, and today was especially bad." However, the next night, she told herself the same thing, and a few months later, she was back to where she'd started.

In a vacuum, without healthier habits in place, most people will return to their old habits. It is not due to a lack of willpower, or laziness; it is more akin to a wagon wheel falling back into a well-worn rut in the ground. It's just what you are familiar with. That is why it is critically important that during the time when you are most motivated to manage your weight, you work to identify your reasons for overeating and put long-term strategies in place to combat them.

After starting to work with Alison, we identified ways that she might directly address the triggers at work, to potentially improve the situation. She asked coworkers how they managed their boss's demands and received some helpful suggestions. She let her boss know that she needed expectations and deadlines to be more clearly communicated. In addition, she started employing coping strategies that didn't involve food. She started a ritual of coming home from work, washing her face with a warm washcloth, putting on cozy loungewear, and lying down on the bed for 20 minutes, closing her eyes and listening to an audiobook. After unwinding for a bit, she would go downstairs and make dinner. These changes enabled her to permanently eliminate her nightly habit of drinking wine and snacking before dinner. She lost the 10 pounds that were making it hard to button her pants, and, most importantly, she was able to keep the weight off for good.

The Five-Step Transformation Challenge

In order to better understand your triggers for overeating, we will embark on a Five-Step Transformation Challenge. This behavioral self-assessment should be taken slowly and carefully, with plenty of time to reflect on each phase. We recommend working through this chapter according to the following schedule:

Step 1. Read about common triggers for overeating and the stories of people who learned how to manage their triggers in order to lose weight. Complete the questionnaire and reflect on the discussion.

Step 2. Read about people with various degrees of eating "restraint" and explanatory styles. Consider the questions and discussion.

Step 3. Read about people struggling with eating disorders. Again, consider the questions and discussion.

Step 4. Learn to recognize depression or other mental health concerns. Complete the questionnaire and consider your score.

Step 5. Relax, step back, and observe yourself. Ask the three questions presented in Step 1 every single time you eat or are tempted to eat.

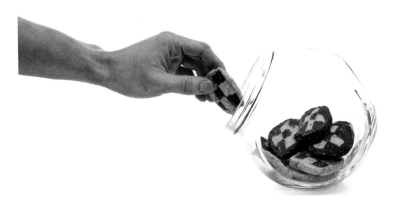

Step 1. Assess Problematic Eating

First, we will take a whirlwind tour of a number of situations and experiences that can lead to problematic eating. For someone who is trying to lose weight, we consider "problematic eating" to be eating when not physically hungry (note: this excludes eating proactively because you won't be able to eat later and are trying to prevent extreme hunger), choosing foods that aren't healthy, or eating portions that are too large. We will share stories of patients in situations that resulted in problematic eating. Your job is to picture yourself in the patient's place and decide whether it is a problem area for you. There are only two rules: first, you must be completely honest with yourself, and second, if you are not sure whether the situation described is a problem area for you, assume that it is.

To begin, there are three important questions that we encourage all people to ask themselves before eating in order to better understand their triggers.

Even without doing anything else, simply asking yourself these three questions whenever you have a desire to eat will almost certainly result in a significant improvement in your eating habits and your relationship with food.

AM I ACTUALLY HUNGRY?

Many times, people want to eat when they are not physically hungry. They are tempted to eat because they see food that looks appetizing, because of their mood, because their friends encourage them

BOX 5-2

Get in the habit of asking yourself these questions every single time you eat:

1 Am I actually hungry?

2 Is this the best choice I could make?

3 Do I need more, or do I just want more?

to eat or drink, because they're tired, or because they've been thinking about food. Other times, they are legitimately hungry, but they are tempted to choose unhealthy foods or to eat portions that are too large because something else is going on (for example, they are sad, tired, with friends). If you aren't sure whether you are really hungry, a good test is to offer yourself an apple, or something else healthy. If it sounds unappealing, it may be that you are wanting to eat for reasons other than true hunger. Later in this chapter, we will explore common triggers for eating when not physically hungry, or for eating beyond satiety.

IS THIS THE BEST CHOICE I COULD MAKE?

By *this*, we don't mean the very best nutritional option available, but rather, is this the best, rational choice for you? In order to answer that question, you need to think about whether the food is something you *really* want and whether it is likely to be worth the extra calories. Consider whether eating the food would satisfy a craving or cause the craving to intensify? Would not eating the food leave you feeling truly deprived and unhappy? How would you feel physically after eating the food—energetic or sluggish? Is there something healthier that could be satisfying? The point is to make very deliberate, conscious decisions about food rather than impulsive, mindless decisions about what to eat. An added benefit of thinking critically about whether to indulge is that you are much less likely to feel deprived if you decide for yourself that a food isn't worth the added calories, physical discomfort, or potential for additional cravings. There is something very different about considering the pros and cons and determining, "I don't want that [doughnut, cake, sandwich, bag of chips, etc.]" versus telling yourself, "I can't have that."

DO I NEED MORE, OR DO I JUST WANT MORE?

As you are eating, check in with yourself and determine whether you are still hungry. The goal is to eat until your hunger is satiated, not until you are full or stuffed. Ask yourself, "Do I *need* to keep eating because I'm still hungry, or do I just *want* more because it tastes good and it's enjoyable to eat?" Listen to your body and teach yourself to stop when you are no longer hungry. This may be hard to do and takes practice. It can be helpful to immediately brush your teeth or chew gum after a meal to cleanse your palate and remove any food particles from your mouth that could cause you to continue craving more. It's also a good idea to engage in a distracting activity to take your attention away from the meal. Sometimes people tell us they are genuinely not sure whether they should eat more. They've eaten what appears to be an appropriate portion, but they still feel hungry. We advise these people to step away from the table, distract themselves with another activity for 15 minutes or so, and then reevaluate. It

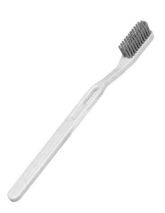
Brushing your teeth may help you curb your craving

is true that it can take time for your blood sugar to go up and for your brain to get the message that you've had enough to eat. If you are dining with others, we suggest you pause, push your plate away, and drink a glass of water or a cup of tea or coffee before deciding whether to eat more. In a restaurant, the remainder of the meal could be boxed up and taken home.

There may be times when you choose to eat when you are not hungry. This is often the case with dessert. This is okay, provided it's an infrequent occurrence. In this case, it's important to eat especially mindfully. Eat as if you are a restaurant critic, or a judge on a reality baking show. Savor each bite, pay attention to the texture and the flavor, and try to limit your portion. You will get the most "bang for your buck" out of the very first bite—that is the bite that will answer your curiosity about what the food tastes like. Nearly 100% of your attention will likely be on that bite. However, as you continue eating, it's normal for your attention to wane. You will pay attention to the conversation of your tablemates and your taste buds will start to become habituated. You may begin to eat on autopilot. This is a good point to stop. Share the dessert with a dining companion, set it aside to enjoy another time, or throw it away.

TRIGGERS THAT CAN CAUSE OVEREATING

Before elaborating on the things that can trigger people to eat when they're not physically hungry, it's worth noting that triggers do not happen in isolation and hunger is on a continuum from "not hungry" to "starving" and everything in between. For example, you may be somewhat hungry but capable of making it to the lunch you planned without any additional snacks. However, if something stressful happens and then a friend offers you a cookie, you might be very tempted to eat it due to the coalescence of multiple triggers.

BOX 5-4

Avoid the top four vulnerability factors for overeating:

1 Sleep deprivation

2 Hunger

3 Physical sickness

4 Intense emotion (for example, being sad, mad, scared)

ENVIRONMENTAL TRIGGERS

Many of us are fortunate enough to live in areas where food is readily available. We live in places where there is food for sale in nearly every gas

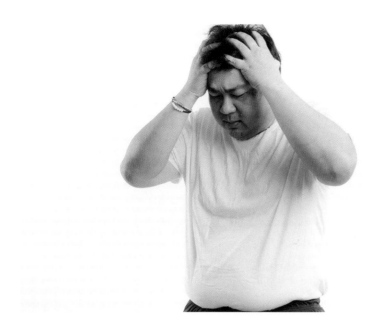

station. There are supermarkets in most towns, grocery delivery services available, and various apps that exist so that you can order food at all hours. We are bombarded by a staggering array of commercial messages advertising tasty (if undernutritious) food choices every day of our lives. There are billboards advertising pizza, commercials touting the latest fast food restaurant burger, and ads for tempting foods, drinks, and places to eat plastered across every avenue of social media. The messages we see and hear in advertising often dovetail with an upbringing that for many of us included such rules as "Clean your plate, there are children starving in Africa," such comforts as "Here's a lollipop to make you feel better," and such rewards as "If you do your homework, you can have some brownies." Add your personal recollections to the list, and you can appreciate how many ways we have learned to misuse food and just how small a role hunger plays in when and why we eat. While people who are not overweight may also eat for reasons other than physical need, they likely do so less frequently, consume smaller portions, or are more physically active, thus minimizing weight gain.

Some environmental triggers are easier to manage than others. For example, we share the case of Vikki, who had the misfortune of living across the street from her favorite grocery store and a number of fast food restaurants. It was a constant source of temptation that was not easy to avoid. She was able to stay on track for the most part by planning her meals in advance and focusing on her reasons for wanting to manage her weight, but she still ended up succumbing to temptation more often than she wanted. After moving to another location, she found it easier to avoid fast food.

If possible, try to reduce your exposure to sights or smells that are triggering. If you can take a different route home that prevents you from driving by your favorite place to get carryout, by all means, take that different route. Doing so may be a surprisingly effective way of avoiding this temptation. Along the same lines, it's important when grocery shopping to make a list and stick to it. Try to avoid buying things you didn't set out to buy or that aren't healthy for you. Some patients find it helpful to shop using cash to help reduce impulse purchases. Other patients find that using home delivery services is a good way to save time and avoid splurge purchases.

If you live with other people, you may need to talk to them about keeping certain foods out of the house, or hidden away. Another option might be to have separate drawers or areas of the pantry. If you are someone who likes to look at cookbooks, watch cooking shows, or follow food personalities on social media, you may want to consider whether these exposures to food are problematic for you. You may be able to switch to watching shows or following chefs that focus on healthy cooking, and you may choose to edit your cookbook library.

The simple truth is that the more you see items that tempt you, the more you will be challenged to avoid eating them. While many people find it empowering to say no over and over again, others find that frequent temptation wears them down and they eventually give in. Your best chance at sticking to your plan is to avoid environmental triggers.

The workplace is another area where people commonly encounter environmental triggers. Smells can waft their way out of shared kitchens and into other employees'

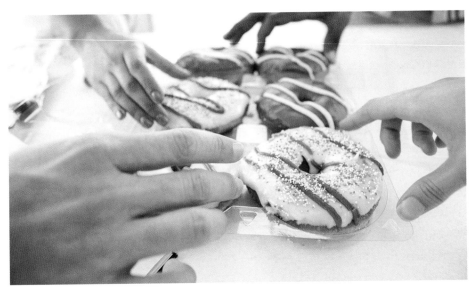

Indulgent foods can be common in the modern workplace

offices or cubicles, and jars of candy can be ubiquitous in certain reception areas. Some of these triggers may be out of your control, but it can at times be worth discussing with coworkers. For example, you may not be the only one who struggles to avoid overeating when management provides a high-calorie catered lunch.

Sometimes it only takes one person to bring about a change to office culture. For instance, Mary found it difficult to avoid the doughnuts and bagels her employer provided on Fridays as a way of showing appreciation for employees. After talking with her coworkers, she realized that they were all struggling with their weight as a result of this gesture of appreciation. Mary told her employer that while she and her coworkers appreciated the gesture, they were concerned about the impact on their health. She asked if perhaps the employer could provide a fruit basket instead, and fortunately, the employer was very receptive and happy to honor her request.

The bottom line is that success requires that you be hypervigilant about the triggers you encounter in your daily life. Your goal is to be in control of your eating, to have a plan and to stick to it, and to not be derailed by triggers in your environment. When you reach your goal, you can experiment by reintroducing stressor foods back into your environment. Some people find that they are able to handle having certain indulgent items in their home; however, the majority find that it's best to always avoid bringing problematic foods into their homes, except on rare occasions. They can still eat unhealthy foods outside of the home where it's potentially easier to acquire and eat only a small portion. One patient told us that she only buys her favorite candy-coated peanuts when she's on the way to a meeting. She will remove one serving for herself and then share the rest with others attending the meeting.

EMOTIONAL TRIGGERS

Some of the more difficult triggers for eating that people must contend with are emotional triggers. Eating food that tastes good works on the reward center of the brain and increases the brain's levels of "feel good" neurotransmitters, including dopamine and serotonin. Eating can have positive psychological and physical effects. The soothing capacity of food was something we likely learned the moment we cried as an infant and received milk, whether we cried due to hunger or not. Culture, in many ways, encourages us to use food as a surrogate for other things. As a result, many people self-medicate with food. They use food to cope with unpleasant emotional states, from boredom to panic, from fleeting disappointment to despair. We even use food to reward ourselves for a job well done or to celebrate a birthday or a promotion. Food is engrained in our emotional and cultural fabrics.

There is evidence that food can be addictive in the same way that drugs are addictive. The potential for a substance to become addictive goes up with the level of distress the person is experiencing at the time. It works the same for drugs, alcohol, and for food. When the brain is looking for relief, it pays special attention to the things that provide relief. It encodes them firmly into memory and begins to ignore any negative consequences associated with consumption. Therefore, when food is used for coping, the potential for addiction is much greater than when consumption is triggered by social situations or by the environment.

We are accustomed to using food in these ways, but not only is it inappropriate, it is often counterproductive. For example, using food to relieve stress may work temporarily, but let's look at it objectively. Say your boss puts pressure on you to do something unpleasant but necessary at work. It's upsetting, you don't want to do it, and you delay by taking a trip to the vending machines. You down a candy bar and diet cola, or even a relatively nutritious snack of yogurt and pretzels. You talk to whoever is near the machine. Soon the day is almost over, so you put off the unpleasant task until tomorrow. Perhaps you will fret about it at home tonight after dinner and eat more. Needless to say, you are not hungry either time. Furthermore, the food has not helped you deal with the stressful situation—in fact, it has distracted you from dealing with the problem altogether. You may not even have enjoyed the extra food. You may not even remember eating it. And you still must do the task assigned by your boss. You have not solved the problem, only added another one. Unfortunately, this is a surefire way to gain weight without really trying.

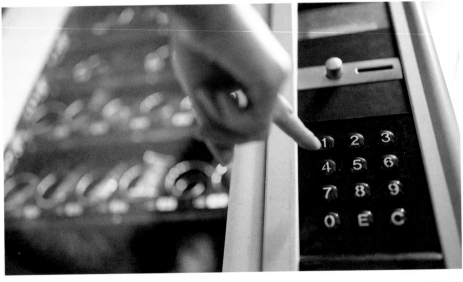

Do you ever find yourself seeking a snack when you are trying to avoid something stressful?

What is the better response? Well, it depends on the circumstances and on your individual coping style. In order to counter emotional triggers, it's critical to be accepting of your own emotional experience. Many patients report having grown up in families where emotional expression was discouraged and emotions were swept under the rug. Sometimes the first step in tackling emotional eating is to work on being more open to your emotional experience and to learn how to tolerate unpleasant emotions. We recommend people work to pinpoint what it is that they are feeling and to validate their emotional experience. Remember that you are human, and you are going to feel happy, sad, disappointed, frustrated, envious, and so on. Our emotional experience is meant to be rich, and the lows are the counterpoint to the highs. Pay attention to your thought process and avoid judging your emotional experience. Try not to be afraid of your emotions. While actions (including speaking) can be hurtful, emotions themselves will not cause harm. Do not use food to distract yourself from your feelings or your problems. As mentioned previously, eating will only provide a temporary fix. One of Dr. Cheskin's patients likes to use the mantra, "If food is not the problem, food is not the answer." Another patient tells herself, "This won't solve my problem; it will just add a second problem." Instead of eating to numb yourself, identify ways to fix the source of the problem. If that isn't possible, then work to find healthier coping strategies.

Again, the first step to avoiding emotional eating is understanding what is bothering you. Then, you can either learn how to cope with the negative emotion or deal directly with the source of the emotion, whether it be a person or a

---

BOX 5-5

Feeling Stressed?

Try these coping strategies:

- Reading
- Watching television
- Listening to an audiobook
- Coloring
- Positive self-talk/ coping statements
- Meditation
- Progressive muscle relaxation

- Yoga
- Going to the movies
- Going to a concert
- Making a to-do list
- Boundary setting
- Time management
- Scheduled time for worrying
- Listening to music
- Exercise

- Sleep
- Taking a shower/bath
- Seek support from a friend
- Problem-solving
- Painting
- Playing a musical instrument

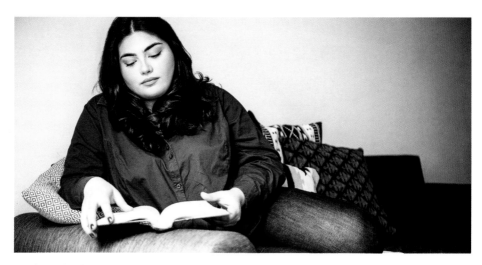
Reading a book can be a helpful way to combat stress

situation. You may have to experiment a bit to find the best techniques for you. Having a flexible repertoire of alternatives to eating in response to emotions will serve you well in your Personal Plan for lasting weight management.

To see how strongly your eating is affected by your emotions, complete the following questionnaire on emotional eating.

In addition to negative emotions, neutral or positive emotions can also trigger overeating. For example, Joe eats when there is nothing better to do. You might say he eats out of boredom. When he gets home from work, he settles in front of the TV and eats. If there's nothing on TV he wants to watch, he may find himself standing by the counter, eating a snack. He usually does this after dinner, but it also happens when he's home during the day. He says he eats because he's hungry, but upon further questioning he reveals that he does not experience physical hunger at all. He is eating because it is his habit to eat when alone.

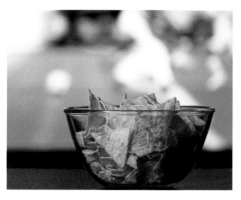
Don't eat when you are distracted

Eating when alone is a common pattern, and eating in front of the TV or computer is a variation on this theme. With TV it is pretty clear why eating is a frequent accompaniment. A large proportion of the commercials are designed to put you in the mood for food. Unfortunately, your body may not need food when you are being urged to indulge. Also, commercials tend to hawk fat-laden convenience foods, perfect for eating on a whim when you are bored and not really hungry.

BOX 5-6

Eating Behavior Questionnaire: Emotional Eating Scale

Directions: Circle the numbered answer that most closely matches your behavior.

Do you have the desire to eat when . . .	Never	Seldom	Sometimes	Often	Very Often
1 You're irritated?	1	2	3	4	5
2 You have nothing to do?	1	2	3	4	5
3 You're depressed or discouraged?	1	2	3	4	5
4 You're feeling lonely?	1	2	3	4	5
5 Someone lets you down?	1	2	3	4	5
6 You're angry?	1	2	3	4	5
7 You're about to experience something unpleasant?	1	2	3	4	5
8 You're anxious, worried, or tense?	1	2	3	4	5
9 Things are going against you or when things have gone wrong?	1	2	3	4	5
10 You're frightened?	1	2	3	4	5
11 You're disappointed?	1	2	3	4	5
12 You're emotionally upset?	1	2	3	4	5
13 You're bored or restless?	1	2	3	4	5

Interpretation: Add the total to get your score, and use the following information to interpret the meaning of your score. For this scale, the average adult who is not overweight scores 17 (men) and 20 (women). Scores higher than 25 may mean that you have a higher tendency to eat in response to emotional cues than most people do.

SOURCE: *Adapted from T. Van Strien, J. E. R. Frijters, G. P. A. Bergers, and P. B. Defares, "The Dutch Eating Behavior Questionnaire (DEBQ) for Assessment of Restrained, Emotional, and External Eating Behavior,"* International Journal of Eating Disorders 5 *(1986): 304. Nederlandse Vragenlijst voor Eetgedrag (NVE). Copyright 1986 by Swets and Zeitlinger, B.V., Lisse. Reprinted by permission of John Wiley & Sons, Inc.*

This is particularly true in the evening when you may already have eaten a perfectly adequate dinner in front of the TV or elsewhere. When is the last time you saw fresh fruits, vegetables, or grains advertised on TV or online? In truth, foods that should constitute the majority of our diet comprise a small fraction of the foods we are urged to consume through advertising. Why? Because staple foods tend to have lower profit margins than convenience foods and are usually generic—no one company stands to profit if we eat more of them.

We suggest you make a new rule in your home that says, "Eating is permitted only in the kitchen or dining room, and only when sitting. No TV, smartphones, or reading material allowed." Make a sign featuring these rules and post it on the refrigerator and cupboard. Other benefits of not eating while distracted by a screen or reading material: there's no mess, and you get to enjoy the taste of your food.

BOX 5-7

Five Strategies to Combat Cravings

1 **Delay.** Most cravings are relatively fleeting. The majority only last 15–20 minutes. Tell yourself to wait and revaluate later. If a craving isn't terribly strong, you might plan to indulge the craving later in the week. This raises the odds that the craving will pass unindulged, or will at least reduce the frequency of indulging.

2 **Distract.** Cravings are at least partly mental, so if you can engage your mind in something else, it can lessen the craving.

3 **Divert.** Sometimes chewing a strong piece of sugar-free gum or brushing your teeth can be enough to divert your attention to a different taste. Or you may find that there's a much healthier way to indulge your craving, like having a piece of fruit rather than a piece of candy.

4 **Visualize.** Most cravings build over time, peak, and then recede. You may find it helpful to visualize yourself surfing such a wave, riding out the craving. It's important to note that most people give into a craving right before they're about to get over the hump. They feel like the craving is getting worse, and they must indulge it to get it over with. This is false; most cravings will go away on their own with time.

5 **Decide.** Oftentimes, the most difficult part about the craving is the indecision about whether or not to indulge it. You feel torn between your goals and your desire. However, relief will come as soon as the decision is made, whether you decide to have the craved food or not. Simply telling yourself, "No, not today," can be enough to end the craving.

Planning what to eat, preparing it, feeding yourself and others, making something new with any leftovers, then thinking about the next meal—all this can relieve boredom by taking up a good part of the day. We have learned to make all these activities enjoyable rather than simply a necessary part of life. There is nothing inherently wrong with letting food become "something to do." It is only a problem when it leads to undesired weight gain or serves to reduce our motivation to find *other* satisfying, useful, or enjoyable things to do with our free time. It is also a problem if it leads to more eating or otherwise keeps you focused on food when you want to lose weight. This is the key to solving the eating out of boredom problem: *substitute something you find more satisfying, useful, or enjoyable for the food or food-related activity.*

The concept is to replace the easy, inappropriate response to boredom (eating) with an appropriate response. The specifics of the appropriate response depend on your individual needs and desires. They also depend on your willingness to try new things.

JOURNALING ACTIVITY: To-Do Lists

To generate a list of personally appropriate responses to boredom, turn to a blank page of your journal and make two columns: one titled "To-Do List—at Home" and the other "To-Do List—Outside." Make a list of the things you need to do (take out the garbage, wash the car) as well as things you've always wanted to do (make a quilt, take karate lessons, volunteer at the hospital). Keep this list updated, crossing out things you have completed or lost interest in and adding others as you think of them. These things can be personal goals and goals you can undertake with your family. For example, if you are the parent of young children, you may have limited personal time. However, you might consider something like visiting local parks more often as a family. Whenever you find yourself reaching for food when you are not physically hungry, look at your list and pick something else to do.

For those times when you are *extremely* tempted to eat inappropriately, it is probably best to pick something from your *outside* to-do list, because it will get you out of the house, far from temptation and boredom. Of course, you should avoid outside activities that are primarily food related, like going to the supermarket. Also avoid outside activities that include temptations to eat when you're not hungry— such as visiting your parents if they ply you with rich

Head outside if you are tempted to eat when you aren't hungry foods. Usually, once you have gone and done your outside activity, the time for eating inappropriately will have safely passed. However, we recognize that not everyone has the flexibility in their lives to respond in these ways or that certain situations (such as the workplace) give us less latitude than others. When you can't drop what you are doing and do something from your inside or outside to-do list, we ask you to problem-solve using the examples and principles we've introduced thus far. For example, stepping away from a tempting food situation even briefly, to use the restroom or get a glass of water, can help you restore your resolve to avoid eating when you don't want to. Making or slowly sipping a fragrant glass of unsweetened herbal tea can also help you control cravings.

If you are tempted again when you return from an outside activity or tried an alternative coping strategy (if you aren't able to get outside), it will probably now be an appropriate time for you to eat. You will have successfully converted an inappropriate eating episode into an appropriate one. Also, you will undoubtedly have spent your time more productively and enjoyably than if you had eaten out of boredom. Savor that accomplishment, and you will soon find it easier and easier to change your habit of eating inappropriately in this way.

When you are moderately tempted to eat inappropriately, when it seems like there is nothing more interesting to do, you should try something on your at-home to-do list. Here, you should also avoid picking food-related activities, such as straightening out the kitchen, and any other specific activities that often tempt you to eat, such as calling someone who upsets you. Food cravings usually don't last very long. Most people say 15 to 20 minutes is how long such urges last, so you don't need to complete a 1,000-piece jigsaw puzzle to get past the danger. Set a timer to see if your immediate craving lessens after the 20 minutes has passed. If you are already doing something on your to-do list, keep your momentum going, even after the timer has gone off.

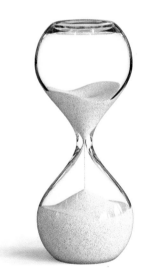

How about the specifics of your to-do list? If you are having trouble coming up with things, or even if you are overflowing with ideas, it can be helpful to subdivide the two columns into different categories of things to do. Consider things you enjoy, satisfying tasks, and things you've always wanted to do (or used to do).

Your list can be as broad as your imagination. Some of these activities can work really

A craving might lessen if you wait before giving in

well to help you resist immediate temptations. The last category is not useful for immediate distraction but is critical in controlling the source of some of the problem, which is not being busy doing things you find enjoyable or worthwhile. You do not have to make every moment of your life interesting, but it can have a wonderful effect on your outlook, as well as your eating behavior, if you broaden your scope of activities and keep your to-do list handy and fresh.

Again, we realize that for many people, such as parents of young children or people with very demanding jobs, the options they have to distract themselves from unnecessary eating are more limited. However, such folks still need distractions, just more efficient ones. When you find yourself tempted to eat, ask yourself what you can do instead to redirect your mental focus away from food.

AVOID REWARDING YOURSELF WITH FOOD

Finally, it is very common for people to eat when they feel happy. They use food to celebrate and to reward themselves. Gayle is a good example of this phenomenon. She believes she eats a fairly nutritious diet most of the time. At the end of a long day, though, she feels like she needs a little reward. In fact, sometimes it can become a bigger reward. She often looks forward to her food reward, thinking about it during idle moments and planning what it will be. Just the thought of it can cheer her up. "Food makes me happy. I really enjoy certain foods," she relates. Unfortunately, she sometimes gets a bit out of control with her food reward. A slowly savored square of dark chocolate is easily replaced by a handful of cookies. These episodes do not qualify as binges because she does not feel particularly guilty or try to hide her eating. Her "eating as a reward" is not in response to hunger, though, and undoubtedly contributes to her weight problem.

As with most of these eating patterns, using food as a reward, or food as happiness, is part of our culture and thus can be difficult to undo. Therefore, it would be wiser to try to modify the response. That is, instead of rewarding or pleasing yourself with rich foods, are there other rewards that you can learn to enjoy as much? For

BOX 5-8

Things that I enjoy
- Reading
- Knitting
- Walking
- Games
- Phone call to friend
- Going to the library

Things that are tasks but satisfying
- Straightening out sock drawer
- Making a to-do list
- Running an errand

Things that I have always wanted to do, or used to do
- Take a class
- Swim
- Meet people
- Join a choir
- Volunteer at a school or animal shelter
- Visit a local park

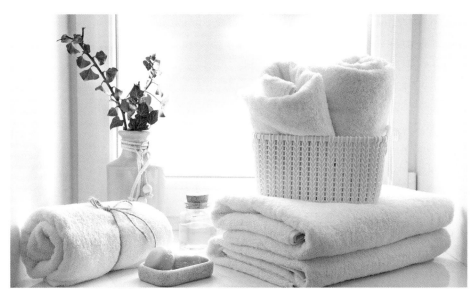

Consider ways to relax and treat yourself in ways that don't involve food

example, after a long day, a relaxing shower might offer another way to decompress and treat yourself. Alternatively, you could simply modify the ingredients and quantity of the food reward so as to reduce the impact on your calorie consumption.

First, though, it may be worthwhile for you to examine the whole concept of rewards. We use rewards almost instinctively as a way to induce ourselves or others to perform in desired ways. Rewards can be external (things like food, money, prestige) or internal (pride, satisfaction, a sense of safety or control). Generally, internal rewards are more effective long-term motivators. For example, a pay raise may keep you temporarily in a job you dislike, but you'd probably accept less pay and do a better job in a position where you were made to feel valued and respected.

The first question to ask yourself if you habitually use food as a reward is, "Reward for what?" If the answer is that you frequently suffer frustrating, unhappy days at work or at home, you may not need a food reward if you can make even a small, positive change in something that is making your life more difficult than it needs to be. It is impossible to guess your precise situation, but some general suggestions may be helpful. First, decide which things you can potentially change, and which things you are unable or unwilling to change. For those things you can change for the better, now is the time to plan it out, preferably in writing (for example, "I'll sign up for a computer course to see if I like that better than what I'm currently doing" or "I'll speak to my significant other about how much it would help if he or she did the vacuuming at home"). For those things you currently cannot or will not change, now is the time to accept them and plan more productive ways of dealing with less than ideal situations. (For example, "My boss's attitude is her problem. It's sad, in a way. Perhaps I should pity her instead of resenting her.")

Identifying the sources of "hard days" and improving the situation can be a major undertaking, which may take some time to enact. Do not underestimate the benefit of even a small improvement in your hard day, though. Such an accomplishment is a powerful internal reward: it can prove to you that you can have a positive impact on your day, your eating habits, your food preferences, and just about anything else you set your mind to.

For dealing with food as a reward for good days (and as a reward for hard days you cannot or do not wish to change), modifying your response can be helpful. Make and keep a list of more suitable rewards. Use them instead of food. What constitutes a suitable reward is up to you. The specific thing is not important and might be quite small. What's important is that you will enjoy it. The rewards you choose should not be used *instead* of eating anything. Rather, they are added to the reasonably portioned and nutritious meal you will eat when you are *physically* hungry. Although it may not strike you as much of a treat, a walk or other form of physical activity is in many ways an excellent reward. This is because the emotional stresses of a hard day can be relieved very nicely by doing something purely physical. The advantage to this form of rewarding yourself is that it both relieves stress and increases fitness while helping you to lose weight. Finally, if all else fails and you occasionally continue to use food inappropriately as a reward, use the techniques of portion control and calorie counting to minimize the impact of this habit and fit it into the budget of your Personal Plan. Instructions for devising this budget are given in detail in the next chapter.

> **BOX 5-9**
>
> ## Nonfood Rewards to Consider
>
> - Bubble bath
> - Small present (such as a magazine or a fuzzy pair of socks)
> - Phone call to a friend
> - Favorite TV show

SOCIAL TRIGGERS

Another common reason for making unhealthy food choices is a temptation to eat what friends are eating, or as a result of direct pressure from friends and family. Socializing with friends and family very frequently takes place over a meal. It's enjoyable, efficient, we need to eat anyway, and it's often viewed as a way of killing two birds with one stone. However, dining out, or even at a friend's home, usually involves larger portions and richer foods than you would prepare for yourself at

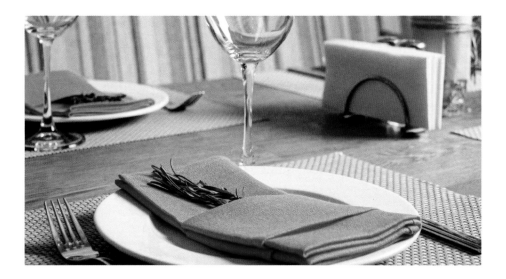

home. In addition, when others prepare your food, you have a lot less control over the amount of oil, butter, and salt that goes into it. While we don't recommend that you avoid socializing, we do recommend that our patients take a hard look at how frequently they are eating or drinking outside of their home. It may be worth considering if there are ways of socializing that could be incorporated into one's schedule that do not involve food.

For example, Marcus is a hard-driving, gregarious businessman who packs most of his extra weight around his middle. He never used to think about his diet at all, and he never had to until the rude intrusion of a heart attack at age 51. He tends to

BOX 5-10

Less Foodcentric Social Activities

- Concert
- Theater
- Meeting for a walk
- Meeting for a hike
- Exercise class (such as taking yoga with a friend)
- Movie
- Bookstore

- Bible study
- Book club
- Dance lessons
- Art class
- Social painting
- Museum
- Art show
- Game night (board games, bunco, poker, etc.)

- Meeting for coffee or tea (can be noncaloric at least)
- Shopping
- Spa (massage, pedicure, etc.)

eat a balanced, nutritious diet at home, thanks largely to his health-conscious spouse, but he has trouble controlling his diet in social situations, especially parties and business lunches. At parties, he can be found at the buffet table, inhaling huge quantities of rich appetizers. "I just like food," he states with assurance. As an afterthought, he adds, "And eating and drinking is part of my job. I have to keep my contacts happy."

While Marcus's eating problems occur largely in business-related situations, many people report similar problems in purely social settings. Experiments in which people's eating habits are observed has shown that eating with others tends to increase the total amount of food consumed. This is called "social facilitation of eating" and applies equally to many animal species. It also applies to people who drink alcoholic beverages. The larger the number of people present, especially family or friends, the larger the meal consumed. On average, meals eaten with other people are 44% larger than meals eaten alone, even though the composition of the meal is about the same. There is also the influence of whom one is eating with—eating with people who exhibit poor habits is likely to reinforce our own less desirable impulses, while eating with people who are very conscious of portions and good food choices will exert a beneficial influence on your eating. Thus, the observation that we tend to look like our close relatives and friends; social networks are often as influential as genetic factors.

Social facilitation seems to occur in all types of eating situations—breakfast, lunch, dinner, and snacks; in restaurants and at home; on weekends and during the week. It might seem that a person who overeats socially could reduce the amount consumed by eating alone, but while avoiding social and business eating situations can be effective during the action phase of your Personal Plan, it is not a useful maintenance technique, since it would adversely affect the quality of your life. Also, as discussed in the third example, eating alone when bored may be a far greater problem.

There are alternatives: If you are hosting the event, you have a greater degree of control than if you are a guest. For instance, you may be able to have a very enjoyable party or productive business meeting that does not occur during a mealtime. Coffee and other beverages, preferably nonalcoholic, may be all that is needed. If the event does need to include a meal, because you control the menu, you can follow the low-fat and portion-control guidelines discussed in chapter 6. As you will see, this does not mean that the food will be tasteless or boring.

If you are a guest, you still have a number of tools at your disposal that will help you to keep within the dietary guidelines of your Personal Plan. For instance, you can find out in advance what will be served. Even if you do not feel comfortable making special requests to fit your diet, you will at least know what to expect and can plan accordingly.

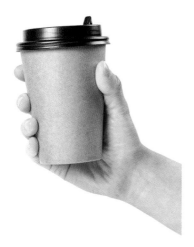

Coffee or tea is a great choice for a meeting or gathering

If the food to be served is likely to take you off your diet plan, eat something substantial that is consistent with your plan just prior to leaving for the event. While having recently eaten is not a guarantee that you will not eat more, it will help you to maintain control. If you must travel a good distance to the event, plan ahead and bring food with you for the ride. If you are tempted during the event, go ahead and sample the foods you crave so that you will not feel too deprived. Even the most fat- and calorie-laden foods can fit into your Personal Plan if you get the most out of a small portion by savoring it over a prolonged period of time. Choosing low-fat and low-calorie foods, however, will allow you to eat larger volumes and fill up earlier.

When your host or others urge you to consume more than you should, you may find it difficult to refuse. Depending on your personality, any of the following responses can be very effective:

Feigning shock: "Please, not more! I know how delicious your cooking is—if I start I can't stop."

White lie: "I already tasted it. It's wonderful."

Direct approach: "I'm really trying hard to lose weight. I know you just want me to enjoy myself, but it's easier when I'm not tempted."

More humor: "If I eat another thing I will explode. It will not be a pretty sight."

Delay/distract: "I'm good. I'll have some later" or "I love your new couch. It's so comfortable."

Escape to the restroom: "Excuse me. I'll be back in a minute."

In business settings, sometimes the problem is how to refuse not food but alcoholic beverages. Try saying this next time: "I'd love to, but it puts me right to sleep lately," or "Thanks, but I'm going to save my calories for the entrée."

Perhaps the most useful way to learn how to deal with eating in social and business situations is to change your perception of the event. What is the primary reason for social or business meetings? Is the eating the important thing going on, or is it something else? Clearly the main reason for having a social gathering or business lunch is to meet with people you like, or at least wish to have like you. In other words, it is important that you recognize that such gatherings are primarily social or business events with food present, rather than eating events with people present. This may seem obvious, but our behavior often makes it seem like we are there primarily to eat. Instead, it is helpful to remind yourself right before entering the house or restaurant that you are here to catch up with the lives of your dear friends, or to make a good impression on a business associate, or whatever your reason is. Have a plan for the event, like: "I need to talk to Joe, Mary, and Rob especially." Focus on your party plan, and the food will remain secondary.

DEALING WITH SABOTEURS

Social triggers can make trying to lose weight more difficult; however, social *support can make weight loss infinitely easier. What do you do, though, when someone very close to you is not supportive of your efforts to lose weight?* Janet has had trouble keeping her weight at a reasonable level since she was a teenager. Many members of her family have weight problems. She was overweight when she married at age 21, but now, at age 32, she weighs 55 pounds more than she did then. She and her husband, Oliver, have no children. Janet works in an office and Oliver in a factory. She tries to watch her diet and recently considered buying a treadmill, but Oliver objected to the cost, saying: "You're never going to use it, anyway. Just use willpower and stop eating so much." She is interested in lowering the amount of fat and carbs in her diet, but her

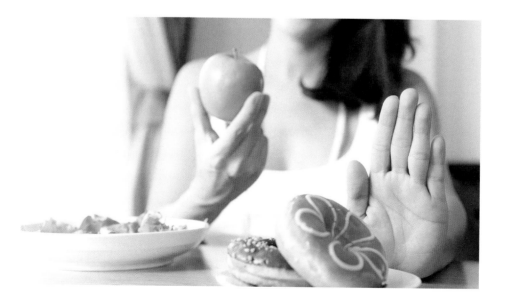

BOX 5-11

Watch Out for Sabotage

Examples include:

- **Eating tempting foods in front of a dieting partner, relative, or friend.**

- **Encouraging the dieter to "take a break" from the diet or splurge.**

- **Giving false sympathy:** "I don't know how you can eat that diet food, poor thing."

- **Giving negative messages about learning to manage one's weight:** "Aren't you hungry?" or "Exercise is boring."

- **Giving negative messages about the dieter:** "You've tried this before; what makes you think this time will be any different?" or "Why can't you just eat less?" and sometimes, "You're too thin" (assuming you are not) or "I like you better heavier."

husband insists on "meat and potatoes." He says he wants to help her lose weight, but he often brings home chocolate and candy bars. Chocolates are hard for Janet to resist, and she eats them when her husband is not around because she is embarrassed. Oliver seems to be able to eat them every day as snacks and not gain an ounce.

There are as many variations on this theme as there are couples like Oliver and Janet. The broad outline is similar—one partner has a weight problem and wants to do something about it; the other, who may or may not have a weight problem, is a saboteur. Intentional and unintentional sabotage can be difficult to distinguish from each other. Bringing home rich desserts for a partner who has trouble resisting them, for example, can be a misguided expression of the "food is love" theme we've all learned, or a conscious or unconscious act of hostility.

You need to learn how to recognize all these forms of sabotage, and how to deal with them effectively. To a certain extent, how you deal with sabotage will depend on the nature of the relationship and communication style you have with the saboteur.

 JOURNALING ACTIVITY: Sabotage

First, how to recognize sabotage. You should observe, and record in your journal, all episodes of dietary and behavioral deviation from your desired diet and behavior. Write down the date and time, the nature of the deviation, and what prompted you to eat. An example of this log is shown below. This log will be useful not just for detecting sabotage but also for detecting other conditions that derail your efforts during the action and maintenance stages of your Personal Plan.

BOX 5-12

Date and Time	What I ate	Why I ate
5/6/96, 2:30 p.m.	1 Big piece of chocolate cake	Feeling upset with Mark; cake left over from birthday celebration

Not all sabotage can be detected in this way. The subtle messages do not usually lead directly to deviations—rather, they undermine self-esteem and self-control. The verbal and body language can be detected by listening critically to your own feelings in reaction to these messages. Do you feel embarrassed by the other person's comments and want to hide your eating? Does something the other person says make you feel angry, or sad, or alone and misunderstood? Even if you do not respond negatively to these messages, you should be aware of their potential negative effect on your motivation for controlling your weight and adhering to your Personal Plan. You need to develop a way of dealing with sabotage appropriately, keeping in mind that the appropriate response varies from one person to another and one situation to another.

For people who are not important to you, you can simply recognize the hidden message behind such statements as "You're too thin," "Aren't you hungry?," and "I could never eat that way," and ignore them. Recognize that you are probably witnessing the saboteur's jealousy or insecurity about their own weight or eating habits. The statements are then unlikely to influence your behavior negatively, or distract you from the commitment you have made to your Personal Plan. If you are feeling insecure at the time you hear a sabotage line, the message can be more harmful, even if the person is relatively unimportant to you. For these occasions, it is particularly important for you to "consider the source." If it's your style to show no pain in public, you will want, again, to ignore the sabotage or just say no (that is, "I'm not hungry"). If you prefer the direct approach, you can say, with a smile, "Yes, I am hungry, but I am committed to making positive changes in my life. Let's talk about something else."

For a person who is important to you, sabotage is usually better dealt with openly and completely. It is best to assume, at least initially, that the sabotaging words or deeds are unintentional. The saboteur may even be laboring under the mistaken belief that he or she is being helpful to you, that the statements or actions will motivate you in some way to stick to a diet. Thus, it may come as a surprise to the saboteur that you do not appreciate his or her "support."

Your primary aims must be to stop the sabotage and, if possible, to replace it with true support. Assume that this person has good intentions and guide these good intentions into something useful to you. Start with a genuine statement of appreciation for the expression of caring and desire to help you in the difficult task of losing weight and changing lifelong habits. This is likely to be well received and may make the saboteur less defensive about your request for a different form of help. Even for the suspected intentional saboteur, this approach is still recommended. Only when the intentional saboteur does not respond to your reasonable requests and gracious assumptions of good intentions should you resort to other measures.

After starting with your statement of appreciation, what should you do next? This depends on the exact nature of the offense. An interaction might go something like this:

Janet: You know, Ollie, I wanted to tell you that I appreciate how you want to help me lose weight and keep it off.

Oliver: Well, sure, I know how much it bothers you.

Janet: And you also don't get down on me when I gain weight.

Oliver: Well, I know it's hard for you and it doesn't bother me.

Janet: Can I ask you to do something that would help me a lot?

Oliver: Sure.

Janet: You know how I love chocolate and cookies and stuff; it's really hard for me to resist them, and I seem to gain weight very easily when I eat them. You're so lucky that you don't seem to have this problem.

Oliver: Uh huh, but I just don't eat any more than I need; I just stop eating when I'm not hungry.

Janet: I guess I eat mostly when I'm *not* hungry, so it's hard to know when to stop. But what I wanted to tell you, since I know you want to help me any way you can, is that it would really help me if there wasn't anything around the house to tempt me for a while. Will you take the cookies and stuff and maybe put them in your car, or bring them to work and only eat them at work or in the car? I know you like them, so this way you could have all you want without making it hard for me.

Oliver: No sweets at all at home?

Janet: Well, I've got an idea . . . You know those sweet fruit fig bars that you sometimes eat?

Oliver: Yes, but you hate them.

Janet: Exactly. Let's buy a lot of them to keep at home. I really appreciate your help.

Oliver: No problem. Hey, what's for dinner?

Janet: Well, while we're on the subject, let's talk about the meat and potatoes thing . . .

You'll get the best results when you know what you'd like the saboteur to do, and bring it up in a gentle but direct manner, preferably at a time separate from the incident, rather than in the heat of the moment. This approach does not work in all cases, but it is worth a try. Notice how Janet defuses Oliver's implied criticism ("I just stop eating when I'm not hungry."). Instead of rising to the bait, she concedes that she has a problem and goes right back to her plan of asking him to help her with it.

Sabotage does not generally end after a single such encounter, even when the encounter goes well. Because sabotage is usually habitual, good follow-up is essential. Just as you may struggle to change your own habits, the well-intentioned saboteur is also likely to slip back into his or her old habits.

To avoid such potentially tense encounters, follow up your initial discussions with verbal reinforcement of your gratitude for the help you are receiving: "You've been really good about not bringing sweets home. I really appreciate it." Other possible reinforcers of your saboteur's good behavior include regularly sharing your success and delight with how your Personal Plan is going, praising the saboteur in front of family or friends, or giving him or her a hug, a small present, a note, or whatever seems appropriate to you. Don't hesitate to ask for help from your partner or others in your social network—only you know the best ways others can support your efforts to make lasting changes in your lifestyle.

For the intentional saboteur who is close to you, it may be reasonable to start with the approach outlined earlier. First, you may be mistaken about the saboteur's intentions. Second, even if you are correct, you may still succeed in changing his or her behavior, despite the initially poor intentions. You are basically providing the intentional saboteur with a face-saving way to change his or her behavior without blame.

If this approach does not succeed, and the sabotage continues, a more direct labeling of this behavior is needed. This doesn't have to be a hostile approach, but you must make it clear to your saboteur that you have pointed out the problem in the past, do not see a change, and find this puzzling and frustrating. Be prepared to hear some very negative things. When someone is accused of dishonorable behavior, he or she will often respond by attacking the accuser, rather than taking responsibility for his or her actions. You must not rise to this bait. Your requests are quite reasonable, and you must remain focused on them. The fact that your saboteur says he or she finds you weak or pitiable is indeed an issue to be dealt with, but it is not your problem. He or she needs to come to terms with that kind of feeling, but it will more likely be resolved by supporting you than by sabotaging you. This is not an easy encounter, but it may need to happen for you to have a reasonable chance of carrying out your Personal Plan. If such encounters are frequent or unproductive, you may want to try couples counseling, which can do a lot to improve communication between partners.

You may choose to accept sabotage rather than deal with it directly. This is the only viable option in some relationships. In such cases, you must be prepared to enlist support from others—family, friends, colleagues—and to detach yourself from the nonsupportive person in your environment.

Finally, in dealing with the problem of intentional or unintentional sabotage, be aware of one very important aspect. The sabotage may relate to the underlying reasons for your desire to lose weight. It is common to want to lose weight because of a disapproving significant other. This is a negative, external influence, and not the best motivator in the long run. If this kind of influence forms an important part of your motivation, you must step back and rethink your reasons for wanting to lose weight. Reread chapter 2, and focus on internal motivators for better weight control.

A NOTE ABOUT FAMILIES

Your eating habits, as we have seen, tend to follow predictable patterns. They are embedded in other habits you may have, like watching television in the evening or buying a particular brand of bread. However, if you live with other people, your eating habits are probably not yours alone. Your habits are intertwined with those of your family members.

Families are about relationships, and psychologists define a close relationship as one in which important habits of the people involved are interlinked—the closer the relationship, the more habits people share. Say that your evening routine usually includes walking the dog, picking up the kids, and taking out the trash; think of the disruption that is caused when you go out of town for a week, just in the evenings alone. Now, imagine what will happen if you change your eating behavior *every single day, for the rest of your life.* You are likely to have a profound influence on the eating behaviors of the people close to you, and those people may react to the changes with anger and frustration.

We recommend getting the people you live with involved in your lifestyle changes. Without their help, change may be impossible. Studies of people with high blood pressure, for example, have shown that they are much more likely to take their medications when close family members are given information about hypertension and instructions about the patient's diet and medications. Your success at sticking to your Personal Plan depends on your ability to collaborate effectively with those around you. Getting your family involved in your plan may not be easy, but if all of you work together on this effort, you will make it a shared project and build a shared commitment to your weight loss. That doesn't mean that your family has to go on the diet with you or that they have to increase their physical activity. It just means that they should understand and agree to certain new behaviors like cooking without butter or excusing you from doing the dishes so you can exercise. In the end, the entire household will be rewarded with a trimmer, more vibrant you—one who will be around much longer.

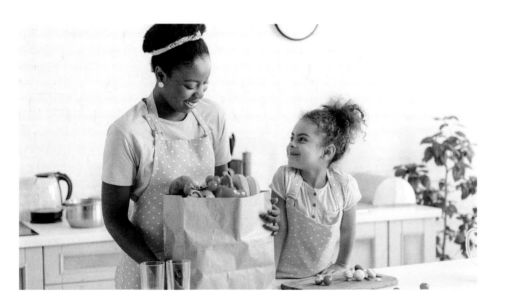

PHYSICAL TRIGGERS

One of the most common physical triggers for overeating is hunger. We recommend eating when hunger gets to a 5 to 7 on a 0 (no hunger) to 10 (famished) scale. One caveat is that if you are about to enter a meeting, or other situation where you might not be able to eat for an extended period of time, you should probably be proactive and eat even if you aren't yet significantly hungry. This is preferable to waiting until you are ravenous and at risk for overeating.

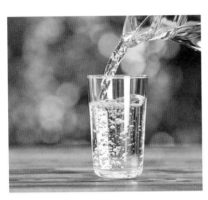

Are you hungry or thirsty?

Another common physical trigger is thirst. As the body starts to become dehydrated, before thirst is perceptible, the body often senses that the body has a need. We liken it to the "check engine" light coming on in the car. It's not specific, so it's often misinterpreted as hunger. In order to prevent this from happening, it's a good idea to keep a water bottle handy and to drink at will throughout the day. Not everybody needs six to eight glasses of water, but most people need more than they get. Increased water consumption can be helpful for other reasons. It can stop water retention, reduce or prevent constipation, and help you feel less hungry.

Hormones are another important trigger. Many women experience cravings during different parts of their menstrual cycle. These cravings can lead to increased caloric intake via sweet foods like chocolate and salty foods like chips. Tracking one's menstrual cycle can be a good way to better understand how your hormones affect your cravings. This knowledge may empower you to ignore your cravings, or may allow you to better plan for them.

For example, Lisa marks her calendar each month with the days she expects to experience PMS symptoms, which include strong cravings for chocolate. Lisa makes sure that she has a low sugar hot chocolate available to satisfy this craving. She also plans pampering activities, such as getting a manicure, to help manage her mood during this time. Menopause also causes a number of hormonal fluctuations that can affect sleep, mood, cravings, hunger, and satiety.

Cortisol, the body's stress hormone, is another big player in the cravings department. Cortisol release is the body's "flight or fight" response, and it is associated with carbohydrate cravings. This is because carbohydrates are the fastest, easiest source of fuel for your body to access. When you are under physical or mental stress, your body is likely to release cortisol and experience increased carbohydrate cravings. Your body doesn't understand that you don't need a sugary soda in order to fight or flee your boss.

SLEEP

Sleep has a huge impact on weight, yet it's often over-looked. It's very important to consider how much sleep you are actually getting as well as the quality of that sleep. In recent years, sleep has been found to have a significant impact on a number of hormones, including ghrelin, leptin, and cortisol. Collectively, these hormones create the "perfect storm"—they can, respectively, make you hungrier, less satiated by what you eat, and more likely to crave carbohydrates. When people begin to track their sleep, using a Fitbit, Garmin, or other movement tracking device, or even a simple pencil and paper log, they are often surprised by how little they sleep. As a result, when people begin to track their sleep, they often begin to make positive changes to their sleep habits.

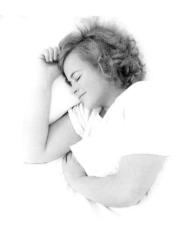

In addition to having a physiological effect on hunger, satiety, and cravings, lack of sleep often weakens your motivation or resolve. You may be more likely to feel cranky and sluggish, and therefore choose a food that is comforting, like a scone along with your coffee. Later in the day, you may find yourself eating to stay awake. It is important to note that in men with a neck size larger than 17 inches, the incidence of sleep apnea is 80%. For women, a neck size larger than 16 inches is also a significant risk factor for sleep apnea. If you fall in that category, or if you snore, gasp in your sleep, or are especially tired despite getting a good amount of sleep, ask your doctor about a sleep study.

If you are not getting the amount of sleep you need, identify the reasons and do what you can to make a change. If you simply can't get more sleep, say, you have a super early plane flight, be aware of the effect this will likely have on your eating. Pack healthy snacks, and be ready to soothe yourself without food if needed. Wake yourself up with a cup of coffee (but resist the extra-large white chocolate mocha with whipped cream), or take a brisk walk.

JOURNALING ACTIVITY: Sleep

We know that lack of sleep can impact both sides of your energy balance equation—causing you to crave sweets on the food intake side and feel less likely to want to be active on the exercise (expenditure) side. Sometimes sleep challenges are caused by medical conditions or prescriptions; if this is the case, you'll want to still make a point to rest in lieu of sleep. This is why it is so important to come up with a nighttime routine that you can enjoy, to support you in having enough sleep of the right quality (or to relax you in lieu of sleep if it is difficult to come by).

BOX 5-13

Sleep Tips

- **Sleep schedule.** Wake up and go to bed at about the same time on work nights and nonwork nights. Bedtime and wake time should not differ from one day to the next by more than two hours.

- **Prioritize sleep.** You can't sleep seven to eight hours unless you are in bed for at least seven to eight hours. Keep an eye on the clock and make sure to finish whatever needs to be done earlier in the day so you can get to bed on time. Avoid starting projects (such as laundry) when bedtime is approaching.

- **Weekends.** Don't sleep in on weekends to "catch up" on sleep. This makes it more likely that you will have problems falling asleep at bedtime.

- **Naps.** If you are very sleepy during the day, nap for 30 to 45 minutes in the early afternoon, if possible. Don't nap too long or too late in the afternoon, or you will have difficulty falling asleep at bedtime.

- **Sunlight.** Spend time outside every day, especially in the morning, as exposure to sunlight, or bright light, helps to keep your body's internal clock on track.

- **Exercise.** Exercise regularly. Exercising may help you fall asleep and sleep more deeply.

- **Bedroom.** Make sure your bedroom is comfortable, quiet, and dark. Make sure also that it is not too warm at night, as sleeping in a room warmer than 75°F will make it hard to sleep. Consider using a fan for white noise or ear plugs.

- **Bed.** Use your bed only for sex and sleeping. Don't read, watch television, or listen to music on your bed.

- **Pets.** No matter how much you love them, keep them out of your bedroom, or at least your bed. Pet owners who sleep with their pets are more likely to suffer from sleep deprivation than those who do not sleep with their pets.

- **Bedtime.** Keep the same bedtime. Let your body and mind get used to a predictable routine. Make the 30 to 60 minutes before bedtime a quiet or wind-down time. Relaxing, calm, enjoyable activities, such as reading a book or listening to soothing music, help your body and mind slow down enough to let you sleep. Do not watch TV, clean, pay bills, exercise, or get involved in "energizing" activities in the 30 minutes before bedtime. Put away your digital screens, which interrupt your natural circadian rhythm.

- **Snack.** Eat regular meals and don't go to bed hungry. A light snack before bed is a good idea; eating a full meal in the hour before bed is not.

- **Caffeine.** Avoid eating or drinking products containing caffeine after 2 p.m. and in the evening. These include caffeinated sodas, coffee, tea, and chocolate.

- **Alcohol.** Ingestion of alcohol disrupts sleep and may cause you to awaken throughout the night.

- **Smoking.** Smoking disturbs sleep. Don't smoke for at least an hour before bedtime (and preferably, not at all).

- **Worry.** Write persistent thoughts and worries down in a notebook and then put them out of your mind. Review the notebook in the morning and take action if appropriate.

- **Frustration.** If you can't fall asleep after 15–20 minutes, get out of bed and read something relatively boring until you feel sleepy.

- **Relax.** Engage in calm activities (for example, reading, listening to music) and relaxation exercises (such as deep breathing, meditation, progressive muscle relaxation, or guided imagery) to help ready your body for sleep.

ADAPTED IN PART FROM: *J. A. Mindell and J. A. Owens (2003).* A Clinical Guide to Pediatric Sleep: Diagnosis and Management of Sleep Problems. *Philadelphia: Lippincott Williams and Wilkins.*

Sleep Questionnaire

Answer the following questions in your journal to help you reflect on your current sleep and nighttime routine so you can decide if you would like to include goals in these areas in your Personalized Plan of Action.

If you were to wave a magic wand and create the perfect nighttime routine, what would that look like for you?

When you think of this magic nighttime routine, and making it a reality, what barriers or obstacles come up for you?

Which barriers and obstacles do you think you could remove from your nighttime routine? What would that look like?

How would you feel about making these changes and improving your routine?

How would it feel to not make these changes and continue your nighttime routine as is?

What is the cost of not choosing to make these changes?

Reflecting on your answers, what goals would you like to set (if any) for your nighttime routine?

SMOKING

Smoking cessation is a trigger for overeating that falls under both physical and emotional headings. There is evidence that smoking cessation might temporarily slow metabolism a bit, as well as remove a common "go-to" stress management activity. Take Ralph, for example. He was always on the "husky" side, but he never really felt he had a weight problem until he quit smoking. In one year, he gained more than 35 pounds. He is not sure why, since he doesn't really feel like he is that much hungrier now than when he was a smoker. He has never been physically active and eats a moderately high-fat diet, but he has never been worried about his weight until this recent weight gain.

For reasons that are not completely clear, most people gain some weight after they quit smoking. The average weight gain in the year after quitting is 6 pounds, but many people gain much more than that. The nicotine in cigarettes does increase metabolism, so there's a possibility that metabolism slows when smoking stops, but the effect is brief and is probably not the major factor in the weight gain, especially for those who gained more than the typical amount. An important and—fortunately—controllable factor is the tendency to use food as a substitute for cigarettes. Initially the mood-elevating effect of certain foods may help to soothe cigarette cravings in recent quitters. Later, eating may simply be a substitute behavior. Eating distracts the person and relieves stress the way cigarettes used to.

It can be difficult, but it is not impossible, to minimize the "bathroom scales" effect of quitting smoking. First of all, decide whether you are going to simultaneously quit smoking while trying to lose weight, or if you are going to change one habit at a time. Suggestions for both options are discussed at the end of chapter 10. For most people, it is more important, from the perspective of risk to your health, to quit smoking than to lose weight. Your health care provider can help you form a plan to quit smoking if you do decide to quit while losing weight.

Second, try to figure out whether you are, indeed, using food as a cigarette substitute; how and when you are most prone to do so; and what kinds of foods you are you most likely to employ. For example, for smokers, smoking after a meal is a common ritual. Now that you've quit smoking, do you substitute desserts or other snacks for your after-meal cigarette? Smoking cessation may depress mood, and some former smokers use sweets to elevate their mood or satisfy their cravings for cigarettes. Indeed, there is strong evidence that sweets do elevate mood, probably by affecting levels of a chemical neurotransmitter in our brains called serotonin. Eating small amounts of sugary foods such as hard candies or chewing gum can

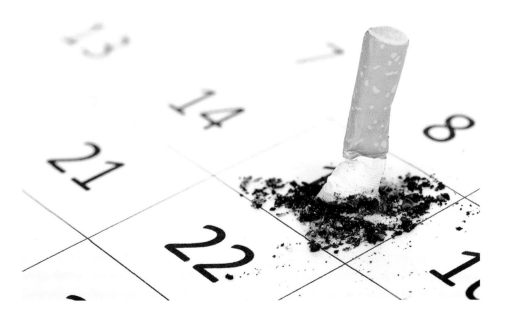

satisfy this desire for sweets without adding unwanted pounds. Try chewing gum after meals. While traditional sweets such as cookies, cake, and doughnuts are indeed sweet-tasting, they derive far too many calories from fat and are poor choices for a cigarette substitute. Better choices are sugar-free gum, crunchy vegetables, and diet drinks.

Third, to combat both the tendency to eat more and the mood-depressing effects of smoking cessation, try increasing the amount and level of your physical activity (see chapter 8).

MENTAL TRIGGERS

Sometimes you don't need to see or smell food in order to be tempted. You don't need someone to offer you a treat. All you need is to think about it, and you want it. Many of our patients describe themselves as "foodies." They love to think about food and enjoy watching the Food Network and perusing cookbooks and cooking websites. They read about new restaurants and think about new foods they'd like to try. It's fine to enjoy your food, and we actually think that a passion for cooking can be helpful for weight management, provided that you are open to modifying recipes to making them healthier. However, a heavy focus on food can be

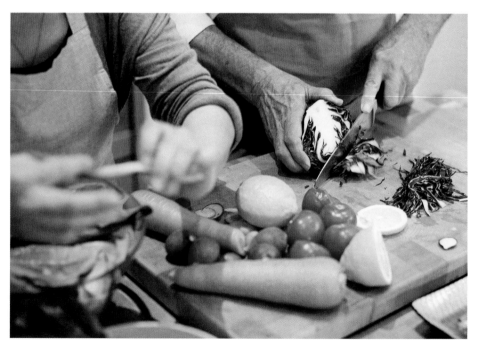

If you like to cook, focus on healthy recipes

problematic if weight control is a goal. We recommend trying to branch out and cultivate other interests, to take some of the focus off of food. We also recommend coming up with strategies and effective self-talk to help combat cravings.

Under the heading of mental triggers, we would also include sabotaging thoughts. These are the things that you say to yourself that give you the green light to move forward with behaviors that you later regret. Sabotaging thoughts can negatively affect your ability to lose weight in many ways. They can destroy your confidence in your ability to be successful and can derail your eating, keep you from exercising, and so forth. Remember Alison from the beginning of this chapter? She gained back the 10 pounds she had lost as a result of this sabotaging thought: "I know this [drinking wine and snacking after work] caused me to gain weight before, but I'm only going to have a drink tonight. I'm not going to do it every night, and today was especially bad." However, the next night, she told herself the same thing, and a few months later, she was back where she'd started.

One very effective strategy, outlined by Judith Beck in *The Beck Diet Solution,* is to first identify the sabotaging thoughts that get in the way of your goals and then to formulate helpful responses or comebacks to the problematic thoughts. If Alison had done this, she might have told herself, "I want wine right now because I am stressed; however, drinking in this situation runs a high risk of reinforcing an old unhealthy habit. Maintaining my weight loss is very important to me, so I need to find something else to help me unwind. I'm going to try taking a nice long hot shower and see if that relaxes me before I decide about the wine." If Alison had responded in this manner, it's quite likely that she would have been able to avoid the wine all night and would have later felt happy and empowered by the fact that she'd made a better choice.

SELF-TALK AND SELF-COMPASSION

Your self-talk is a term that describes how you are communicating with yourself in your "inner monologue" or that "voice inside your head." This inner voice can be supportive or critical, depending on the habits you have built.

HABIT AS A TRIGGER

Habit is often an overarching trigger. All of the previously mentioned triggers can morph into habits if they occur consistently. Do any of your eating behaviors reflect the force of habit? Eating while watching TV is often a conditioned or habitual

BOX 5-15

The following assessment by Dr. Kirsten Neff will survey the way you communicate with yourself in tough times, which is also called self-compassion. Learning to be less mean and more kind and compassionate with yourself as you lose weight can help you be more accepting of yourself throughout the process of losing weight—for example, during plateaus when the scale doesn't change or during slip ups from your plan of action.

Procedure: Please read each statement carefully before answering. To the left of each item, indicate how often you behave in the stated manner, using the following scale:

Almost Never   **Almost Always**

1   2   3   4   5

____ 1. I'm disapproving and judgmental about my own flaws and inadequacies.

____ 2. When I'm feeling down, I tend to obsess and fixate on everything that's wrong.

____ 3. When things are going badly for me, I see the difficulties as part of life that everyone goes through.

____ 4. When I think about my inadequacies, it tends to make me feel more separate and cut off from the rest of the world.

____ 5. I try to be loving toward myself when I'm feeling emotional pain.

____ 6. When I fail at something important to me, I become consumed by feelings of inadequacy.

____ 7. When I'm down and out, I remind myself that there are lots of other people in the world feeling like I am.

____ 8. When times are really difficult, I tend to be tough on myself.

____ 9. When something upsets me, I try to keep my emotions in balance.

____ 10. When I feel inadequate in some way, I try to remind myself that feelings of inadequacy are shared by most people.

____ 11. I'm intolerant and impatient toward those aspects of my personality I don't like.

____ 12. When I'm going through a very hard time, I give myself the caring and tenderness I need.

____ 13. When I'm feeling down, I tend to feel like most other people are probably happier than I am.

____ 14. When something painful happens, I try to take a balanced view of the situation.

____ 15. I try to see my failings as part of the human condition.

___ **16.** When I see aspects of myself that I don't like, I get down on myself.

___ **17.** When I fail at something important to me, I try to keep things in perspective.

___ **18.** When I'm really struggling, I tend to feel like other people must be having an easier time of it.

___ **19.** I'm kind to myself when I'm experiencing suffering.

___ **20.** When something upsets me, I get carried away with my feelings.

___ **21.** I can be a bit coldhearted toward myself when I'm experiencing suffering.

___ **22.** When I'm feeling down, I try to approach my feelings with curiosity and openness.

___ **23.** I'm tolerant of my own flaws and inadequacies.

___ **24.** When something painful happens, I tend to blow the incident out of proportion.

___ **25.** When I fail at something that's important to me, I tend to feel alone in my failure.

___ **26.** I try to be understanding and patient toward those aspects of my personality I don't like.

Scoring Your Results

1 After you complete the test (item 19), separate your responses as follows:

Positive Items	Negative Items
Self-Kindness Items: 5, 12, 19, 23, 26	Self-Judgment Items: 1, 8, 11, 16, 21
Common Humanity Items: 3, 7, 10, 15	Isolation Items: 4, 13, 18, 25
Mindfulness Items: 9, 14, 17, 22	Over-identified Items: 2, 6, 20, 24

2 Add the scores from the positive items (self-kindness, common humanity, mindfulness), then write the total here: _____

Reverse scores on the negative items (that is, 1 = 5, 2 = 4, 3 = 3, 4 = 2, 5 = 1), then write the total here: _____

3 Add the two scores (positive and negative) and divide by 26 to get your self-compassion score (average).

4 Reflect on your score and whether you want to add a commitment to improving your self-compassion (self-talk) in your Personal Plan of Action.

Neff, K. D. (2003). "Development and Validation of a Scale to Measure Self-Compassion." Self and Identity 2:223-250. https://self-compassion.org/wp-content/uploads/2015/06/Self_Compassion_Scale_for_researchers.pdf.

TABLE 5-1

Potential stressors that trigger eating and strategies to reduce their effect

Stressors	Goals	Strategies
Environmental • Seeing food • Smelling food	• Reduce exposure to stressors • Modify your reaction to stressors	• Remove trigger foods from your home and work environment • Ask family or friends to keep treats out of sight
Emotional • Sadness • Anger • Anxiety • Boredom • Frustration • Stress • Happiness • Reward	• Deal with challenging emotions without relying on food for comfort	• Reduce distraction while eating • Label emotions to increase your awareness of what you are feeling • Learn to accept and tolerate some unpleasant feelings • Practice changing negative emotions into more helpful ways of thinking • Use coping strategies (such as listening to music, taking a walk, getting a massage, watching a movie, spending time with a friend). Increase your involvement in activities that bring you joy and satisfaction • Improve time management and organizational skills to reduce stress
Mental • Thinking about food • Situations in which you want to eat like "everyone else"	• Think differently about food • Identify and change unhelpful ways of thinking • Learn how to restructure unhelpful thoughts (for example, "It's not fair")	• Use thought-stopping techniques (imagine a big red stop sign and don't allow yourself to continue with that train of thought) • Utilize distraction techniques • Alternately, use acceptance strategies (for example, "I wish I could have bacon every morning, but it's not good for my heart. It's disappointing, but I need to make some changes.")

Stressors	Goals	Strategies
Social • People who urge you to eat • Situations in which you want to eat like "everyone else"	• Realize how social contexts affect your eating habits • Learn to cope with feelings • Ask your friends and family for support • Please yourself, not others	• Practice being assertive and saying no when others offer you food • Order carefully and eat slowly when dining with a group • Shift your focus from feelings of deprivation to feelings of pride for having made a healthy decision
Physical • Hunger • Thirst • Fatigue • Hormones • Frustration • Stress • Happiness • Reward	• Increase awareness of the mind-body connection • Eat mindfully • Have a greater understanding of what's going on with your physiology	• Know the difference between being tired, thirsty, and hungry • Recognize that hunger is not an emergency • Learn to identify between hunger and cravings and how to manage both (for example, acceptance, distraction, relaxation techniques, planned indulgences)

response. Likewise, eating when coming home from work often hearkens back to having a snack when coming home from school as a child. A morning routine, such as having a scone with a cup of coffee, may have started one day and just continued.

Ivan is a good example of someone who struggles with eating out of habit. Ivan eats "three squares" a day, without fail, like clockwork. He rarely snacks, but his meals tend to consist of large portions with second helpings. He may be hungry when he starts eating, but he will often continue eating past the point of fullness. He is likely less aware of how much he's eating because he always eats while watching TV. "I guess it's just a habit," he volunteers.

Ivan is engaging in ritual eating—that is, eating on a rigid schedule or in a stereotyped pattern. This is only a problem if it is combined with eating in excess of caloric needs.

What should be done about a ritual eating pattern? If you believe you may be eating out of habit, when you are not physically hungry, you may want to try the following: For people who are on a normal daytime-awake, nighttime-sleep schedule, it is usually best to eat a nutritious breakfast such as those described in the next chapter. Do this even if you are not hungry. Research has shown that eating breakfast provides health advantages such as improved blood sugar control and better appetite control. It may also decrease the tendency to overeat later in the day.

For the specific habit of eating pastries, doughnuts, breakfast sandwiches, and other foods in your car while commuting to or from work, an effective tool is to plan ahead. Prepare fast, nutritious breakfasts and snacks the night before. Schedule this preparation time as a weekend errand. Buy fresh fruits, whole grain breads, jams or jellies, fat-free yogurt, and fat-free cheese, and put breakfast-size portions in the refrigerator. Ideally you will get up ten minutes earlier and eat these breakfasts at home. Or, you can continue to rush and grab a bag of nutritious car food on your way out the door. In either case, you will be less likely to eat the doughnuts and may well find that your energy level is higher and lasts longer. Be as consistent as possible when working to form a new habit; the more consistent you are, the more quickly the habit will be adopted. I recommend making a firm commitment to whatever plan you lay out for yourself; be strict with yourself and don't allow excuses to get in the way.

Step 2. Understand Different Eating Approaches

Now that you are familiar with the common reasons for problematic eating, it is time to turn your attention to some basic behavioral concepts that may help you understand the ways people, including yourself, approach their eating. Here we will explore the concepts of restraint, self-efficacy, and explanatory style. Try to decide which concepts may be most important to you and build the suggested actions into your Personal Plan whenever possible.

RESTRAINT

Your level of restraint in eating is graded on a continuum. It is not that you are either restrained or not restrained; instead, it's a question of how much and what consequence your level of restraint brings. We all have our own habitual levels of restraint that we must learn to deal with. Simply defined, restraint is the degree to which a person consciously controls his or her food intake.

Luisa and Clara are sisters with different levels of restraint. Both Luisa and Clara weigh about 180 pounds and are about 5 feet, 6 inches tall, but this is where the similarity ends. Luisa has been concerned about her weight since early adolescence and has been on numerous diets. She has had some successes but inevitably regains the weight she loses within a year or two. She tries to be careful about what she eats, has learned a lot about good nutrition, and has adopted a low-fat, high-fiber diet—sometimes. She often skips breakfast and eats very little for lunch because she is trying to watch her weight. She reads food labels and often refuses foods with a high fat content. Such vigilance drains her, however, and she has an unfortunate tendency to lose control of her eating in the evenings and on weekends. When this happens, she is often truly hungry because of the high degree of restraint she has exercised earlier in the day.

Clara does not understand how her sister can eat this way. Clara has never tried to control her urge to eat. It's not that she purposely eats to excess, but she always responds to her desire to eat. She has always eaten what she likes, when she likes, and in the quantity she desires, without giving much thought to the consequences—that is, until recently, when she developed some medical problems and was strongly advised by her physician to lose weight.

If you haven't guessed by now, Luisa exemplifies high-restraint eating and Clara, low-restraint. A fascinating experiment was done with high- and low-restraint eaters that illustrates the paradoxical consequence of high restraint. Subjects in a study were offered as much ice cream as they wanted under three separate conditions. First, they were told to eat all the ice cream they desired in one sitting. Second, the subjects were instructed to eat one scoop of ice cream (a "preload"), after which they were offered as much ice cream as they desired. Third, they were told to eat a preload of two scoops of ice cream, then were offered as much additional ice cream as they desired.

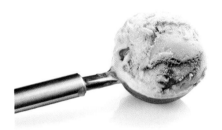

The results? The low-restraint eaters, as expected, ate much more ice cream under the no-preload condition than the high-restraint eaters. After the one-scoop preload, however, the high-restraint eaters ate *more* ice cream than the low-restraint eaters, who felt more full after the preload ice cream and so ate less.

After the double-scoop preload, the high restrainers ate slightly *more* than they had eaten after the single-scoop preload, and the low-restraint subjects ate even less.

How can we explain this? The low-restraint eaters were responding appropriately to fullness cues, while the high-restraint eaters suppressed the urge to eat under the no-preload condition. But when required to eat a preload, the high-restraint eaters

---

BOX 5-16

Eating Behavior Questionnaire: Restraint Scale

Directions: Circle the numbered answer that most closely matches your behavior.

	Never	Seldom	Sometimes	Often	Very Often
1 When you have put on weight, do you eat less than you usually do?	1	2	3	4	5
2 Do you try to eat less at mealtimes than you would like to eat?	1	2	3	4	5
3 How often do you refuse food or drink offered to you because you are concerned about your weight?	1	2	3	4	5
4 Do you watch exactly what you eat?	1	2	3	4	5
5 Do you deliberately eat foods that are not fattening?	1	2	3	4	5
6 When you have eaten too much, do you subsequently eat less to avoid becoming heavier?	1	2	3	4	5
7 Do you deliberately eat less to avoid becoming heavier?	1	2	3	4	5

experienced "release of restraint" and ate more than the group that doesn't control their intake at all. This is the same phenomenon that many people experience when they stray from a restrictive diet. Once they stray, they figure, "Well, I blew it, so I might as well eat the rest of this cheesecake." Clearly, this response is unhelpful. The lesson here is that when it comes to restraint, *moderation is the key.*

How can this understanding of restraint help you achieve a good balance? First, look at the pattern of your own eating. Is it closer to Luisa's or to Clara's? The Restraint Scale (below) can help you answer this question. If you are a restrained eater like Luisa, In addition to having a physiological effect on hunger, you may need to loosen your restraint a bit (we will discuss how later in this chapter). If you are an unrestrained eater like Clara, you may want to impose some restraints on the situations or habits that have contributed to weight gain. Recognize also that few people

	Never	Seldom	Sometimes	Often	Very Often
8 How often do you try not to eat between meals because you are watching your weight?	1	2	3	4	5
9 How often in the evenings do you try not to eat because you are watching your weight?	1	2	3	4	5
10 Do you take your weight into account in deciding what to eat?	1	2	3	4	5

Interpretation: Add the total to get your score, and use the following information to interpret the meaning of your score. For this scale, the average adult who is not overweight scores 18 (men) and 24 (women). A score of 30 is usual for overweight women. If you scored higher than 35, this suggests that you exercise a high degree of restraint over your eating.

SOURCE: *Adapted from T. Van Strien, J. E. R. Frijters, G. P. A. Bergers, and P. B. Defares, "The Dutch Eating Behavior Questionnaire (DEBQ) for Assessment of Restrained, Emotional, and External Eating Behavior," International Journal of Eating Disorders 5 (1986): 304. Nederlandse Vragenlijst voor Eetgedrag (NVE). Copyright 1986 by Swets and Zeitlinger, B.V., Lisse. Reprinted by permission of John Wiley & Sons, Inc.*

are pure Luisa or pure Clara. There may be times when you are highly restrained and other times when you exercise no restraint. Probably the most useful way to use your understanding of restraint is to analyze each situation that comes up with restraint in mind. Then consciously decide how much restraint is appropriate.

As with most behaviors, though, our restraint (or lack of it) is recognized most readily in retrospect. What was your immediate response to the question of whether your eating patterns are most like Luisa's (restrained) or like Clara's (unrestrained)? If you feel that you are overly restrained, it is time to look at the pattern of your daily food intake. Do you eat mostly in the evening, or do you spread out your meals evenly? If you tend to consume most of your calories later in the day, eating a bigger breakfast or lunch or enjoying a midmorning or midafternoon snack may be useful. Most people's energy needs are highest during the early and middle portions of the day anyway, so that's when your body can make best use of the energy produced by food. If you make this switch to less restraint earlier in the day, you will be less likely to overeat late in the day or evening.

The highly restrained eater is also likely to pass up favorite foods entirely, leading to feelings of deprivation later and loss of control. Try using tasty substitutes for favorite foods (for example, substitute a moderate-sized portion of fat-free and sugar-free frozen yogurt for premium chocolate ice cream), or use small portions of favorite foods. This can help prevent problems late in the day. Of course, if you know that you are someone who would be very dissatisfied with one of the substitute foods suggested, another approach that works better for some people is to choose something healthy like a large salad as your main meal and allow a small portion of a favorite food (such as macaroni and cheese) on the side. If you take this approach, just be aware of which foods you will not be able to handle as a side portion ("trigger foods"). The key is to satisfy the craving with a small portion but not to keep going and eat more and more.

The unrestrained eater, on the other hand, may benefit from a period of self-monitoring, or keeping a food diary (see chapter 6 for information about this tool). Learning about portion sizes and how to control portions (also in chapter 6) is also useful for this person. The idea is to achieve a moderate level of restraint for both the unrestrained and the highly restrained eater. This means exercising restraint every time you eat but being aware of your physical and emotional needs.

EXPLANATORY STYLE AND SELF-ESTEEM

Another important influence on your eating behaviors is your explanatory style. Recognizing that few people are all one way or all the other way, we can still find it useful for our discussion to divide people into two general categories of explanatory style.

The first type of person tends to explain life in terms of external, hard-to-influence forces. They answer the question "Why haven't I been able to lose weight?" with statements like, "Because the world conspires against me (the stresses of my life, my unsupportive family, my job and the long hours)," or "My metabolism must be off, because I can just smell a piece of cake and gain weight," or "I just can't exercise because I don't have the time, and besides, no one has explained to me what kind of exercise to do," or "I just can't resist things that taste good, even if I'm not hungry." Psychologists call this explanatory style "external locus of control," or "external" for short. It means the tendency to explain problems in terms of forces, places, or people that are largely outside your personal control.

The second style, as you may have guessed, explains life in terms of internal, controllable forces. For such individuals, the same question, "Why haven't I been able to lose weight?" produces this kind of answer: "Because I have not stuck with what I intended to do. The stresses of my life do not make it any easier, but I need to see if I can reduce them, or work around them. If my metabolism is slow, I should find out whether this can be offset by eating differently or exercising more."

While few people exclusively use one or the other explanatory style, you probably have a sense of how you usually respond to problems. To see how you rate when it comes to responding to external eating cues, complete the external eating questionnaire below. There are pros and cons to each kind of response. Certainly, if there is a problem you truly can do nothing about, it is not helpful to approach it as something you believe you should be able to fix. An example of this might be a coworker who dislikes you because of your religion or race. While you may need to coexist with this person, believing that you can change your coworker's opinion by behaving a certain way, or that you are somehow responsible for their opinion, is probably less desirable than simply saying, "It's not my fault; he's just prejudiced and insecure."

On the other hand, if the problem is that you haven't been able to lose weight, the external style is probably not going to result in long-term behavior change. The external explanatory style allows you to make excuses for your current situation, and for not trying to change. The internal explanatory style is best for successful weight loss, because it puts the responsibility squarely within you—you are the person who can make this work.

The only potential drawback to an internal explanatory style in weight management is the tendency to be too hard on yourself when things do not go perfectly. Those who employ the internal explanatory style may blame themselves for everything and view anything less than unqualified success as a kind of failure. This belief is all the more damaging because of the notion that it is due to a personal failing—a lack of strength, perhaps. While it is probably best not to blame the outside world when weight loss doesn't proceed according to your Personal Plan, it is also best to keep the problem in perspective and not blame yourself entirely. That is, accept responsibility for small and large deviations from your plan, but don't dwell on them or attribute them to giant failings in your character. For example, it is useful to accept that your actions at the party resulted in an estimated 1,000-calorie deviation from your plan and erased three days of stellar adherence; it is not useful to conclude that you are a bad person who is not capable of change.

If you tend toward the external explanatory style, it can be helpful to start examining your thinking and see whether you can reframe your approach a bit, at least as it applies to weight loss. For example, if you find yourself thinking that a food problem is outside your control, or that you cannot change a particular eating behavior,

Eating Behavior Questionnaire: External Scale

Directions: Circle the numbered answer that most closely matches your behavior.

	Never	Seldom	Sometimes	Often	Very Often
1 If food tastes good to you, do you eat more than usual?	1	2	3	4	5
2 If food smells and looks good, do you eat more than usual?	1	2	3	4	5
3 If you see or smell something delicious, do you have a desire to eat it?	1	2	3	4	5
4 If you have something delicious to eat, do you eat it right away?	1	2	3	4	5
5 If you walk past the bakery, do you have the desire to buy something delicious?	1	2	3	4	5
6 If you walk past a snack bar or a café, do you have the desire to buy something delicious?	1	2	3	4	5
7 If you see others eating, do you have the desire to eat?	1	2	3	4	5

ask yourself whether this is really so. Perhaps you just need to develop a new strategy for dealing with it. This book is full of strategies and tools that address specific problem areas such as portion control or distracting yourself when you are tempted to eat out of stress or boredom. If you pick and choose the most relevant ones for your situation, your Personal Plan of Action will help you prove to yourself that you are in control, and that it is usually not necessary to blame others.

SELF-EFFICACY AND SELF-ESTEEM

Self-efficacy is the belief that you can make specific changes in your life. Weight management self-efficacy, then, is the belief that you can manage your weight effectively. Self-esteem is a broader, less well-defined concept concerning your estimation

	Never	Seldom	Sometimes	Often	Very Often
8 Can you resist eating delicious foods?	1	2	3	4	5
9 Do you eat more than usual when you see others eating?	1	2	3	4	5
10 When preparing a meal, are you inclined to eat something?	1	2	3	4	5

Interpretation: Add the total to get your score, and use the following information to interpret the meaning of your score. For this scale, the average adult who is not overweight scores 26 (men) and 27 (women). If you scored higher than 35, this suggests that you respond more than most people to external eating cues.

SOURCE: *Adapted from T. Van Strien, J. E. R. Frijters, G. P. A. Bergers, and P. B. Defares, "The Dutch Eating Behavior Questionnaire (DEBQ) for Assessment of Restrained, Emotional, and External Eating Behavior," International Journal of Eating Disorders 5 (1986): 304. Nederlandse Vragenlijst voor Eetgedrag (NVE). Copyright 1986 by Swets and Zeitlinger, B.V., Lisse. Reprinted by permission of John Wiley & Sons, Inc.*

of your own worth as a person. Many people confuse these concepts, but it's very useful to maintain the distinction between them. While the level of self-efficacy is usually similar to the level of self-esteem, this is not always the case. A person can have low self-efficacy and high self-esteem, or vice versa, and any gradation in between. This means that even a person who has high self-esteem may believe that losing weight is beyond his or her control. Or, a person can have generally low self-esteem but still believe that controlling weight is within his or her power.

We find that many people with weight problems suffer from low self-esteem and low self-efficacy, but we are not sure why this is so. It is clear that society's prejudices contribute to the low self-esteem of many people with obesity. But it is probably not true that low self-esteem *causes* weight problems (aside from the relationship between low self-esteem, depression, and eating for comfort). Low weight management self-efficacy, on the other hand, in an individual who is genetically or environmentally susceptible to excessive weight gain will make it far more difficult for that person to control his or her weight. Even if your self-esteem is high, you may have learned through experience that you are generally unsuccessful at maintaining a stable, healthy weight. This contributes to even lower self-efficacy in a continuous downward spiral.

While the evidence is scant, it also makes sense that continued lack of success in weight control may adversely affect your general level of self-esteem. Obviously, both of these consequences are undesirable. Lack of weight management self-efficacy and low self-esteem jeopardize the outcome of a weight control plan in a phenomenon called a "self-fulfilling prophecy." In other words, if you don't believe that you can be successful, you won't be. And, if you are initially successful despite a lack of belief in your own abilities, the success may be jeopardized by negative thinking such as: "It can't be true. I'm going to mess it up somehow." When the first signs of relapse occur, they may be greeted almost with relief, because relapse is the expected outcome for the person burdened with low self-efficacy or low self-esteem.

If your self-efficacy with regard to weight control is low, is there anything you can do to improve it? Yes. You can change your mindset. If you develop a belief in your ability to achieve and maintain a healthy weight, and combine that belief with the proper tools, your chances of success will be vastly improved.

How can you adopt a more positive mindset? First, do things that require no change in mindset but will establish the conditions for success. These include recognizing appropriate motivators and having a coherent plan. Thus, the first step in improving your level of self-efficacy with regard to successful weight management is to finish reading this book and, in the process, develop your Personal Plan of Action.

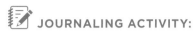

Build upon Past Success

Next, you must begin to pay attention to your successes, no matter how small. Let's assume for the moment that your weight management self-efficacy is about as low as it can be. You may be having sabotaging thoughts and telling yourself things like: "This is too hard. I keep messing up. Maybe I just can't lose weight." Even at this minimal level of confidence, there is always some positive experience to build on in the path to successful weight management. Think back over the past decade or two: Was there any time when you achieved a modicum of success at maintaining a stable, healthy weight, even if it was very brief? If so, you have proved that you can do it. Formulate a healthy response that you can keep repeating to yourself, such as "I am striving for progress, not perfection. When I make mistakes, I will learn from them. I have made important changes and seen some results. I just need to stick to it."

What were you doing correctly at that time? How is it that you were able to do it then? Can you reinstitute at least one of the conditions that enabled you to be successful in the past? Perhaps you were more physically active, or your stress was under better control, or you believed in your ability more at that time. A change of mindset can often be achieved by recalling past successes and applying some of the same attitudes to the present.

Even when there is no past success to build on, there are examples of desirable behaviors that serve the same purpose. For example, if you have a craving for a specific food (chocolate cake) or tend to eat to excess under a specific condition (for example, your mother's telephone calls upset you), can you think of the last time you did *not* eat the entire chocolate cake, or did not eat but instead got out of the house to clear your mind? You almost certainly can think of such an occasion.

What you'll find is that there are times when you *are* able to stop eating chocolate cake before you are stuffed or do something other than eat in response to emotional stress. Your job now is to recognize and accept this ability, to analyze what you did *right* and build on it.

Over the next ten times the temptation or stress occurs, perhaps you can aim for the modest goal of behaving in a successful

BOX 5-18

Take a moment now to write down the specifics of the occasion below or in your journal:

_____
_____
_____
_____
_____
_____

way one time out of ten. As you know, if you can do it one of the ten times, you can surely do it two out of ten times. Pay attention to what you do right, mimic it, and improve on it. Pretty soon you will have yourself believing that you can do it right three or four or even nine out of ten times. Even if you do only slightly better than you used to, this is important—you must recognize that it is important and give yourself credit. Your weight may not change significantly from small changes in mindset, but building on effective, successful behaviors is very important for maintaining a new, lower weight.

The third phase in improving your mindset about weight management is to learn how to talk to yourself. A key ingredient for success is learning to be your own best booster. Some people are already good at this, but many people, unfortunately, have learned instead to be their own harshest critic. The causes of this maladaptive attitude are various. They include excessively high personal expectations, negative childhood experiences, and self-protection. The causes really don't matter as much as the fact that such an attitude doesn't get people very far toward their goals in life. The old concept of a self-fulfilling prophecy comes into play when we are overly self-critical and predict our own failure.

The best way to change how you talk to yourself is to just do it. Remarkable as it may seem, just saying positive things to yourself will help silence the critical voice within. Learn to give yourself a break, and you will lift a great burden from your shoulders. You may even improve your self-efficacy, self-esteem, and weight control.

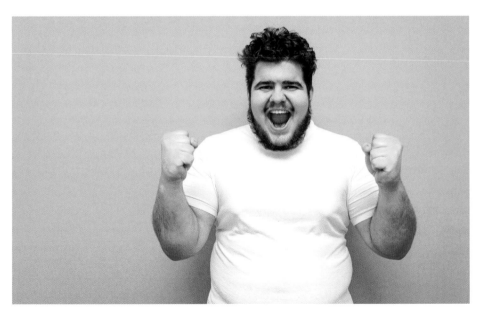

Be a cheerleader for yourself

Step 3. Spot Binge Eating Disorders

Now we will visit with Zahra. Zahra is very conscious of her weight. She was never very overweight, but she comes from a family where being thin was important. She gained weight after her daughter was born and she quit her job as an office clerk. She is a very restrained eater and rarely eats much around other people. Several times a week, however, she binges. These binges are not the same as what we have previously described as simple overeating. What Zahra does is eat, in a couple of hours, much more food than normal, while alone at home. She feels as if she cannot stop eating and then feels guilty or sad afterward. She is very afraid, both of the binges and of gaining more weight. She is currently 190 pounds and stands 5'5" tall. Zahra came in for help in losing weight. As part of her assessment, she was given a binge eating questionnaire. If you see some aspects of yourself in Zahra, complete the questionnaire below.

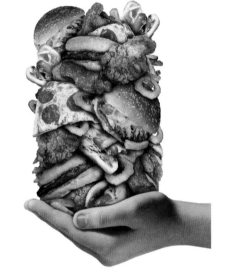

In brief, binge eating disorder is defined by having two or more episodes per week of binge eating: a distinct episode of excessive, rapid food consumption, in private, that you are unable to stop, accompanied or followed by a negative emotional state like sadness, anger, or guilt. If you feel you may meet these criteria for binge eating disorder, you are not alone. Studies of overweight women who see a doctor for treatment, for example, suggest that up to 30% meet the criteria for a diagnosis of this eating disorder. Men commonly experience binge eating disorder as well.

If you think you might have binge eating disorder, you need to seek professional help from a mental health professional or physician skilled in the treatment of eating disorders. While it is beyond the scope of this book to detail the techniques used in treatment, successful treatment does exist. Some of the techniques used by experts include stimulus control, cognitive and interpersonal therapy, and sometimes medications. While the Personal Plan you are building will be helpful to you, you will only succeed if you also seek the in-person opinion of an expert about this particular problem.

If binge eating disorder is accompanied by purging (via self-induced vomiting, laxative or water pill misuse, or excessive exercising), it is called bulimia nervosa. If your BMI is normal and you are unhappy with your weight, or have an intense fear of gaining weight, causing you to restrict your calorie intake to lose more weight, you could have a condition called anorexia nervosa. Binge eating, bulimia nervosa, and anorexia nervosa can seriously affect your health. You need to seek help, and we urge you to do so.

BOX 5-19

Binge Scale Questionnaire

Binge eating is defined as the rapid consumption of a large quantity of food (more than most would consider normal), usually within less than two hours. Often a person who binges feels out of control, fearing that he or she will not be able to stop eating. Once the binge ends, that person often feels guilty and depressed.

1 How often do you binge eat?
 a Seldom
 b Once or twice a month
 c Once a week
 d Almost every day

2 What is the average length of an eating episode?
 a Less than 15 minutes
 b 15 minutes to an hour
 c 1 to 4 hours
 d More than 4 hours

3 Which of the following statements best applies to your binge eating?
 a I eat until I have had enough to satisfy me.
 b I eat until my stomach feels full.
 c I eat until my stomach is painfully full.
 d I eat until I can't eat anymore.

4 Do you ever vomit after a binge?
 a Never
 b Sometimes
 c Usually
 d Always

5 Which of the following statements best applies to your eating behavior when binge eating?
 a I eat more slowly than usual.
 b I eat about the same way as I usually do.
 c I eat very rapidly.

6 How much are you concerned about your binge eating?
 a Not bothered at all
 b Bothers me a little
 c Moderately concerned
 d A major concern

7 Which of the following statements best describes your feelings during a binge?
 a I feel that I could control the eating if I chose.
 b I feel that I have at least some control.
 c I feel completely out of control.

8 Which of the following statements describes your feelings after a binge?
 a I feel fairly neutral, not too concerned.
 b I am moderately upset.
 c I hate myself.

9 Which of the following phrases most accurately describes your feelings after a binge?

a Not depressed at all
b Mildly depressed
c Moderately depressed
d Very depressed

Scoring: The questionnaire helps distinguish people who meet criteria for binge eating from people who do not, even if they occasionally binge eat. While an expert is required to make a diagnosis, you should be aware that you may have an eating disorder if you answered the above questions in the following manner:

1 C or D

2 B, C, or D

3 C or D

4 B, C, or D may indicate bulimia nervosa (see below)

5 usually C

6 C or D

7 B or C

8 B or C

9 B, C, or D

SOURCE: *R. C. Hawkins and P. Clement, "Development and Construct Validation of a Self-Report Measure of Binge Eating Tendencies,"* Addictive Behaviors 5 (1980): 219-226. Reprinted by permission of Elsevier Science Ltd., Oxford, England.

Step 4. Identify Depression

Now you will assess yourself for a condition that can affect your perception of the world and your life, as well as your ability to develop and adhere to a Personal Plan: depression. As mentioned earlier in the chapter, depression is common among people with weight problems or eating disorders, regardless of whether it predates or follows weight gain. The symptoms and signs of depression include some things you might expect, such as crying spontaneously, along with others that you might not, such as change in appetite and waking up early in the morning.

Depression Questionnaire

During the past two weeks, how often have you been bothered by any of the following problems?	Not at all	Several days	More than half the days	Nearly every day
1 Little interest or pleasure in doing things	0	1	2	3
2 Feeling down, depressed, or hopeless	0	1	2	3
3 Trouble falling or staying asleep, or sleeping too much	0	1	2	3
4 Feeling tired or having little energy	0	1	2	3
5 Poor appetite or overeating	0	1	2	3
6 Feeling bad about yourself—or that you are a failure or have let yourself or your family down	0	1	2	3
7 Trouble concentrating on things, such as reading the newspaper or watching television	0	1	2	3
8 Moving or speaking so slowly that other people have noticed? Or the opposite—being so fidgety or restless that you have been moving around a lot more than usual?	0	1	2	3

The Patient Health Questionnaire (PHQ) is the most commonly used screening tool in primary care to help determine whether someone is suffering from depression, and to what degree. It is currently the most validated and reliable depression tool, and it is recommended by the US Preventive Services Task Force to help primary care providers diagnose depression more effectively. Circle your honest response to each of the following questions, even if you do not think you are depressed. Depression is treatable, and it is a shame to suffer needlessly. Depression is the most common psychiatric problem in the United States, and many instances go undiagnosed for years.

During the past two weeks, how often have you been bothered by any of the following problems?	Not at all	Several days	More than half the days	Nearly every day
9 Thoughts that you would be better off dead or of hurting yourself in some way	0	1	2	3

Directions: Circle the number for each statement which best describes how often you felt or behaved this way during the past two weeks.

Scoring: Add the numbers for each item you circled to get the total number of points.

Total Score: _____

Interpretation:

Total score 0–4: Minimal depression, may not need depression treatment

Total score 5–9: Mild depression

Total score 10–14: Moderate depression

Total score 15–19: Moderately severe depression

Total score 20–27: Severe depression

While scoring lower than 5 is not a guarantee that you are not depressed, you are much less likely to suffer from clinical depression than if you score well above 5. If you scored higher than 5, you may have some degree of depression, and you should seek help from a qualified professional—a psychologist or a psychiatrist or another physician. Among the treatments available for depression are various medications and psychotherapy.

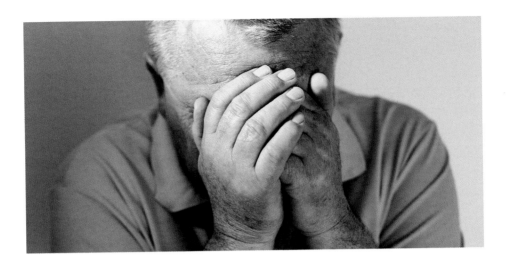

As discussed previously, other mental health conditions, such as anxiety, post-traumatic stress disorder (PTSD), ADHD, bipolar disorder, and so forth, can also have a huge impact on your ability to manage your weight. If you feel like your mood is interfering with your day to day life (e.g., causing problems at home, work, school, etc.), or affecting your ability to manage your weight, it is worth discussing your concerns with your doctor or a mental health professional. Again, these conditions are very common, and addressing them can significantly improve your quality of life and make it a lot easier to lose weight as well.

Step 5. Observe Yourself

Now that you are familiar with a wide variety of concepts important to changing eating-related behavior, it is worthwhile to engage in a period of careful self-observation. Self-observation (also called self-monitoring) is a good way to make yourself more aware of your current habits so you can focus your efforts in designing and carrying out your Personal Plan. As an added benefit, this period of self-observation will help you develop the habit of monitoring your behavior, both during the action phase of your Personal Plan and during the relapse-prevention phase (the rest of your life). It has been shown in research studies that successful long-term weight management is more likely among people who self-monitor than among those who do not.

How do you monitor your eating behavior? There are two aspects to the process: monitoring what you eat and monitoring the circumstances of your eating. Chapter 6 will help you monitor what you eat, covering the basic nutritional information you need to become an educated "consumer." Monitoring the circumstances of your eating is your task for the next three days. The Three-Day Eating Record (also in chapter 6) will help you do this.

Here's an example of a completed record for one day:

The idea is to eat in your usual manner. Do not try to eat "well" for the purposes of this exercise. Ideally, you will gain a better sense of the situations, time of day when you eat, and things that cause you to eat. You will also see the time pattern of your eating. As discussed previously, there are specific ways to change your eating habits for each situation if necessary.

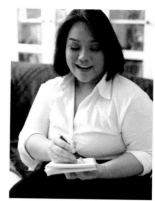

What should you do with these monitoring forms? This depends on what you are most interested in monitoring. Once you have gained a better understanding of where your problem areas are, it is wise to focus on monitoring just one or two types of problem situations at a time. For example, you may decide to focus your monitoring on how you respond to stress at work, or how you deal with boredom. If so, your monitoring would focus on the times of day these are problems. You could keep track of exactly what you eat at those times and how well and often you substitute other activities for the inappropriate eating cues you are monitoring.

If you have a mathematical bent, you can even track frequencies of different behaviors. What percentage of stressful events leads you to overeat? Are you showing ongoing improvement? Are there new substitute behaviors you have thought of that can be added to your repertoire? By becoming a student of your own behavior, you will have the best chance of making permanent changes in your eating pattern and lifestyle. As you will see in the diet and exercise chapters that follow, monitoring can be used to gain control in these areas as well.

BOX 5-21

Day/Time	Type of Meal/Snack	Where Eaten	Circumstances
Monday			
8:30 a.m.	**Breakfast:** coffee	Kitchen	Rushed
8:50 a.m.	**Snack:** doughnut	Car	Passed store, looked good
Noon	**Lunch:** diet soda, candy bar	Cafeteria	Not hungry—no time, stressed
5:30 p.m.	**Snack:** leftovers	Out of refrigerator	Very hungry
6:00 p.m.	**Dinner:** pizza	Den, in front of TV	Tired, didn't want to cook

THE WATCH TRICK

Let's say you have learned, either from past experience or from this period of self-monitoring, that you need to stop eating when you are under stress at work but are not physically hungry. Eating is a habit that can briefly relieve stress and provide pleasure. Unfortunately, the relief is fleeting—and worse, it does nothing to address the source of the stress. In fact, it adds another stress in the form of a weight problem. How do you go about changing such a pattern of eating?

One of the greatest obstacles to stopping a habit like this is lack of awareness of the behavior while it is occurring. In other words, people say that they often don't realize they are eating as a stress reliever until it is too late—the snack has already been consumed. If there was a way to recognize the situation while there is still a chance to do something else instead of eating, the task of changing this and similar habits (such as eating out of boredom or eating as a reward) would be much easier. We suggest a unique technique that may work for you. It's called the "watch trick" and serves as a tap on the shoulder to help you recognize inappropriate eating and choose how you are going to respond.

Here's how to use it. If you are like many people, you wear a watch. (If not, buy or borrow one.) The beauty of a watch is that you tend to look at it periodically. In fact, you are likely to look at it at exactly those times when you are about to eat in response to inappropriate cues.

For example, you are bored. What time is it? How much longer until the show starts on television? Or, you are under stress at work—there's time pressure and an undesirable task to be done. Do I have to do it yet, or should I grab a snack first? What time is it?

Now we need a signal, a tap on the shoulder. Your watch is slightly annoying to you every time you lift your arm because *it is on upside down!* The 12 is on the bottom; the 6 is on the top. This is a gentle reminder to watch, not so much what you eat but why you eat and whether your eating is being driven by bodily needs or by one of those inappropriate eating cues like stress or boredom. It is a reminder to be mindful of what is going on for you physically and emotionally in that moment.

Once alerted by the watch to the fact that you are considering eating, you can step back a moment and analyze the situation. First, are you physically hungry? If so, you are well justified in eating and should eat something. With your new awareness of your body's signals, you can eat without guilt because you will be eating appropriately, in response to your body's stated needs.

On the other hand, if you see your upside-down watch and remember that you recently ate or are not physically hungry, you are now aware that there is something else driving your urge to eat. Often you will be able to figure out what it is, or at least put it into one of the major categories of eating cues or "triggers" described in Step 1 of the self-assessment in this chapter. If you can figure out what is causing you to want to eat when you are not hungry, you can now choose what to do about it.

If you typically use a cell phone to tell the time and don't have a watch, an upside-down Fitbit is a good alternative. Or you can wear something you are used to having on but wearing it in an unexpected way (say a bracelet on the opposite arm) or even keeping a rubber band on your wrist (to remind you like an upside-down watch would).

 JOURNALING ACTIVITY: **Stress**

The most appropriate response in most cases is to address the issue head-on. Stress? What can you do to address the source? Even writing down in your journal, "I am stressed because of X" is a more effective stress reliever than temporarily avoiding the issue by eating. Better still, write down a plan to deal with the source of the stress. Boredom? As discussed, pick something to do from your lists of alternative activities. Do the same if you are using food as a reward.

With this tap on the shoulder, you have a choice. You can choose to go ahead and eat when you are not hungry, with all the lasting consequences it brings you (and such fleeting benefits). Or, you can recognize that you don't *need* to eat at this moment and do something else. Urges to eat tend to last for only 10 or 15 minutes, so if you distract yourself briefly, the urge will usually pass.

Remember, you do not have to be perfect in your adherence to the plan described previously. For example, if only half the times you were about to eat in response to an inappropriate cue you caught it in advance and responded appropriately, you will have a very important advantage in weight maintenance, now and after you have completed the action phase of your Personal Plan. This is because the difference between gaining weight and maintaining a stable weight is usually only 100 calories or less per day. Consistently cutting out an unneeded cookie or two a day is the difference between weight gain and stable weight.

One other factor is worth emphasizing. In some ways, it gets easier to avoid inappropriate eating the more experienced you become at monitoring yourself, using either the "watch trick" or other means such as keeping food records. This is because appropriate eating and appropriate responses to stress, boredom, and the like are learned habits. Respond appropriately to a stressful situation a few times in a row instead of eating, and you will find that this is a far more satisfying response than eating. You will find that you are in much better control, not only of your eating but of your stress as well. This is a reward that eating cannot provide, and this reward will make it increasingly easy to respond appropriately.

Put Your Assessments to Work

You have now performed a thorough self-assessment of your eating-related behaviors, and you have learned a few techniques to address triggers for overeating. If you have completed the assessments faithfully and honestly, you have learned some things about your eating habits that will help you lose weight and, more importantly, keep it off for the long haul.

Your Personal Plan of Action can include a collection of miscellaneous behavioral tools that can help you gain control of your eating. Not all of them will work

---

BOX 5-22

Behavioral Change Tools

1 Use smaller plates for meals. They hold less and look fuller with less food.

2 Serve yourself a reasonable portion of food for each meal and forbid seconds. Help yourself stick to this by cleaning up the kitchen and putting away serving dishes before you start eating. Serving dishes left out on the table, counter, or stove are a source of temptation.

3 If you are still hungry after a reasonably sized meal, have a noncaloric cold or hot drink or a piece of fruit or sugar-free gum. Get busy at once doing something unrelated to food. If you are still hungry later, have another noncaloric drink, stick of gum, or piece of fruit.

4 Slow down your eating pace to allow the satiety signal to get through. Chew your food completely (this also aids digestion). Put down your eating utensil between each bite of the meal.

5 Limit where you eat to one room of your home—preferably the kitchen or dining room.

6 Do not allow eating in front of the television. Do not do other things while eating. Concentrate on the eating.

7 Enjoy much smaller but more frequent servings of the foods you like. A sliver of chocolate cake, consumed slowly and in small bites, savoring it as it melts in your mouth, will give you better "value" for your calories.

8 Buy only single serving sizes, not economy sizes, of foods that you have trouble controlling your intake of.

9 Brush your teeth immediately after eating. This may inhibit you from snacking soon after the meal (particularly dinner).

for everyone all of the time, but all of them can be helpful in the right setting. Pick a few that make sense to you.

Eventually, you will integrate the behavior change aspects of your Personal Plan with the diet and exercise aspects. To do this, it is vital that you recognize that behavior change is the essence of changing your eating habits and becoming more physically fit. If you temporarily restrict your diet and engage in lots of exercise in order to lose weight but do not make permanent changes in the kinds of food you eat, portion sizes, and the amount of physical activity you get, the weight loss will be only temporary. In order to maintain weight loss, you need to make permanent changes in three areas of your lifestyle: behavior, nutrition, and activity level.

As you read the next chapter, keep in mind that your aim is to make behavior changes you can stick with, without deprivation, for the rest of your life.

Action Items

- If you haven't already, complete the following questionnaires that were included within this chapter:
  - Eating Behavior Questionnaire: Emotional Eating Scale
  - Sleep Questionnaire
  - Eating Behavior Questionnaire: Restraint Scale
  - Eating Behavior Questionnaire: External Scale
  - Binge Scale Questionnaire
  - Depression Screening Tool: The Patient Health Questionnaire (PHQ)

- Review your assessments for depression, binge eating disorder, and other mental health concerns, and seek help if there is a problem.

- Weight loss journal
  - Come up with a list of flexible responses to use when faced with inappropriate eating cues. Brainstorm a list of activities to do inside and outside your home.
  - Take some time to recall any past successes you have had at avoiding temptations or managing your weight. Recall the conditions of those successes and your mindset at the time. Consider how you can apply those attitudes to your current weight loss efforts.
  - Select and write down a few behavioral tools that can help you gain control of your eating.

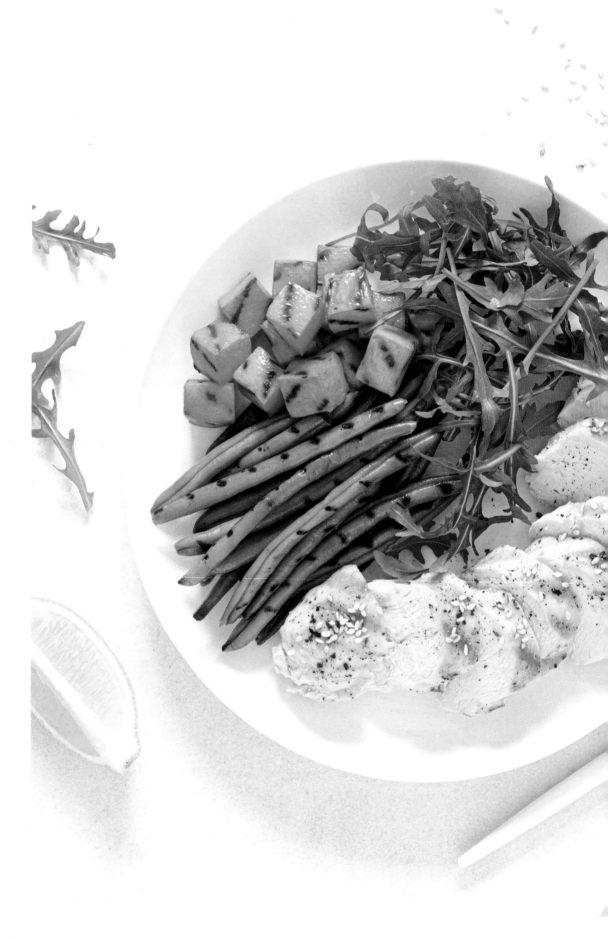

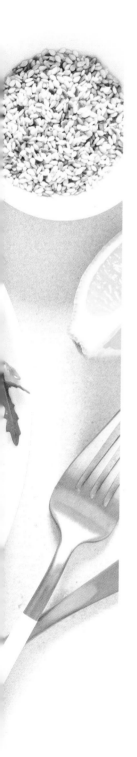

CHAPTER 6

Designing Your Dietary Plan

IN THIS CHAPTER, WE WILL:

- **show** how modern American food culture promotes weight gain,
- **identify how to spot** a fad diet,
- **describe** the qualities of a healthful diet,
- **review the major** food groups as defined by the United States Department of Agriculture (USDA),
- **discuss** portion size information as defined by the USDA,
- **review which foods** should be consumed liberally and which should be limited,
- **offer strategies** for identifying healthy portion sizes,
- **identify how savoring** small portions of rich foods can provide the same level of satisfaction as large ones,
- **conduct a daily** energy audit to help you determine your caloric needs,
- **review samples** of healthy daily food choices for a variety of daily calorie goals,
- **conduct a three-day** dietary evaluation, and
- **provide strategies** for changing your daily food choices to match your energy needs and weight loss goals.

THE UNITED STATES IS CURRENTLY IN A STATE of calorie overload. Our greatest food imbalance is excess dietary energy—too many calories. The human body has an intense, built-in, biological drive to consume everything available, to "store up" in anticipation of a time when resources aren't plentiful. In the days when food was scarce, that drive was an important asset for survival. But many people now live in an environment where energy-rich food is abundant and easily accessible. The problem of hunger for many Americans has been replaced with the problem of never being hungry.

Over the past 100 years, as the science of nutrition has developed, so has the food industry's ability to produce and market great quantities of highly palatable, highly caloric, and highly convenient foods. These foods are created through the addition of fat, sugar, salt, and the processes of refinement, preservation, and packaging. "Ultra-processed" foods are marketed to those of us who want tasty, but simple, grab-and-go food choices to accommodate our ever-busier lifestyles. As these convenience foods became increasingly available, consumer demand has continued to grow. We are now often at a point where we expect, and are accustomed to having, nearly any type of food we choose immediately at our fingertips. While we are prone to nutrition shortages, many Americans are not faced with the same sort of food shortages of the old days and have become conditioned, often since childhood, to prefer the highly craveable taste of these processed foods.

Eating More, Getting Less

Not only is plenty of tempting food *available*, but plenty of it is also routinely *offered* to us. The past three decades have seen a gradual shift toward larger portions, larger single-serve packaging, and greater availability of food. We widely accept the practice of eating just about anywhere. There are cupholders on lawn mowers, fast food in airports and malls, and vending machines in the library. These are just some of the influences in our environment that lead us to consume additional, and usually unnecessary, calories throughout the day.

FIGURE 6-1

Nutrition facts label

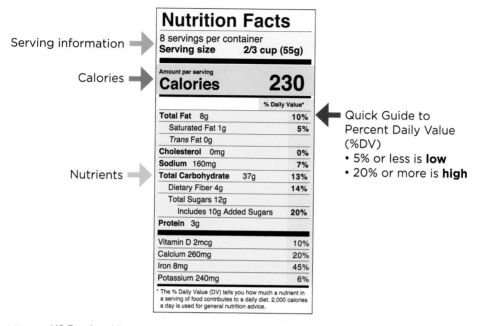

Serving information →

Calories →

Nutrients →

Nutrition Facts

8 servings per container
Serving size   2/3 cup (55g)

Amount per serving
Calories   230

	% Daily Value*
Total Fat 8g	10%
Saturated Fat 1g	5%
Trans Fat 0g	
Cholesterol 0mg	0%
Sodium 160mg	7%
Total Carbohydrate 37g	13%
Dietary Fiber 4g	14%
Total Sugars 12g	
Includes 10g Added Sugars	20%
Protein 3g	
Vitamin D 2mcg	10%
Calcium 260mg	20%
Iron 8mg	45%
Potassium 240mg	6%

* The % Daily Value (DV) tells you how much a nutrient in a serving of food contributes to a daily diet. 2,000 calories a day is used for general nutrition advice.

← Quick Guide to
Percent Daily Value
(%DV)
• 5% or less is **low**
• 20% or more is **high**

SOURCE: US Food and Drug Administration

While the number of calories we consume is on the rise, the quality of our nutritional intake is on the decline. For example, many women routinely consume less than the recommended dietary allowance for calcium, iron, vitamins A and C, and fiber, and yet many of those same women appear *over*nourished because of excess caloric intake and the resulting excess body fat. Eating too many calories also tends to result in taking in more sodium, sugar, alcohol, cholesterol, and saturated fat than is healthy. So, while many people have plenty available to them, they are not all choosing nourishing foods. Even as the availability of things to eat has increased, many neighborhoods are considered food deserts, since fresh fruits, vegetables, and other nonprocessed foods are scarce or entirely absent. This is especially true when the only local "market" is a convenience or corner store.

As a result of living in an environment where large quantities of food are ever-present, we have the opportunity to eat far too many calories while many of those calories are not accompanied by the critical nutrients we need and are too high in others. This is why our food climate is frequently called "obesogenic," meaning that our current environment is one that, for many people, contributes to obesity and makes weight loss challenging.

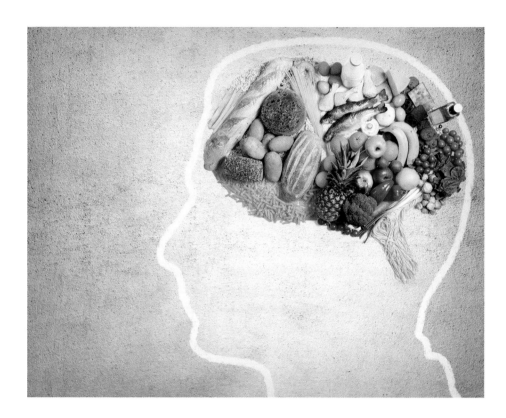

The average American today consumes twice as many meals prepared by a restaurant or outside of the home compared to 30 years ago; simultaneously, these meals and snacks have grown both in size and calorie content. For many families, the sit-down restaurant meal is no longer a once-in-a-while celebratory treat, but an everyday convenience. Quasi-restaurants (not fast food but not a formal restaurant) like Panera, Chipotle, and Starbucks go completely unrecognized as a potential source of excess calories because they are not the typical fried-food joint like McDonald's or Wendy's. They may market themselves to be a healthful choice, but often the number of calories is equal to, or can exceed, traditional "fast food."

As our environment has become more obesogenic, figuring out what a healthy diet means is often a source of confusion. Entire industries promoting various trendy diets and weight loss supplements have only added to the challenge of figuring out what to eat and when. We receive mixed messages throughout the day: eat at these restaurants and make these unhealthful food choices, but lose weight with these diets and magic pills.

However, note that gaining excess weight occurs over time, and so does the adoption of healthful eating patterns and subsequent weight loss to achieve a healthy body weight. Let's take a look at fad diets, "good" diets, and recommendations for beginning your lifestyle changes to achieve a healthy weight. Then, in the chapters to follow, we will present you with information about food groups, nutrition basics, and how to incorporate your dietary lifestyle changes into your Personal Plan.

FAD DIETS

Fad diets over the years have led to a multi-billion-dollar-a-year weight loss industry. Just like the fashion fads of big hair and shoulder pads, fad diets might look good at the time, but they just don't last. While they may provide motivation to get started losing weight, fad diets often lead to burnout because they don't lead to the desired effect, or it becomes too hard to eat that way for long periods of time.

It's likely that you've tried a diet or two (or more) throughout your life so far. Over the years, we've seen many fad diets come and go, and our patients often feel stranded in a sea of overwhelming information of questionable validity. Fad diets are masterful at appearing scientific and credible by using terminology and medical jargon, and they are written in such a way to convince you that *this* is the

---

BOX 6-1

Fad Diets

Learn to spot a fad diet with these red flags:

- **Blames a single nutrient** or food group for weight gain (such as carbohydrates, gluten, fat, dairy)

- **Promotes a single food** or restricts foods (for example, the Keto diet, the "cabbage soup diet," Slim Fast meal replacements, juice cleanses)

- **Does not mention** potential risks

- **"Guarantees" weight loss** in an unrealistic time period ("10 pounds in 1 week")

- **Makes promises of "easy"** weight loss or that fat will "melt off"

- **Promotes a very low-calorie** consumption (for example, less than 1,000 per day or the recommended daily intake for age and gender)

- **Requires purchase** of special products or monthly subscription

- **Claims to alter genetics** or metabolism

- **No plan for weight maintenance** after losing weight

answer you have been waiting for all along. However, it is clear as we look back on diets like the "blood type diet," the "cabbage soup diet," and numerous "detox" diets that their claims are usually just that: claims.

WHAT'S A "GOOD" DIET?

So, what's a "good" diet? The truth is, there is no one magic answer. A healthy approach to weight loss must combine several key components: nutrition and food choices that provide both nutrient adequacy and calorie deficit while at the same time being "livable" or "sustainable" in your daily lifestyle. That combination will look different for different people.

Our experience has shown that developing a *sustainable weight loss lifestyle* will require making food choices that fit your lifestyle, as well as making small, gradual changes that promote healthful, low-calorie food choices.

For instance, Jasmine was used to eating take-out dinners three to five times a week because she was too busy to shop and cook. We suggested she practice measuring portions and tracking her intake (noticing the calorie contribution of her usual take-out foods). She realized that multiple take-out meals were contributing more calories than she could afford in a given week. It became more important to her *not to eliminate* all take-out meals for the sake of weight loss but *to practice carefully choosing smaller servings of lower-calorie items* when she does do take-out. Over time, she gradually reduced the number of take-out meals she regularly relied on.

This gradual but intentional lifestyle change takes practice and time. We would not expect you to pick up a musical instrument the first time and be able to play Beethoven's Concerto No. 5, nor do we expect you to make perfect choices every day and have immediate weight loss success. So, say goodbye to fad diets, and let's start developing the skills you will need to improve your current lifestyle.

How often do you eat at restaurants or away from home? Take a moment to add up the number of times you went out to eat this past week (including for snacks and drinks, like lattes, soft drinks, or alcohol). Are there times you could pack a lunch or make a "to-go" snack for yourself from home this week instead? Small decisions like this will add up throughout the week and cut down on excess calories.

The most current "good" dietary recommendations are the USDA's Primary Dietary Guidelines, which reflect federal nutrition policy distilled from a wealth of scientific information. These guidelines promote greater intake of some nutrients and discourage overconsumption of others. They also indicate the importance of shifting gradually away from our obesogenic tendencies as well as incorporating personal/cultural food preferences.

Though simply stated, these directives form a complete picture of self-managed, lifelong eating for good health. To expand on them somewhat, the USDA offers key recommendations to provide further guidance on how people can follow the five guidelines.

By following these guidelines, the person who is at a reasonable weight can maintain that weight and increase his or her chances of avoiding many illnesses. For someone whose calorie imbalance has resulted in obesity, these guidelines can also easily incorporate a plan for reducing weight as well.

It is never too early or too late to start making healthier choices. It is also never too hard. It may require more searching, especially if you don't live near a

The Guidelines

1 **Follow a healthy eating pattern across the life span.** All food and beverage choices matter. Choose a healthy eating pattern at an appropriate calorie level to help achieve and maintain a healthy body weight, support nutrient adequacy, and reduce the risk of chronic disease.

2 **Focus on variety, nutrient density, and amount.** To meet nutrient needs within calorie limits, choose a variety of nutrient-dense foods across and within all food groups in recommended amounts.

3 **Limit calories from added sugars and saturated fats and reduce sodium intake.** Consume an eating pattern low in added sugars, saturated fats, and sodium. Cut back on foods and beverages higher in these components to amounts that fit within healthy eating patterns.

4 **Shift to healthier food and beverages choices.** Choose nutrient-dense foods and beverages across and within all food groups in place of less healthy choices. Consider cultural and personal preferences to make these shifts easier to accomplish and maintain.

5 **Support healthy eating patterns for all.** Everyone has a role in helping to create and support healthy eating patterns in multiple settings nationwide, from home to school to work to communities.

SOURCE: *page xii of https://www.dietaryguidelines.gov/sites/default/files/2019-05/2015-2020_Dietary_Guidelines.pdf*

Key Recommendations

Consume a healthy eating pattern that accounts for all foods and beverages within an appropriate calorie level.

A healthy eating pattern includes:

- **a variety of vegetables** from all of the subgroups—dark green, red, and orange; legumes (beans and peas); starchy; and other;

- **fruits,** especially whole fruits;

- **grains,** at least half of which are whole grains;

- **fat-free or low-fat dairy,** including milk, yogurt, cheese, or fortified soy beverages;

- **a variety of protein foods,** including seafood, lean meats and poultry eggs, legumes (beans and peas), and nuts, seeds, and soy products; and

- **oils.**

A healthy eating pattern limits:

- **saturated fats and trans fats,** added sugars, and sodium.

Key recommendations that are quantitative are provided for several components of the diet that should be limited. These components are of particular public health concern in the United States, and the specified limits can help individuals achieve healthy eating patterns within calorie limits:

- **consume less than 10%** of calories per day from added sugars;

- **consume less than 10%** of calories per day from saturated fats;

- **consume less than 2,300 milligrams** (mg) per day of sodium; and

- **if alcohol is consumed,** it should be consumed in moderation—up to one drink per day for women and up to two drinks per day for men—and only by adults of legal drinking age.

In tandem with the recommendations above, Americans of all ages—children, adolescents, adults, and older adults—should meet the Physical Activity Guidelines for Americans to help promote health and reduce the risk of chronic disease. Americans should aim to achieve and maintain a healthy body weight. The relationship between diet and physical activity contributes to calorie balance and managing body weight. As such, the Dietary Guidelines includes a Key Recommendation to:

- **meet the** *Physical Activity Guidelines for Americans.*

SOURCE: *page 15 of https://www.dietaryguidelines.gov/sites/default/files/2019-05/2015-2020_Dietary_ Guidelines.pdf.*

well-stocked indoor market or outdoor farmer's market, but healthy foods surround us just as the unhealthy ones do. It is true that it requires more planning and preparation time to consume foods in their healthiest state (unprocessed, most nutrient-dense forms). Many of us have become so accustomed to ready-made meals that we have budgeted little time to plan, shop, and prepare healthy meals and snacks. The choice to eat healthfully revolves around whether you are willing to *spend the time* it takes to care for your body by fueling it with the calories and nutrients it needs. It also means a mindset shift for many people. Meal planning and preparation need not be considered a chore. Many people find that shopping for fresh ingredients, especially if you have access to locally grown items, can be a source of fun and exercise. Trying out new, healthy recipes can also be a fun challenge and even a time for relaxation.

USDA Dietary Guidelines

However, we understand that big lifestyle changes don't happen overnight. The USDA guidelines specifically recommend a more *gradual* transition. It is important to begin with small, reasonable, achievable tweaks to one's routine. In making small gradual changes, most people find more success on a daily basis without feeling like they have to "give up everything that tastes good" for the martyrdom of weight loss. In this fashion, many people can be far more successful in not just their daily food choices but also in the long-term commitment to adhering to a healthy eating pattern than those who try more drastic "crash dieting" techniques.

The USDA has organized foods into groups according to the major nutrients each food provides. These groups are: grains, fruit, vegetables, protein, and dairy. Throughout the rest of this chapter, we'll first discuss carbohydrates and then look at the five major food groups more closely. As you read, consider how you can incorporate dietary changes into your Personal Plan of Action.

A NOTE ABOUT CARBOHYDRATES

Carbohydrates, or "carbs," have gotten a bad rap lately. Strenuously avoiding carbs has become the predominant trend in many popular diets (such as Keto or Atkins), replacing even fat as the bogeyman for many weight-conscious people. Are all carbs to be avoided? Can you eat carbs and maintain a healthy weight? The answers to these questions are no and yes, respectively. However, you need to make thoughtful choices about the carbs you include in your diet. Let's cut through the hype and explore carbs in more detail.

Carbohydrates can be found in foods across all five of the USDA's five food groups. Yes, even the protein group. Carbohydrates come in all shapes and sizes and have different effects on our health. *Carbohydrate* gets its name from its chemical composition, which is carbon plus hydrogen and oxygen (H_2O), or carbo-hydrate. This food group is essential for our brain and body functions, but not all carbohydrates ("carbs" from here on out) are created equal. Carbs are divided into starches and fiber (complex carbs), and sugars (simple carbs). Though we need all of them to survive and function, we need to use them wisely and knowledgeably.

Starch

Starchy foods include some vegetables (such as potatoes, corn, and squash), legumes (beans and peas), and grains (both whole and refined). With the exception of refined grains, these are all considered complex (or "good") carbs because they are unprocessed, take energy to digest, provide essential nutrients and vitamins, and tend to be higher in fiber and lower in sugar content. Whole grains (such as oats, items made from whole wheat flour, and brown rice) are complex carbs because they contain fiber, vitamins, minerals, and starch. Refined grains (such as pastas and breads made with white flour) contain just starch and thus are nutritionally poor.

Sugar

Sugars include honey, maple syrup, white and brown sugars, milk sugars (lactose), and fruit sugars (fructose). Sugars are absorbed directly into the bloodstream. They elevate blood sugar quickly, and an excess is associated with insulin insensitivity, or diabetes. Sugars should be limited.

Fiber

Fiber passes through your body without being digested. Consuming fiber will therefore provide a sense of fullness without adding calories. It can also lower your blood sugar and cholesterol. High-fiber foods include legumes, vegetables and fruit, nuts, and whole grains.

TABLE 6-1

Types of carbs

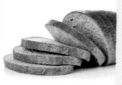 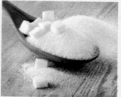 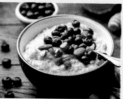

Type of Carb	Starches	Sugar	Fiber
Examples	• Starchy veggies like corn, pota- toes, and winter squash • Beans, peas, and lentils • Grain foods	• Fruit sugar (fructose) • Milk sugar (lactose) • White, brown, and powdered sugar • Corn syrup • Maple syrup • Honey • Molasses	• Beans, peas, and lentils • Veggies and fruits—especially ones that have skin or seeds that you eat • Nuts, such as pea- nuts, walnuts, and almonds • Whole grain foods
Health Tip	Choose whole grains: Whole grains contain fiber, vitamins, minerals, and starch. Refined grains contain just starch.	Limit sugars: Of the three types of carbs, sugars cause the biggest jump in your blood sugar.	Get enough fiber: Fiber passes through your body without being digested, so it fills you up without adding calories. It can also lower your blood sugar and cholesterol.

SOURCE: *https://www.cdc.gov/diabetes/prevention/pdf/t2/participant-module-22_more_about_ carbs.pdf, pp. 3–5.*

BOX 6-3

Daily Fiber

Try to get 25 to 30 grams of fiber each day. Check the nutrition facts label to see how much fiber an item contains. Many of us don't get enough fiber. If you need to boost your fiber intake, increase it slowly, over time. And drink plenty of water. This will help prevent an upset stomach. It's best to get your fiber from food, instead of from a supplement. That's because food has many nutrients besides fiber, such as vitamins and minerals.

As you can see, not all carbs are created equal, and many foods with carbs are an important part of a healthy diet. However, refined grains and sugars should be limited. Many processed "convenience" foods are mostly these "bad" carbs since they offer little to no nutritional benefit.

In general, the average American eats far more carbohydrates every day than the body needs to function well. Our usual carbohydrate intake comes from a disproportionately large amount of refined grains and added sugars rather than from nutritionally rich whole grains, fruits, vegetables, and dairy products. In light of reducing total calorie intake for the prevention of weight gain or to encourage weight loss, it is safe to say that nearly everyone could benefit from reducing their carbohydrate intake from the unhealthy sources.

The question then becomes "How low do I go?" First, let's look at a few food items so you can gauge how many carbs you might be eating in a day.

If you had oatmeal, orange juice, milk, a granola bar, an apple, a cup of rice, and some zucchini over the course of a day, it would total 152 grams of carbs. (It's easy to look up carbohydrate content of foods using any free fitness or food tracking mobile app, like MyFitnessPal.)

As a short-term weight loss technique, many popular diets encourage a carb intake of less than 50 grams per day. This will usually result in

BOX 6-4

Carb Counts for Common Foods

1 cup of oatmeal = 30 grams

1 cup of 1% milk = 13 grams

1 cup of orange juice = 26 grams

1 granola bar = 18 grams

1 apple = 20 grams

1 baked potato = 25 grams

1 cup of white rice = 36 grams

1 zucchini = 9 grams

a fairly efficient weight loss. However, an eating pattern that significantly restricts grains, fruits, some vegetables, and most dairy is usually hard to adhere to for a long time. It is also possible to create specific nutrient deficiencies by lack of intake from these important food groups. As a long-term lifestyle, a more moderate carb restriction is usually easier to adhere to, and an eating pattern that includes several servings per day from the "healthy carb" group will also be more nutrient dense.

Dr. Cheskin's patients have been very successful when they have employed a moderate carb restriction (90–100 grams per day) for the purpose of intensive weight loss, followed by a gradual and conservative increase in healthy carbs (in accordance with the person's individual weight maintenance needs).

GRAINS

Breads, cereals, rice, tortillas, and pasta, among other food items, provide energy in the form of complex carbohydrates and are good sources of B vitamins, minerals, and fiber. Using Choose My Plate as a guide, these carbohydrates typically fall into the "Grain" group.

As we noted in our discussion on carbs, the grain group contains both *whole grains* and *refined grains*. When choosing grain products, look for "whole grain flour" listed as the first or second ingredient on the food label. Good sources of

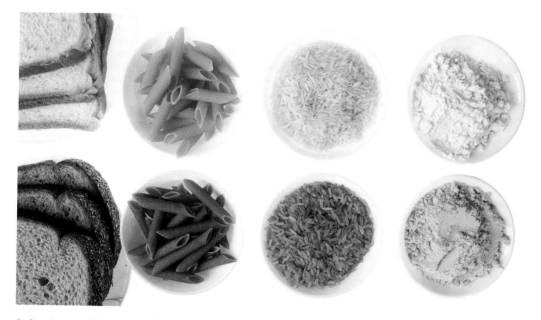

Refined grains (shown in the top row) generally have a lighter appearance than whole grains (shown in the bottom row)

What Is a Whole Grain?

Most grain products are first processed by grinding the grain kernel into a flour. When the entire edible part of the grain kernel is used, all nutrients within the grain are incorporated into the final product. We call this a whole grain product. Therefore, you receive all the B vitamins, which include thiamin, riboflavin, niacin, and vitamin B6, as well as fiber, and other minerals including iron, magnesium, and zinc. The current US food supply, however, heavily favors refined grain products. Refined grains are made from flour that has been milled into a finer, smoother consistency, resulting in a sweeter flavor. Many of the important nutrients in the initial whole grain, however, are lost in the milling process. You may recognize "enriched" refined grain products, which is an attempt to add back in the lost nutrients, but this process is generally incomplete.

whole grains include wheat, corn (including popcorn), brown/wild/red rice, barley, buckwheat, bulger, oats, millet, rye, quinoa, teff, and farro. At least half of your daily grains should come from *whole* grain sources.

FRUIT

Fruits contribute vitamin C, vitamin A, potassium, folate, and fiber to the diet. They are also relatively low in calories and provide energy from both their simple and complex naturally occurring carbs. Fruits are low in fats and added sugars but are bulky with water and fiber. They are all derived from plants.

It is best to eat fruit in its original form, with its skin or seeds, to get the fiber content that is necessary for healthy digestion. Limit fruits that have been canned or frozen in syrups, which contain added sugars. Fruit juices, even those without added sugars, should also be limited because most are void of their natural fiber content.

VEGETABLES

Vegetables are generally low in calories, provide energy mostly from complex carbs, and are good sources of vitamin A, vitamin C, vitamin K, folate, magnesium, iron, potassium, and fiber. Vegetables cover a wide spectrum of foods, from the usual suspects—potatoes, carrots, broccoli, and celery—to legumes (black beans, garbanzo

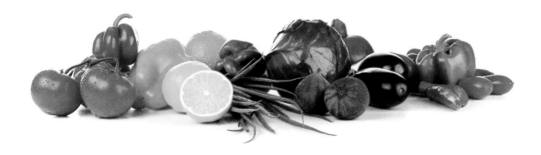

beans, lentils, and soy products like tofu), hominy, artichokes, asparagus, cucumbers, eggplant, mushrooms, okra, and zucchini.

Like the fruit group, vegetables are nutrient dense and should be eaten in their original form as much as possible—with skins and seeds if possible, and baked or grilled instead of fried. Use caution when sautéing vegetables in fats or oils, which can add excessive calories to an otherwise low-calorie food group. Limit canned or jarred vegetables in oils and with added sugars, like baked beans, coleslaw, potato salad, and marinated artichoke hearts.

PROTEIN

The protein group is traditionally derived mostly from animal sources and includes foods such as poultry, fish, beef, pork, eggs, milk, and cheese. However, alternative protein sources are becoming more widely available and include beans, nuts, seeds, quinoa, soy, and even vegetables and grains.

In addition to protein, all of these foods include high levels of iron, zinc, and vitamins D and B-12. However, higher-fat options (beef, pork, whole milk) should be treated with caution as they can contribute high levels of artery-clogging saturated fat and dietary cholesterol. Therefore, selections from these groups should be

BOX 6-6

High-Volume Foods

The same way we can look at nutrient density, we can also consider "energy density." When losing or maintaining weight, the goal is to eat the largest amount or volume of food for the fewest number of calories. Fruits and vegetables are great examples of foods with low energy density; they provide fewer calories with more volume, as opposed to foods with high energy density with lots of calories even in small quantities (for example, french fries). By increasing the volume of your eating, you can make healthy food choices, eat fewer calories, and feel fuller while slowly losing weight. High-volume foods like fruits and vegetables often contain high proportions of water and fiber, both of which contribute to the overall feeling of fullness. These foods are associated with increased satiety, visual satisfaction, textures, and overall meal satisfaction.

limited in order to limit saturated fat intake. In the case of milk, fat-free or reduced fat selections are now readily available.

Thus, plant-based protein sources such as legumes, soy, nuts, and seeds can provide high quality protein at a lower cost, with the added benefit of being cheaper and more environmentally sustainable. The types of fat contained in some of these products tends to be more polyunsaturated and monounsaturated and are not associated with elevated total cholesterol and LDL cholesterol.

Whether he or she selects animal-based or plant-based proteins, a person must take care not to take in more protein than is needed. Protein, especially from animal sources, can be a costly source of calories. In general, using a 2,000-calorie limit, between 50 and 175 grams of protein (10% to 35% of one's total calories) is acceptable. Based on kilograms of body weight, the average adult should eat 0.8 grams of protein (slightly more for athletes and the elderly).

Most Americans get plenty of protein in their daily diets. During intensive weight loss, a slightly elevated protein intake is known to sustain lean muscle mass, as well as to provide noticeable satiety after each meal, resulting in less hunger throughout the day. However, beyond this phase, there's no benefit to overdoing it. Excess protein can provide excess calories, as well as overburden the liver and kidneys. Overdoing it may also contribute to the development of osteoporosis, because excess protein intake makes the body excrete too much calcium in the urine.

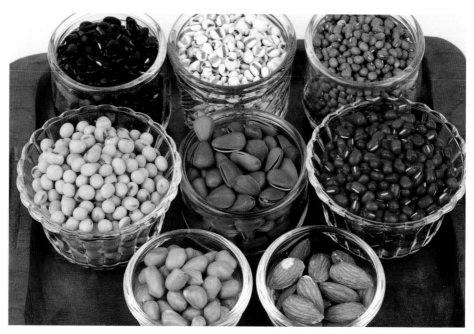

Plant-based protein sources include legumes, soy, nuts, and seeds

When choosing protein sources that align with your personal and cultural preferences, it is best to eat a combination of different protein sources because each contains different essential amino acids, which are required for muscle growth, repairing body tissues, digestion, and cellular health. Legumes (beans and lentils) lack the amino acids methionine and tryptophan, but they can be paired with a grain that contains these two. Together, the balance of different protein sources covers all nine essential amino acids.

Beware of higher-fat sources of protein: marbled meat, peanut butter, poultry skin, ribs, sausage, bacon, hot dogs, and bologna. As we begin to use the USDA's food groups to create a weight loss plan that is right for you, we will encourage use of only the leanest protein sources.

DAIRY

The dairy group (milks, yogurts, and cheeses) provides high levels of protein, iron, zinc, and calcium as well as vitamins D and B-12. But within this group, the higher-fat options also contribute high levels of fat, including artery-clogging saturated fat and dietary cholesterol. Lower-fat and fat-free versions of nearly all dairy

BOX 6-8

Protein Supplements: Do You Need Them?

A protein powder might be helpful for increasing the protein content of a single meal (like a smoothie with fruit, kale, and almond milk, which is rather high in carbs, low in protein, and may leave you hungry long before lunchtime). But protein powders are not usually the cheapest way to increase your protein intake. Go for lean sources of protein-based foods like lean beef, poultry, fish, egg, tofu, light cheeses, low-fat Greek yogurt, and cottage and ricotta cheese. Combine brown rice with black beans or oatmeal and low-fat milk of your choice for a plant-based source of all the amino acids you need.

products are readily available, as well as lactose-free milk for those with lactose intolerance, and these options still provide all the important nutrients. It is worth noting, though, that commonly used dairy substitutes such as almond milk, rice milk, and coconut milk, while providing a white-colored liquid suitable for a bowl of cereal or coffee whitener, do not contain the same levels of protein, calcium, and other nutrients provided by cow's milk.

FATS AND OILS

The fats and oils category is technically not considered a food group by the USDA. However, these ingredients are included in many standard food prep techniques and contribute such a large number of (often hidden) calories to our daily intake that we cannot go without recognizing them.

Fat is found in both animal (for example, ribeye) and plant substances (for instance, avocados). Every kind of fat, including olive oil, butter, beef, lard, coconut oil, and corn oil, whether liquid or solid, has about 9 calories per gram. Carbs only have 4 calories per gram. This means a lot of fat calories can fit in a small package. A five-inch baked potato might have 200 calories, but a much smaller

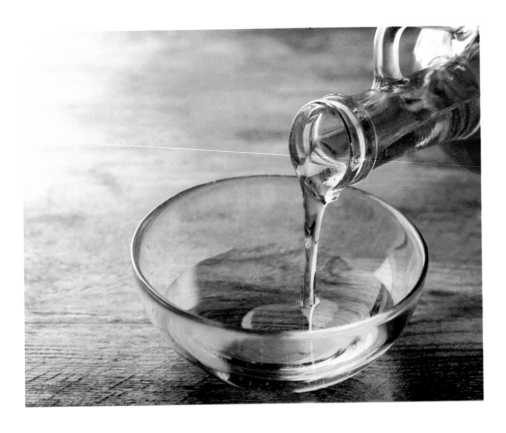

tablespoon of margarine to go on top could have the same amount, and every single calorie from margarine comes from the fat content (that is, calories from fat).

Think about two glasses of milk, each 8 ounces: one whole milk (3%) and one skim milk (0%). The whole milk contains 8 grams of fat and has 146 calories, but the skim milk is nearly fat-free with only 90 calories. The amount of milk is the same in each glass, but the removal of fat from the whole milk cuts the calories significantly when compared with the skim milk.

Many food components contribute flavor to our foods, including salt, sugar, acids, herbs, and spices, but the addition of fat in combination with these components is especially appealing to most of us. Fats often have flavors of their own, which tend to carry through or boost other flavors. Fats also impart desirable textures to foods such as tenderness in baked products, crispiness in fried foods, moistness or juiciness in meats, and smoothness in candies and frozen desserts. Fatty foods are the most likely to be overeaten, often beyond the point of fullness, and can make you want to eat even when you're not hungry. Think about how many times your stomach has growled when you smelled sizzling bacon, or how often you eat a rich dessert even when you "don't have room for it." Many foods that are high in fat content, particularly those that are combined with sugar or salt, or both, are often eaten for fun or comfort rather than for fuel or nutrient density.

High-fat foods are not just tempting to our senses. Recent evidence indicates that high-fat meals seem to be less filling than high-carbohydrate meals. In other words, we don't feel as full during or right after a high-fat meal as we do when the meal is high in carbs or protein, or we may feel equally full despite a large difference in total calories. This combination of sensory appeal and delayed or reduced fullness can result in eating too many calories without realizing it. For some people, eating a high-fat, high-calorie meal doesn't suppress the amount of food they consume at the next meal. Since automatic adjustments in food consumption may not occur during the high-fat meal itself, and the high-fat meal may not be compensated for later, total calories for the day will often be higher than needed.

When too many calories are eaten but the calories come from carbs rather than fat, the body tends to burn off some or all of the extra calories through a slight increase in metabolism. Conversely, extra calories from fat do not promote an increase in metabolism and are quickly and efficiently stored as body fat; 97 calories of an extra 100 calories consumed as fat *will* be stored. When extra calories come from both carbs and fat, most of the carbohydrate calories are used first, either right away or sometime later, between meals, because they are easily removed from temporary storage in the liver, and because we may be inefficient at converting them into fat. However, extra fat is automatically transported into semipermanent fat storage and is only burned during prolonged physical exertion or after carbohydrate stores are depleted—in other words, when you go on a calorie-deficient diet.

High-fat foods trigger consumption of too many calories and promote weight gain for these four reasons:

1   One gram of fat provides more than twice as many calories as an equal amount of protein or carbohydrate (one gram of fat contains 9 calories, while the same amount of protein and carbohydrate each contains 4 calories).

2   Fat adds an appealing flavor and texture to food, which makes us want to eat more of it. We are evolutionarily designed to like fat because it helped us survive in times of famine.

3   The more fat there is in a meal, the less likely we are to balance daily caloric intake with daily caloric needs.

4   When excess calories are eaten, carbs are burned first, while fat is efficiently stored (another survival tactic), particularly when you are inactive.

In summary, fat contributes to weight gain because it tastes so good that we tend to eat more than we need. It has more than twice as many calories per unit weight as other food sources, and our bodies prefer to store fat rather than to burn it, particularly when we are inactive or excess calories are present—or both.

By switching to a lower-fat way of eating, we can eat just as much as, and sometimes a little more than, we usually do and avoid progressive weight gain. For most people, lowering overall fat intake automatically promotes the selection of more healthful foods. For some people, the result is a substantial decrease in total calories and, thus, weight loss. Using fat-budgeting (which means limiting fat calories to between 15% and 25% of total caloric intake) along with a high-nutrient, portion-controlled food plan and physical activity, helps most people achieve gradual but significant weight loss with minimum deprivation.

When weight loss is a goal, total daily calorie intake is always part of the picture. Fats (no matter what the source) are simply very calorie dense. High-fat foods are also commonly foods we think of as "ingredients" (like the olive oil we use to sauté veggies) or part of the way we prepare other foods (such as spreading cream cheese on a bagel, topping a burrito with sour cream and guacamole, or adding cream to coffee). As a result, our total intake of high-calorie fats can go unrecognized throughout the day. Even though we may be choosing all the right kinds of fats, the calorie contribution is still a concern. So, take it easy—fat calories add up fast.

A WORD ABOUT SATURATED FATS

We recommend you begin replacing saturated fats with monounsaturated and polyunsaturated fats. But what is saturated fat, exactly? Any fat that becomes solid at room temperature is typically considered saturated fat. The more saturated, the more solid. Saturated fats include butter, coconut oil, beef fat, shortening, palm oil, pork fat, and chicken fat. Alternately, unsaturated fats (that is, monounsaturated and polyunsaturated fats) are typically liquid at room temperature. Unsaturated fats include avocado oil, olive oil, some fish oils, canola oil, peanut oil, and other vegetable oils.

The USDA recommends that no more than 6% of our total calories should come from saturated fats because they are linked to increases in total cholesterol and "bad" LDL (low density lipoprotein) cholesterol levels, so when choosing between cooking oils or food products, stick to unsaturated fats like avocados, nuts, and olive oil. You can also practice quick fixes to reduce the amount of saturated fat in your diet by taking off the skin of chicken, cutting out the fat on pork and beef products, and choosing lean meats. Take a moment to review your eating habits and ask yourself: Are there saturated fats I can replace or modify?

SALT

Sodium is an element of sodium chloride, commonly known as salt. Sodium has important functions in the body. People can easily consume adequate amounts of salt just by choosing the recommended types of foods from the major groups, and they can easily overdo the salt in an unhealthy way by adding it to foods either in cooking, using high-sodium ingredients, seasonings, and sauces, or consuming a lot of processed foods, which tend to be high in salt. To avoid consuming too

---

BOX 6-9

Calories in Common Fat Sources

2 tablespoons cream in your coffee = 100 calories

2 tablespoons cream cheese on your bagel = 100 calories

15 almonds = 100 calories

1 tablespoon mayo on a sandwich = 100 calories

2 tablespoons regular salad dressing = 120 calories

2 slices of bacon on your salad = 100 calories

1 tablespoon olive oil for sautéing = 120 calories

much salt, temper your temptation to season with salt from the shaker, and avoid eating (or at least limit) the following foods, which contain excess sodium:

- cured and pickled foods;
- highly processed and salted snacks;
- canned vegetables and soups;
- instant flavoring packages, especially included in "meal kits";
- cheeses;
- soy sauce; and
- condiments.

You also may wish to consider buying low-salt or no-salt versions of many of your favorite condiments.

For people who retain excess amounts of water or who have high blood pressure, it is especially important to control sodium intake. It's important to keep in mind, too, that while it is easy to consume too much sodium, sodium *does not* contribute energy or calories to the diet and does not cause a person to gain fat weight. Controlling sodium intake may help you control how much water you retain (bloating) or help you control high blood pressure (an important enough reason), but it will not help you lose excess body fat. In fact, reducing salt *too much* can interfere with your weight reduction success; if you restrict salt to the point where your food doesn't taste good, that may make it harder for you to stick to a weight reduction food plan. Of course, creative use of other flavorings and spices can make low-salt foods much more appealing. A healthy sodium intake is 1,500 milligrams for most adults and no more than 2,300 milligrams in one day.

"EMPTY" CALORIES

On a daily basis, most of our intake should include the most nutrient-dense food choices in order to maximize nutrient adequacy for a minimum number of calories. However, "empty" calories, though not a food group themselves, are all too often part of our regular diet. Empty caloric foods tend to be higher in fat, higher in sugar, and have few nutrients or no nutrients to offer. In general, ultra-processed foods all fall into this category because they contain highly refined grains or starches like corn starch or potato starch. Alcohol, soda, and candy ("junk food") fall into this category because they provide calories but no nutritional value.

In the USDA's food planning guide, the category of empty calories, while not a food group in itself, refers to the small number of daily calories that an individual can choose to spend on any food at all. These empty calories can be spent on "splurge" foods, higher-fat or higher-sugar selections, or additional servings of nutrient-dense foods. The crucial point is that most of us can only afford a few empty calorie foods, and in moderation. The vast majority of us are already getting far too many (often without even realizing it).

We are often asked about artificial sweeteners—are they good or bad? Most sweeteners are actually perceived to be much sweeter than regular sugar, and we just don't have great evidence one way or another in human research to say what the effects are on the body. Recent studies have suggested there is a link between drinking more than two artificially sweetened drinks per week and an increased risk for stroke and heart disease in women. If you are substituting sugary beverages with artificial sweeteners, it is recommended you limit how long this substitution is used and transition to water or drinks without sugar.

Also, there are plenty of naturally occurring sweeteners that may even provide some nutritional benefit, especially if it comes from a fruit source (like raspberries or oranges). We have seen many patients wean themselves off added sugar and artificial sweeteners, and after some time of abstinence, it is usually difficult for them to go back to high-sugar drinks and foods. So, if you must add an artificial sweetener to your drink during weight loss, it is better to do that than to partake in "empty" added calories of real sugar, but know that no added sugar is really best for your body's insulin and metabolism regulation in the long run.

ALCOHOL

The Centers for Disease Control and Prevention advises no more than seven standard drinks for women per week and 14 for men. A standard drink refers to a 1.5-ounce shot, a 12-ounce beer, or a 5-ounce glass of wine. (Binge drinking is having four or more drinks on a single occasion for women or five or more drinks on a single occasion for men.) However, if you are trying to lose or maintain weight, we recommend limiting your intake even further.

Eliminating or cutting back on alcohol can help you to control overall calories and therefore body weight. Alcoholic beverages contain few, if any, necessary nutrients and many calories—many *empty* calories. Each gram of alcohol has 7 calories. This is more than sugar, at 4 calories per gram, and nearly as much as fat, at 9 calories per gram. Also, in mixed drinks, the beverage combined with the alcohol (such as soda, cream, or fruit juice) often contributes hundreds of extra empty calories, either as carbs or fats. Only in the case of fruit juice are key nutrients contributed.

There's a "one-two punch" that often goes along with the consumption of alcoholic beverages—alcohol is most often consumed in a social setting, where high-calorie snack foods or large meals are readily available. Since alcohol lowers defenses (causing disinhibition—a state of no longer being inhibited or restrained), many people eat more of this food than they would under ordinary circumstances. To complicate matters, it seems that the body may slow down its fat-burning processes when alcohol is present. The body seems to prefer to burn alcohol before fat, perhaps in an effort to rid itself of this toxin. While the body is busy burning the alcohol, it's storing away the fat.

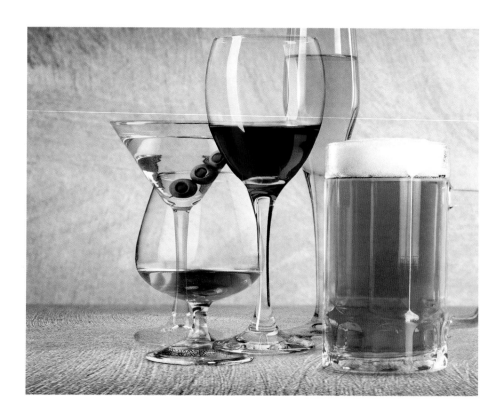

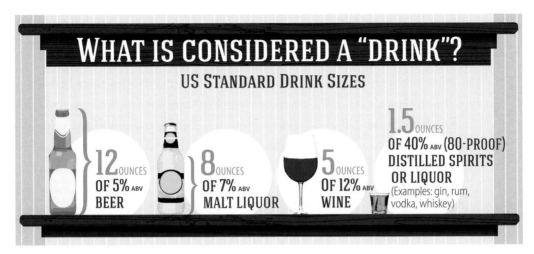

Drinking in moderation (or not at all). **SOURCE:** *https://www.cdc.gov/alcohol/fact-sheets/moderate-drinking.htm*

FLUID NEEDS

Did you know that water is considered the most fundamental essential nutrient? Water makes up 60% of the adult body weight and is a required component of nearly all metabolic functions. It is normal for your fluid status to fluctuate daily, yet it is vital that we continually replenish it. Fluid needs are governed by your

BOX 6-12

But What If I Don't Like Plain H₂O?

- Try sparkling water, Perrier, or seltzer (or dilute by half with tap water if there are too many bubbles)

- Minimize nonnutritive/artificial sweeteners

- Add a lemon, lime, or orange wedge

- Add 1 inch of light cranberry juice or 1 tablespoon of mango nectar, then fill your glass with sparkling water

- Brew herbal tea or green tea (you can brew it hot, add ice, and drink it cold)

- Infuse your H2O with: cucumbers, mint, sliced strawberry, orange wedge, frozen raspberries or pineapple chunks

- Experiment with temperature: hot, cold, or room temperature may make a big difference

- Invest in a water bottle you enjoy drinking from that can help you keep track of intake

sense of thirst, which we commonly mistake for hunger, or overlook entirely. The average adult female requires approximately 9 cups (72 fluid ounces) per day, and the average male needs approximately 13 cups (104 fluid ounces) per day.

Fluid needs can at least partly be met by the fluid contribution of some foods like broth and other beverages, or foods with high water content like cucumbers or fresh fruit. However, in order to meet the standard recommendations, most of us actually need to drink *something* on a regular basis. Our basic physical need for fluid combined with the high-volume effect of fluid on our sense of fullness make daily fluid intake an important component of healthy eating and weight maintenance.

CHOOSE MY PLATE

The Choose My Plate icon (produced by the USDA along with the Department of Health and Human Services) shows how the five major (nutrient-dense) food groups should come together in appropriate proportions to create a template for a typical meal. It is the framework we will use to conduct your daily diet audit.

The order in which the five major groups are positioned on the plate, and their relative position, illustrate dietary *proportionality, variety,* and *moderation*, all of which contribute to overall dietary balance. It is obvious from the large amount of space on the plate dedicated to the vegetables that these foods should figure most prominently in our diets. They serve as the foundation for a healthful way of eating. Grains and fruits compose the next priority. Again, the amount of space dedicated to plant-based foods and healthy carbs means that we should consume lots of the foods in these groups.

FIGURE 6-2

USDA My Plate

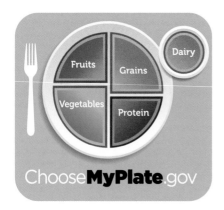

We also see space allocated for smaller amounts of iron-rich and calcium-rich dairy and protein foods. These are foods of both animal and plant origin, such as milk, eggs, meats, poultry, fish, beans, nuts, and seeds. Within these groups, you should aim to consume the leanest, or lowest-fat, selections available.

By choosing from the five major groups, you are most likely to eat a *variety* of foods for basic nutrient adequacy. Using the concept of high-volume eating noted previously, simply by choosing to eat more vegetables, fruits, and grains, you will help increase the likelihood of maintaining or reducing your weight. With some simple modifications and a little practice, most of us can approximate the proportions on the Choose My Plate image when preparing a meal at home. For example, you can eyeball whether the protein on your plate is about the same amount or size as your grain portion.

Foods to Limit or Avoid

Yummy things to eat are simply all around us, every day. From the candy jar on your coworker's desk, to the open bag of chips your kids left out on the counter; from the two bites of potatoes the baby left on her plate, to the grab-and-go snack you saw at the convenience store checkout aisle. It's easy to reach out and pop another bite, taste, snack, or nibble into your mouth. If it isn't part of a meal, or you didn't select it from a food group or even think it through, you might not even have wanted it. But, there it was and . . . pop—in it went. Nonmeal calories add up at an alarming rate and can also go easily unrecognized because we don't ever see them on our plates. Identifying sources of

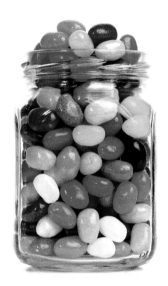

Nutrition Facts: Bites, Licks, and Tastes

Here's an example of how quickly unconscious calories can add up throughout the day:

2 doughnut holes in the break room at work	150
1 handful of nuts because lunch is going to be late	120
5 french fries nibbled from a friend's take-out order	75
4 pieces of crackers and cheese at home before dinner	150
3 bites of mashed potatoes while making family dinner	100
2 bites of leftover chicken while cleaning up dinner	50
2 Oreos before bed	100
Total	745 calories

Tips for Weight Management

View the following as fun challenges that will help you lead a healthier lifestyle:

- Eat no more than one meal per week prepared away from home.

- Drink no more than one 12-ounce soda per day (even that is a lot).

- Cut way back on animal fats and fried and processed foods.

- Fill half your plate with fruits or veggies at every meal.

- Choose whole grains most of the time.

"invisible" calories like these will play an important role in weight loss and keeping weight off long term.

Keep in mind that making healthy food choices for weight loss or maintenance is not just what you *do* eat—it's also what you *do not*. Within the concepts of nutrient density and calorie control, there is not much room for fast food, fried foods, sugary foods, added sugars, sodas, fancy coffee drinks, and the millions of prepared and processed foods that currently make up the bulk of the typical American intake. Although there is nothing wrong with the occasional use of any of these foods, we are simply at a place right now where our population relies so heavily on these calorie-laden choices that anyone who cuts back even just a bit is likely to feel better, have more energy, and even lose weight (or at least stop gaining). Is there any room for birthday cake and pizza? Sure. But not in huge quantities, and not every day.

While the focus of the Choose My Plate icon is on a *meal*, many people overlook the additional contribution of calories consumed *in between* meals. As discussed in chapter 5, snacking in between meals or grazing on food throughout the day can also be important factors to consider when managing your weight. Be aware that eating outside of designated mealtimes, which is often done for reasons other than hunger, can contribute significant unwanted calories that can derail your weight loss efforts. As previously discussed, the influence of our modern food climate encourages these behaviors, and it is important to take steps to reject these negative influences as much as possible.

Eating Healthy Portion Sizes

Many of our patients have said, "I try to eat only heathy foods, but my weight isn't changing." They feel confident that they have already cut back on total fat, reduced sodium intake, limited alcoholic beverages, and significantly cut down on

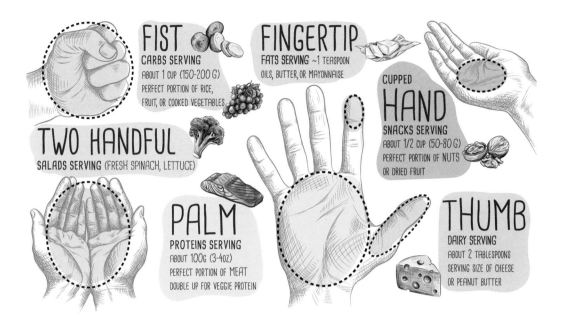

FIST
CARBS SERVING
ABOUT 1 CUP (150-200 G)
PERFECT PORTION OF RICE,
FRUIT, OR COOKED VEGETABLES

FINGERTIP
FATS SERVING ~1 TEASPOON
OILS, BUTTER, OR MAYONNAISE

CUPPED
HAND
SNACKS SERVING
ABOUT 1/2 CUP (50-80 G)
PERFECT PORTION OF NUTS
OR DRIED FRUIT

TWO HANDFUL
SALADS SERVING (FRESH SPINACH, LETTUCE)

PALM
PROTEINS SERVING
ABOUT 100G (3-4OZ)
PERFECT PORTION OF MEAT
DOUBLE UP FOR VEGGIE PROTEIN

THUMB
DAIRY SERVING
ABOUT 2 TABLESPOONS
SERVING SIZE OF CHEESE
OR PEANUT BUTTER

sugar and processed foods. What they may not realize, however, is that they haven't reduced the total calories consumed; in fact, for most Americans, average caloric intake has steadily increased.

The upswing in caloric intake over the past three decades is partly due to a lack of understanding of the size of reasonable portions of food. We have no visual concept of how much is enough. How many calories should be found in a typical meal, and what does that meal look like on a plate? How many calories do we really need? Generally, we have lost track of a visual sense of what healthy portions look like.

The food and restaurant industries in the United States have gradually marketed larger and larger servings and packaging of all kinds of foods, meals, and even sizes of plates, cups, and containers in which our food is served. In terms of calories, most of us have little idea how many calories a single food contributes and are therefore unable to estimate how any food choice might factor into a day of appropriate calorie intake.

For example, when canned soda first became available in the 1940s and 1950s, it was sold in 8- or 12-ounce bottles. Now, the typical vending machine stocks 20-ounce plastic bottles, and we have doubled our rate of consumption since the introduction of plastic bottles and vending machines in the 1970s. Not coincidentally, the rate of obesity doubled along with our consumption habits. If you asked the typical person today if they want a soda, they accept a 20-ounce bottle as normal and refer to an 8-ounce can as "a mini."

Here's another way to look at it. Let's say a woman was gradually trying to lose weight by eating approximately 1,500 calories each day. But if she didn't recognize that just one serving of cheesecake during one restaurant meal can contribute upward of 1,000 calories, she could easily exceed a day's worth of careful food choices by splurging on just one desert! Underlying this common problem is the fact that the slice of cheesecake served probably looked completely "normal." And the fact that it was served as one piece might make her (or anyone) automatically assume it is one serving, and that it is therefore reasonable to eat the whole thing.

If she had been served a slice that was one-third that size, it most likely would have still felt like a special treat and she would likely have felt just as satisfied, but consumed only one-third the calories. But we are so accustomed to seeing huge portions of just about any food that we simply don't consider the math, especially if we've paid for it. Likewise, if she had been told at the outset that the "single serving" of cheesecake would indeed contribute nearly a whole day's worth of calories, she might have chosen differently. This is why the calorie menus available at some restaurants can be so helpful in making decisions that align with daily caloric recommendations. In your weight loss efforts, if you hear yourself saying, "I'm being so careful almost all the time, but I'm just not losing weight," it is possible that this huge-portion phenomenon is affecting you.

Developing an understanding what a single portion looks like is a key skill and will be explained in more detail later (in the discussion of the three-day dietary evaluation). Once again, the USDA's food groups, which are represented on the Choose My Plate icon, also include recommended portion sizes to help target a suggested number of daily calories. It is an important step to notice the discrepancy between the USDA's stated portion and the much larger "expected" or "usual" serving we think of as normal. The recommended number of daily portions from each food group can easily be adjusted to meet personal goals either for weight maintenance or for weight loss.

SAVOR THE FIRST FEW BITES AND THEN PAUSE

The vast majority of us, if we really paid attention, would notice that it is reliably only the first two or three bites of any food that are the very yummiest. The first three bites of that cheesecake would have cost only about 120 calories. The rest is good, but it does not continue to get any tastier. In fact, most of us will continue eating while our attention drifts to other thoughts, so that the remaining portion doesn't deliver the same levels of enjoyment.

By pausing after savoring the first three bites, we would consume far fewer calories and be equally satisfied with just a taste of special treats like desserts.

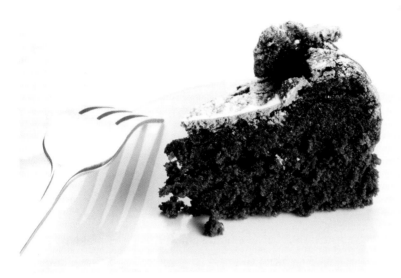

Put your fork down and pause after a bite

This principle applies to almost every food, though especially to hyper-palatable, high-calorie items such as fast food meals, super-sweet desserts, and extra-large sweetened beverages. Take the time to read food labels and restaurant calorie counts. These will help you make thoughtful food choices. However, it still takes a lot of practice and attention to share the meal, take half home, downsize your order, or simply put your fork down when presented with an overlarge serving.

A key step to mastering healthy portions is to start in your own kitchen. Challenge yourself to actually measure each food you serve at your next meal. Start your meal with the number of portions from each food group in the example meal (yes, that's ½ cup of *cooked* pasta for one portion from the grain group). Slowly, and with great attention, consume that meal, enjoying every bite. Wait 20 minutes after you finish, then ask yourself how you feel. Most of us will note that we are pleasantly satisfied (not stuffed), which is an indication of an appropriate level of fullness. Most of us could, however, find room for more if it were still on the plate in front of us. Learning to stop eating after an appropriately sized meal and noticing an appropriate level of fullness are critical steps in long-term calorie control for continued weight loss and long-term weight maintenance.

On the other hand, once you have truly learned that you only need three bites of cake (or whatever indulgence you crave) for maximum satisfaction, it is much easier to factor 120 extra calories into a carefully chosen day so that you can still approximate your weight loss calorie intake. This ability gives you the freedom to factor in small portions of just about any of your favorite foods *once in a while,* so you don't have to feel like you need to always be on a "diet" to lose weight.

Another way to experiment with this concept is to go through your normal day, choose your regular foods and your regular serving sizes. Then commit to leaving one-quarter of every serving on your plate, every time, all day. By the end of the day, you will have saved hundreds of calories without giving up the taste of any of the foods you chose.

The Daily Energy Audit

So, what should your caloric intake be? The figure of 2,000 calories per day you may have heard of is not for everyone; it is simply an average used by the USDA as an example on nutrition facts labels. Each person's daily requirements depend on his or her age, gender, physical activity level, energy used in digestion, and basal metabolic rate, which is the number of calories the body uses at rest to sustain itself. In many medical weight management programs, patients are able to find out what their basal metabolic rate is by breathing into a machine for about ten minutes at rest. This is then used to determine the total *estimated energy require-ment,* or the number of calories you can consume in a day to maintain your weight. Weight loss can then occur if fewer calories are used throughout the day. If you don't have access to this specialized equipment at a medical office to determine your basal metabolic rate, you can use the following information to gauge your activity level and then match your age on the chart in figure 6.3 to find your daily caloric allowance.

First consider your level of daily activity. Which of the following categories best describes you?

Mostly inactive/sedentary. Only activities of daily living (light chores, bathing, eating, dressing). Some walking but fewer than 2,000 to 5,000 steps per day with no intentional exercise. Sits most of the day at work, watching TV, or reading.

Moderately active. Activities of daily living, and mostly standing and walking during the day, including at work (nursing, childcare, waitstaff) or for pleasure (walking the dog, shopping, outdoor chores). Brisk walking three to five miles most days.

Active. Activities of daily living plus walking at least five miles per day (10,000 steps) and intentional workouts three to five times per week. Usually gets at least the weekly recommended 150 minutes (2.5 hours) of aerobic exercise. May do heavy housework, frequent engagement in sports, or physical activity.

Find your activity level and age on the estimated caloric intake chart. If your weight is currently stable, this is the number of calories you are eating on average. If your weight is increasing, then you may be eating more than this or perhaps you've

FIGURE 6-3

Estimated caloric intake chart

	Males				Females		
Age	Sedentary	Moderately active	Active	Age	Sedentary	Moderately active	Active
18	2400	2800	2800	18	1800	2000	2400
19–20	2600	2800	3400	19–20	2000	2200	2400
21–25	2400	2800	3000	21–25	2000	2200	2400
26–30	2400	2600	3000	26–30	1800	2000	2200
31–35	2400	2600	3000	31–35	1800	2000	2200
36–40	2400	2600	2800	36–40	1800	2000	2200
41–45	2200	2600	2800	41–45	1800	2000	2200
46–50	2200	2400	2800	46–50	1800	2000	2200
51–55	2200	2400	2800	51–55	1600	1800	2200
56–60	2200	2400	2600	56–60	1600	1800	2200
61–65	2000	2400	2600	61–65	1600	1800	2000
66–70	2000	2200	2600	66–70	1600	1800	2000
71–75	2000	2200	2600	71–75	1600	1800	2000
76 and up	2000	2200	2400	76 and up	1600	1800	2000

underestimated your activity level. Talk to your health care provider if you think you are within range (or under your limit) and still gaining weight; medications and medical conditions can contribute to this disparity. If you are trying to manage your weight, you can aim to consume the same number of calories while maintaining your activity level. If you are trying to lose weight, you can aim to consume fewer calories or increase your activity level so that you have a caloric deficit. We will talk more about how to increase your activity level in chapter 8.

JOURNALING ACTIVITY:
How Long Will Weight Loss by Caloric Reduction Take?

How many pounds have you decided to lose based on the information you have learned so far in this book? To determine the amount of time it will take to lose this weight at various rates of weight loss per week, multiply the number of pounds you wish to lose (either ultimately or initially) by the factors below.

1 (Number of pounds) multiply by 2.0 = _____ weeks to lose an average of *0.5 pound per week.* (This is the preferred rate of loss if you have fewer than 10 pounds to lose.)

2 (Number of pounds) multiply by 1.0 = _____ weeks to lose an average of *1 pound per week.*

3 (Number of pounds) multiply by 0.67 = _____ weeks to lose an average of *1.5 pounds per week.*

4 (Number of pounds) multiply by 0.5 = _____ weeks to lose an average of *2 pounds per week.*

It's simple, but the more weight you lose per week, the faster you will reach your goal. However, it is important not to choose a rate of loss that results in a calorie level below 1,200 for a woman or 1,500 for a man, since it can be difficult to take in enough vitamins and minerals below these levels.

The tendency is to try to lose as quickly as possible, but many people find that the caloric sacrifice is too high a price to pay. You may want to work your daily calorie level down gradually until you reach the lowest level that is comfortable for you. Gradual loss is usually defined as between half a pound and two pounds per week. If you are a small woman, you can expect to lose half a pound to one pound per week when you follow a well-balanced, low-calorie food plan. If you are a woman with a medium to large structure, you are likely to lose one to two pounds per week. Men's energy needs are often higher than women's energy needs. For that reason, men tend to lose weight more rapidly, commonly two to three pounds per week. Excessive deprivation often makes it less likely that you will be able to succeed in staying on target in your Personal Plan of Action.

 JOURNALING ACTIVITY:
Daily Weight Loss Calorie Budget

Complete the appropriate equation below to decide on your daily weight loss calorie budget based on how much you would like to lose per week.

For an example, we will use José, who is a 30-year-old, moderately active man. José currently eats about 3,200 calories per day and is ready to lose weight. Using the estimated caloric intake chart, José figures he needs 2,800 calories per day to maintain his weight. In order to lose weight, he will have to reduce his caloric intake each day. He will now subtract between 250 and 1,000 calories per day to see how feasible it is to lose at minimum 0.5 pounds per week and a maximum of 3 pounds per week:

1 2,800 calories – 250 calories = 2,550 *calories/day for a loss of 0.5 pound per week*. (This is the preferred rate of loss if you have less than 10 pounds to lose.)

2 2,800 calories – 500 calories = 2,300 *calories/day for a loss of 1 pound per week*.

3 2,800 calories – 750 calories = 2,050 *calories/day for a loss of 1.5 pounds per week*.

4 2,800 calories – 1,000 calories = 1,800 *calories/day for a loss of 2 pounds per week*.

5 2,800 calories – 1,500 calories= 1,300 *calories/day for a loss of 3 pounds per week*.

Note. Any limit at or below 1,000–1,200 calories is to be considered only if you have more than 100 pounds to lose, and then it must be done only under the supervision of a physician.

Try these equations with your own daily estimated caloric intake and ask yourself whether this number of daily calories seems realistic. Keep in mind that the faster you lose, the less time it will take but the stricter you must be and the more difficult it may be to sustain this challenge, especially in the beginning. You may want to start slower and adjust to a lower-calorie goal as you begin to master lifestyle changes necessary for weight loss or maintenance. Gradual and sustained weight loss usually reflect a thoughtful, careful refining of food habits rather than a "crash diet." The diet you are designing for your Personal Plan of Action is a healthful, nutritionally complete, and sustainable diet. If it is practiced long enough to promote significant weight loss, it can become a permanent lifestyle change.

Now, record your new daily calorie limit for weight loss in your journal so you can add it to your Personal Plan of Action when ready.

Choosing Foods to Match Your Caloric Needs

Eating at least the minimum number of servings from each food group, using a variety of specific food choices, helps ensure healthful levels of all the key nutrients. A nutritious, three-meal-a-day pattern of servings for an 1,800-calorie day might look like this.

By varying the number of servings within the recommended range, total calories for the day can be manipulated to meet individual needs (this is what is meant by *moderation*). By choosing a lower total daily calorie level, the number of recommended servings from each food group can be appropriately modified to create weight loss without sacrificing nutrient adequacy. Total calories can also be manipulated by choosing the foods lowest in fat from each of the five groups and limiting servings to the minimum number recommended.

Match your caloric goal with the following recommended portions or servings for each food group.

The food groups are a helpful guide for a wide range of healthy people who are choosing a balanced diet. All the nutrients are provided in adequate, but not excessive, amounts for maintaining good health while simultaneously balancing energy intake with energy needs to maintain or improve body weight. Food groups help to moderate portion sizes and thereby control total daily calories. A daily goal for each food group also helps weed out many high-calorie, fried, packaged, and processed foods that tend to contribute extra calories without a lot of nutrient value.

You can follow the general guidelines provided by the USDA, but you also need to tailor them to fit your own specific needs and food preferences. Each food group

TABLE 6-2

Sample diet: 1,800 calories per day

Breakfast	1 cup hot oatmeal with ½ cup blueberries	1 serving grain with ½ serving fruit
	1 cup milk	1 serving dairy
	1 egg	1 serving protein
	1 tablespoon fat/oil for cooking	
Lunch	1 slice of bread for a sandwich	2 servings grain
	½ cup raw spinach and ½ tomato	1 serving vegetable
	1 ounce cooked chicken on sandwich	1 serving protein
	1 slice pepper jack cheese	1 serving dairy
	1 banana	1 serving fruit
	water	
Dinner	1 ½ cup cooked wild rice pilaf	2 ½ servings grain
	½ cup cooked zucchini	1 serving vegetable
	3 ounces salmon	3 servings protein
	1 lowfat yogurt cup	1 serving dairy
	2 tablespoons fat/oils for cooking	
	Chamomile tea	
Total		**Grain:** 5.5
		Vegetable: 2
		Fruit: 1.5

SOURCE: *https://www.choosemyplate.gov/resources/MyPlatePlan.*

contains a wide variety of healthy food choices, and those listed as "1 serving" in the third column are just examples of the many food choices you can make. Vary your specific selections using indicated portion sizes for each food to meet your food preferences and cultural tendencies. You can use mobile phone apps to look up exactly how much a serving is of thousands of foods, or do a simple internet search; if the food comes in a package, look at the nutrition facts on the back for "serving size."

TABLE 6-3

Recommended servings for a daily calorie goal of 1,600

Food group	My recommended servings	1 Serving size equals
Grain	5 servings/ounces	1 slice of bread 1 cup of boxed cereal ½ cup cooked rice, pasta, or hot cereal (such as oatmeal)
Fruit	1½ servings/cups	1 cup raw, frozen, cooked, or canned fruit ½ cup dried fruit 1 cup 100% fruit juice
Vegetable	2 servings/cups	1 cup raw, cooked, or canned vegetables 2 cups leafy greens 1 cup 100% vegetable juice
Protein	5 servings/ounces	1 ounce cooked or canned lean meat, poultry, or seafood 1 egg ¼ cup cooked beans or peas ⅛ cup nuts or seeds 1 tablespoon peanut butter
Dairy	3 servings/cups	1 cup milk 1 cup low-fat yogurt 1 cup soy/milk beverage 1.5 ounces natural cheese 2 ounces processed cheese

SOURCE: *https://www.choosemyplate.gov/resources/MyPlatePlan.*

TABLE 6-4

Recommended servings
for a daily calorie goal of 1,800

Food group	My recommended servings	1 Serving size equals
Grain	6 servings/ounces	1 slice of bread
		1 cup of boxed cereal
		½ cup cooked rice, pasta, or hot cereal (such as oatmeal)
Fruit	1½ servings/cups	1 cup raw, frozen, cooked, or canned fruit
		½ cup dried fruit
		1 cup 100% fruit juice
Vegetable	2 servings/cups	1 cup raw, cooked, or canned vegetables
		2 cups leafy greens
		1 cup 100% vegetable juice
Protein	5 servings/ounces	1 ounce cooked or canned lean meat, poultry, or seafood
		1 egg
		¼ cup cooked beans or peas
		⅛ cup nuts or seeds
		1 tablespoon peanut butter
Dairy	3 servings/cups	1 cup milk
		1 cup low-fat yogurt
		1 cup soy/milk beverage
		1.5 ounces natural cheese
		2 ounces processed cheese

SOURCE: *https://www.choosemyplate.gov/resources/MyPlatePlan.*

TABLE 6-5

Recommended servings
for a daily calorie goal of 2,000

Food group	My recommended servings	1 Serving size equals
Grain	6 servings/ounces	1 slice of bread
		1 cup of boxed cereal
		½ cup cooked rice, pasta, or hot cereal (such as oatmeal)
Fruit	2 servings/cups	1 cup raw, frozen, cooked, or canned fruit
		½ cup dried fruit
		1 cup 100% fruit juice
Vegetable	2½ servings/cups	1 cup raw, cooked, or canned vegetables
		2 cups leafy greens
		1 cup 100% vegetable juice
Protein	5½ servings/ounces	1 ounce cooked or canned lean meat, poultry, or seafood
		1 egg
		¼ cup cooked beans or peas
		⅛ cup nuts or seeds
		1 tablespoon peanut butter
Dairy	3 servings/cups	1 cup milk
		1 cup low-fat yogurt
		1 cup soy/milk beverage
		1.5 ounces natural cheese
		2 ounces processed cheese

SOURCE: *https://www.choosemyplate.gov/resources/MyPlatePlan.*

TABLE 6-6

Recommended servings
for a daily calorie goal of 2,200

Food group	My recommended servings	1 Serving size equals
Grain	7 servings/ounces	1 slice of bread
		1 cup of boxed cereal
		½ cup cooked rice, pasta, or hot cereal (such as oatmeal)
Fruit	2 servings/cups	1 cup raw, frozen, cooked, or canned fruit
		½ cup dried fruit
		1 cup 100% fruit juice
Vegetable	3 servings/cups	1 cup raw, cooked, or canned vegetables
		2 cups leafy greens
		1 cup 100% vegetable juice
Protein	6 servings/ounces	1 ounce cooked or canned lean meat, poultry, or seafood
		1 egg
		¼ cup cooked beans or peas
		⅛ cup nuts or seeds
		1 tablespoon peanut butter
Dairy	3 servings/cups	1 cup milk
		1 cup low-fat yogurt
		1 cup soy/milk beverage
		1.5 ounces natural cheese
		2 ounces processed cheese

SOURCE: *https://www.choosemyplate.gov/resources/MyPlatePlan.*

TABLE 6-7

Recommended servings for a daily calorie goal of 2,400

Food group	My recommended servings	1 Serving size equals
Grain	8 servings/ounces	1 slice of bread
		1 cup of boxed cereal
		½ cup cooked rice, pasta, or hot cereal (such as oatmeal)
Fruit	2 servings/cups	1 cup raw, frozen, cooked, or canned fruit
		½ cup dried fruit
		1 cup 100% fruit juice
Vegetable	3 servings/cups	1 cup raw, cooked, or canned vegetables
		2 cups leafy greens
		1 cup 100% vegetable juice
Protein	6½ servings/ounces	1 ounce cooked or canned lean meat, poultry, or seafood
		1 egg
		¼ cup cooked beans or peas
		⅛ cup nuts or seeds
		1 tablespoon peanut butter
Dairy	3 servings/cups	1 cup milk
		1 cup low-fat yogurt
		1 cup soy/milk beverage
		1.5 ounces natural cheese
		2 ounces processed cheese

SOURCE: *https://www.choosemyplate.gov/resources/MyPlatePlan.*

TABLE 6-8

Recommended servings for a daily calorie goal of 2,600

Food group	My recommended servings	1 Serving size equals
Grain	9 servings/ounces	1 slice of bread 1 cup of boxed cereal ½ cup cooked rice, pasta, or hot cereal (such as oatmeal)
Fruit	2 servings/cups	1 cup raw, frozen, cooked, or canned fruit ½ cup dried fruit 1 cup 100% fruit juice
Vegetable	3½ servings/cups	1 cup raw, cooked, or canned vegetables 2 cups leafy greens 1 cup 100% vegetable juice
Protein	6½ servings/ounces	1 ounce cooked or canned lean meat, poultry, or seafood 1 egg ¼ cup cooked beans or peas ⅛ cup nuts or seeds 1 tablespoon peanut butter
Dairy	3 servings/cups	1 cup milk 1 cup low-fat yogurt 1 cup soy/milk beverage 1.5 ounces natural cheese 2 ounces processed cheese

SOURCE: *https://www.choosemyplate.gov/resources/MyPlatePlan.*

TABLE 6-9

Recommended servings for a daily calorie goal of 2,800

Food group	My recommended servings	1 Serving size equals
Grain	10 servings/ounces	1 slice of bread
		1 cup of boxed cereal
		½ cup cooked rice, pasta, or hot cereal (such as oatmeal)
Fruit	2½ servings/cups	1 cup raw, frozen, cooked, or canned fruit
		½ cup dried fruit
		1 cup 100% fruit juice
Vegetable	3 ½ servings/cups	1 cup raw, cooked, or canned vegetables
		2 cups leafy greens
		1 cup 100% vegetable juice
Protein	7 servings/ounces	1 ounce cooked or canned lean meat, poultry, or seafood
		1 egg
		¼ cup cooked beans or peas
		⅛ cup nuts or seeds
		1 tablespoon peanut butter
Dairy	3 servings/cups	1 cup milk
		1 cup low-fat yogurt
		1 cup soy/milk beverage
		1.5 ounces natural cheese
		2 ounces processed cheese

SOURCE: *https://www.choosemyplate.gov/resources/MyPlatePlan.*

TABLE 6-10

Recommended servings for a daily calorie goal of 3,000

Food group	My recommended servings	1 Serving size equals
Grain	10 servings/ounces	1 slice of bread 1 cup of boxed cereal ½ cup cooked rice, pasta, or hot cereal (such as oatmeal)
Fruit	2½ servings/cups	1 cup raw, frozen, cooked, or canned fruit ½ cup dried fruit 1 cup 100% fruit juice
Vegetable	4 servings/cups	1 cup raw, cooked, or canned vegetables 2 cups leafy greens 1 cup 100% vegetable juice
Protein	7 servings/ounces	1 ounce cooked or canned lean meat, poultry, or seafood 1 egg ¼ cup cooked beans or peas ⅛ cup nuts or seeds 1 tablespoon peanut butter
Dairy	3 servings/cups	1 cup milk 1 cup low-fat yogurt 1 cup soy/milk beverage 1.5 ounces natural cheese 2 ounces processed cheese

SOURCE: *https://www.choosemyplate.gov/resources/MyPlatePlan.*

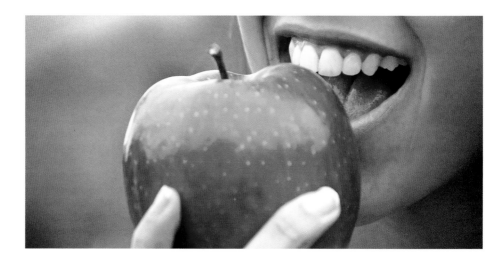

You'll notice that the USDA did not write you a specific menu. One size does not fit all. Your ability or desire to make healthy food choices for the long term often depends on how well you like the pattern you have developed. There's no sense in recommending bananas with breakfast if you don't like bananas, for example. But there are plenty of other fruits that you could choose instead. If, for instance, your cultural background includes serving rice at every meal, there is no sense in recommending that you eliminate rice. But, for the purpose of limiting calories, it is important to recognize that one serving of rice is ½ cup cooked rice so you can compare with your typical serving size. And to incorporate your knowledge of nutrient density, consider using brown rice instead of white. These smaller, stepwise changes can have a profound impact on our long-term ability to make healthy food and calorie choices.

Action Item: The Three-Day Dietary Evaluation

So far, you've figured out your estimated caloric intake needs, how quickly you'd like to lose weight, and your adjusted caloric intake limit to do so. You also know how many servings of the major food groups you should aim for while staying within this new caloric limit. The next step is to evaluate your *current* eating patterns and adjust them to fit with your new lifestyle and healthful eating goals.

Refer back to the daily food record you kept for three days. Or, if you haven't yet done this, pause and for the next three days eat the same way you normally do, but write down *everything* you eat, all day long, using the daily food record, which can be found in the resources section of this book.

Here is an example of Ximena's completed food record for her first day of tracking.

TABLE 6-11

Example food record

Time	All food/drinks	Food group	Servings	Calories
8:00 am	Plain oatmeal, 1 cup	Grain	2	150
	2% milk, 1 cup	Dairy	1	120
	1 large banana	Fruit	1	155
10:00 am	1 glazed doughnut	Un-food/empty calories	1	270
	Black coffee, 1 cup	n/a	n/a	0
12:30 pm	2 slices white bread	Grain	2	140
	2 tablespoon peanut butter	Protein Fats/oils	2 2	186
	2 oz potato chips	Un-food/empty calories Fats/oils	1 1	300
	12 oz cola soda	Un-food/empty calories	1	160
	1 brownie with nuts			233
3:00 pm	25 mini pretzels	Grain	1	100
5:30 pm	2 slices American cheese	Dairy	1	158
	6 saltine crackers	Grain	1	118
	12 oz cola soda	Un-food/empty calories	1	160
7:00 pm	3 oz fried pork chop	Protein	3	334
	1 cup mashed potatoes	Vegetable	1	222
	1 cup green peas, cooked	Vegetable	1	134
	1 teaspoon margarine	Fats/oils	1	34
Total		Grain	6	2974 calories
		Fruit	1	
		Vegetable	2	
		Protein	5	
		Dairy	2	
		Un-food/empty calories	3	
		Fats/oils	4	

SOURCE: *Data from USDA, https://fdc.nal.usda.gov, accessed 3.5.21.*

STEP 1. RECORD FOOD AND DRINK

Using the blank daily food records in the resources section, write down all your food and drinks for three consecutive days, using one food record per day.

STEP 2. MEASURE AND KEEP TRACK

Every time you eat or drink something, write it down immediately instead of waiting until the end of the day. Measure everything accurately (or look up serving sizes either online or using a mobile app). Use standard measuring utensils (teaspoon, tablespoon, cups, etc.), especially for items that you normally pour (cream in coffee, oil in skillet, salad dressing). Do not use measurements like "a bowlful," "a handful," or "one serving." Be as specific as possible. Carrying your food record with you will help ensure that everything is recorded promptly.

STEP 3. ASSIGN FOODS TO FOOD GROUPS

Look at each of your three food records and, line by line, decide which food group the food belongs in (carbs/grains/vegetables/fruits, protein, dairy, "un-food"/ empty calories, fats/oils) and how many servings of the food you ate.

STEP 4. TOTAL AND COMPARE

After you have completed recording your intake for the day, total the number of servings you ate in each of the food groups. Compare these totals with your food group goals for your selected weight loss calorie level. Are the numbers close? If not, ask yourself if you were totally accurate in recording what you ate. Did you eat in your usual fashion? Did you record everything?

STEP 5. REVIEW YOUR CHOICES

Decide what changes you would like to make (in hindsight) to bring your eating habits in line with your calorie and food group portion goals. What foods could you have avoided that added to your caloric intake?

STEP 6. EVALUATE AND PLAN

How often did you eat each day? Did you eat fewer than three times? More than five or six times? If your answer was fewer than three, and this is a pattern for you, then you may be eating too many calories at a sitting. This pattern of infrequent but high-volume consumption is often associated with difficulty in controlling weight. The related habit of skipping breakfast is harmful because excess hunger or a sense of deprivation can cause you to lose control once you do start eating after a prolonged period of restraint. If your answer was more than five or six times, then perhaps you are eating too much by grazing throughout the day. This could be an indication that you do not plan adequate time to prepare and eat healthy, well-balanced meals throughout the day, so you gravitate to quick and easy snack items. It is possible to never feel adequately fed (full), which leads to seeking out the next snack to eat just a short while later. It then becomes very easy for excess calories to accumulate over the day without feeling like you've really eaten "anything big." Grazing is also sometimes a habit people learn as a way of coping with negative feelings such as stress, fatigue, boredom, loneliness, or pain. Grazing is usually a means of experiencing temporary pleasure and is rarely associated with true physical hunger. Eating food when you are not truly hungry is the perfect activity for *gaining* weight.

There's no question that completing this part of the assessment requires some time and discipline, but the effort will yield important information about your eating patterns—it may even reveal information about your food habits that surprises you. Completing the dietary evaluation is crucial for designing your Personal Plan of Action; it will also give you practice in the important weight loss and weight maintenance skill of *self-monitoring*.

FATS AND OILS

Do you have more than four servings of fats and oils? If so, put a line through these items on your daily food record. Look carefully at these eliminated foods. Ask yourself if you can live without them for a while, or whether you can eat a much smaller amount of them or eat them less frequently. Alternatively, is there something you can substitute that may be lower in calories and fat that you can eat the same amount of? Is there another food you could choose instead that would help fill in for a different food group of which you didn't get enough? As previously mentioned, the fats/oils food group is an especially calorie dense, low-volume source of calories. Many of these foods are used as ingredients or in preparation of other foods and can easily go unnoticed. For some, simply reducing these concentrated sources of excess calories can be crucial for initiating weight loss.

DAIRY AND PROTEINS

What do you see in the milk and protein groups? Are you eating more servings than you budgeted for weight loss? If the answer is yes, then again draw a line through each of the extra portions you ate in these two categories. Notice how much closer you're getting to your food group goals? Apart from portions, another point to consider in these two categories is what foods you're eating. Many high-protein, high-calcium foods (protein and milk) are also very high in fat. Can you think of nutritious alternatives you could have chosen that you might like just as well but that don't pack the same high-fat punch? For example, instead of reaching for the ice cream, try a low-fat yogurt cup placed in the freezer for 30 minutes.

FRUITS AND VEGETABLES

On each of your three daily records, add enough vegetables and fruit servings to bring your servings up to the recommend amounts. Chances are good that, so far, you've eliminated some servings of food from the first three groups you looked at, but you've replaced some or all of these foods with servings from bulky, filling fruits and vegetables. Note that little if any food volume has been sacrificed, only fat and calories.

GRAINS

Now look at the grain group. Again, if you're like many people, you may not have eaten enough whole grain breads, cereals, rice, or pasta. Just as in the fruit and vegetable categories, most whole grain foods are very low in fat. On the other hand, you might find that you consumed more than your goal of refined grain products. Adjust each of your food records either up or down to reflect the number of servings you should be eating from this category according to your personal food group pattern. Consider ways to substitute whole grain products instead of refined grain products as you make your adjustments. If you did eat too many servings, then tweak just enough to reach your food group pattern budget. If your servings are too low, use the food tables to help you add satisfying, low-fat, whole grain options to your food choices. Be mindful that it is often the toppings we add to our grain servings that add unnecessary calories. If you did eat the correct number of servings and some of your toppings were high in fat, then consider how to adjust portions or use lower-fat options. Adjust your daily totals for each food record accordingly.

OTHER FOODS

Did you eat any foods that didn't fall into one specific category? Some foods we consider "combo" foods, like pizza. It isn't quite a grain, or a vegetable, or part of the dairy group, but it has components of all of these. Typically, but not in all cases, these combo foods are higher in fat, carbohydrates, and sodium, and they tend to be packaged or processed. Calories and fat content from combo foods can add up quickly.

EATING EVENTS

Look at each eating event over your three-day record. Try to recall the experience. Do you remember feeling hungry? Consider the kind of hunger that's in your stomach, or makes you tremble, or causes light-headedness or a headache? If each day you felt true physical hunger only once, or not at all, then the chances are good that your reasons for eating are not associated with physical need, and that you may tend to eat out of habit or desire. It will be important for you to be reintroduced to the sensation of physical hunger, learn to respond to it in a measured fashion, and plan ahead for its return. You can do this by arranging to eat a meal (light or moderate) within two hours of waking each day and then planning on two or three light-to-moderate meals or snacks every three to four hours thereafter. It's best not to eat during the two hours before you go to bed. This will allow your appetite to return promptly in the morning and can help you stay on track. Of course, if you've missed a meal along the way and you're truly hungry right before bed, then by all means eat something. Try to keep it light, though—just enough to take the edge off.

Now take your three revised food records and average the three days together. First add together all three daily calorie totals, then divide by three. Are the average daily totals for each food group close to your goals for weight loss? If your answer is no, review these steps again to help you adjust your food group selections and portion sizes as needed. If your answer is yes, and your adjusted records are close to your food group budgets, then you now have a Personal Plan of Action for how many servings of enjoyable, low-fat foods to choose on a daily basis to reach your weight loss goal. You will be eating satisfying yet nutritious low-calorie foods.

Tips for Future Diet Modifications

Here are some more quick tips to get you started making small, easily adaptable modifications to reduce your intake of both fats and calories the next time around:

- **Avoid using fat as flavoring in cooking or at the table.**
  - Avoid rich sauces on vegetables and potatoes.
  - Eat bread without butter or margarine.
  - Reduce butter, margarine, and oil in recipes.
  - Eat potatoes without butter or margarine.
  - Eat vegetables without butter or margarine.
  - Bake, broil, or poach fish and shellfish rather than fry them.

- **Limit high-fat meats and meat substitutes (eat one or more vegetarian meals per day).**
  - Use vegetarian tomato sauce on pasta; most marinara sauces are vegetarian.
  - Limit hamburger, most lunch meats, and hot dogs.
  - Eat small (2–4 oz) servings of lean meat at any one time.
  - Eat beef, pork, and lamb infrequently.
  - Eat small amounts of chicken, fish, and beans more often.
  - Eat low-fat cheese or vegetarian pizza.
  - Avoid excessive use of whole eggs, nuts, and seeds.

- **Modify your choices.**
  - Purchase low-fat or fat-free versions of your favorite crackers and chips.
  - Buy low-fat or fat-free cheese (less than 6 grams of fat per ounce).
  - Remove skin from chicken and remove visible fat from meat.
  - Use skim or 1% milk rather than whole or 2%.
  - Eat fat-free frozen yogurt instead of regular ice cream.
  - Replace cream or whole milk in recipes with evaporated skim milk.

- **Use specially manufactured fat-free or low-fat food substitutes, being mindful to avoid such products high in added sugars.[1]**
  - Use cooking spray in baking pans or skillets.
  - Use lemon juice, vinegar, or nonfat dressing on salad.
  - Use fat-free mayonnaise instead of regular. ➡

---

1 Some fat-free or low-fat food substitutes include added sugars used to make up for the taste change that can result from eliminating or reducing fat.

- Use low-fat or fat-free plain yogurt or Greek yogurt instead of sour cream.
- Use fat-free cream cheese on bagels and in recipes.
- Use light or whipped margarine, or fat-free substitutes, instead of butter or regular margarine.
- Replace whole eggs with egg substitutes.

- **Replace one food choice with another.**
  - Spread jelly, jam, or apple butter on toast or bread instead of butter or margarine. (If you have diabetes, you may wish to discuss some different options with your doctor.)
  - Eat fruit for dessert or a snack instead of cakes, candy bars, cookies, or ice cream.
  - Eat pretzels instead of potato chips.
  - Suck on hard candy or chew gum instead of eating a chocolate candy bar.
  - Replace high-fat breakfast meats (bacon, pork sausage) with turkey or chicken sausage.

BOX 6-14

Low-Calorie "Free" Foods

As part of your Personal Plan of Action, you can incorporate "free foods." A free food is any food or beverage that contains less than 20 calories per serving. They contribute very little (if at all) to your daily caloric and fat totals, and some will be counted as servings of vegetables or fruits. The following are examples of these low-calorie free foods:

Beverages
- 1 cup bouillon or broth, fat-free
- ¼ cup fat-free (skim) milk
- Diet soda (12 fl oz per day)

Raw Vegetables (1 cup)
- Spinach
- Romaine
- Onions
- Green beans
- Bell peppers
- Cabbage
- Celery
- Bok choy
- Cucumber
- Hot peppers
- Green onion
- Mushrooms
- Radishes
- Zucchini

Fruits
- ¼ grapefruit
- 1 lemon
- 1 lime
- ¼ cup pomegranate seeds
- ½ kiwi, raw
- ¼ cup orange segments, raw
- ¼ cup blueberries
- ⅓ cup strawberries, halved
- ¼ cup watermelon or cantaloupe
- ½ pear, raw
- ½ peach or plum, small
- ½ apple, small or ¼ apple, medium/large
- 5 grapes

Sweets
- 2 pieces sugar-free hard candy
- 1 sugar-free popsicle
- 1 cup sugar-free gelatin

Additional Foods
- 4 large green olives
- 4 large black olives
- ½ cup tomato juice
- 12 oyster crackers
- ¾ cup air-popped popcorn

Condiments
- 1 tablespoon parmesan cheese
- 2 tablespoons fat-free yogurt
- 1 tablespoon ketchup
- 2 tablespoons fat-free salad dressing
- 3 tablespoons taco sauce
- ¼ cup salsa
- 1 tablespoon sweet-and-sour sauce
- 1–2 tablespoons sugar-free syrup
- 1 tablespoon sugar-free jelly/jam
- 2 tablespoons fat-free whipped topping
- 1 tablespoon fat-free mayonnaise/sour cream
- Mustard

Unlimited
- Sugar-free gum (< 10 calories/piece)
- Spray salad dressing (do not pour)
- Spray butter (do not pour)
- Artificial sweeteners

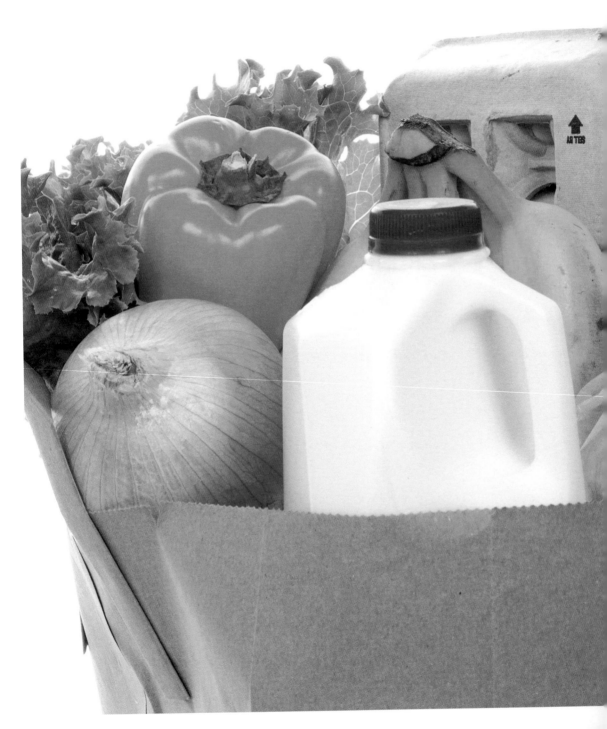

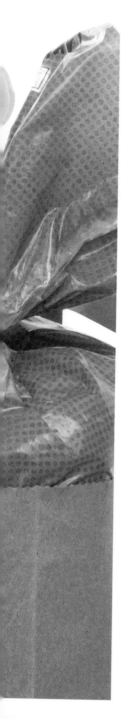

CHAPTER 7

Food Shopping, Meal Planning, and Monitoring Principles

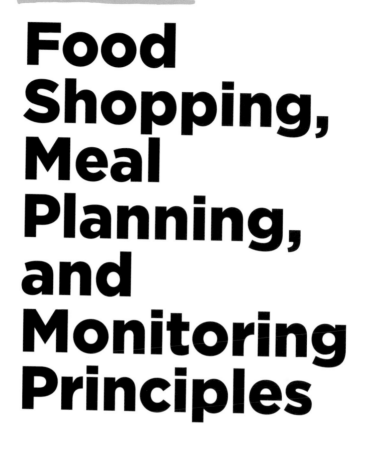

IN THIS CHAPTER, WE WILL:

- **show** you why preparing your own food will help you reach and maintain your ideal weight,

- **provide tips** for making the best choices when food shopping,

- **recommend** staple foods to always have at home,

- **suggest** food preparation strategies and ideas for quick and healthy meals,

- **offer strategies** for how to make smart choices when eating out, and

- **outline** monitoring strategies to help you make optimal food choices for losing weight.

YOU'VE BEEN FOCUSED ON a wealth of basic nutrition facts—food groups, calories, portion sizes, and food records—and can go a long way toward managing your total calorie intake with the tools we have discussed so far. However, in our food climate today, we have become accustomed to letting someone else prepare the majority of our food. To be successful in controlling your calorie intake, nutrient density, and weight management, it is imperative that you make the decision to regain your own personal control over what foods you should and should not select. This will require spending *time* to plan, shop, prepare, and store food.

Many people do not currently allocate enough time for these tasks, perhaps because they don't think of them as a crucial part of their health care. The following tips will help you streamline the process of getting your food from the store to the table in the most efficient and nutritious ways. There is plenty of room for your own personal strategies as well. Although many of these tips may seem basic in print, actually making them happen consistently within the context of your daily responsibilities will take some effort. So, let's take it step by step. Don't be afraid to practice, practice, practice.

Prepare Your Own Food Most of the Time

Current USDA recommendations encourage no more than one meal per week prepared away from home. If you are one of those people who doesn't typically prepare your own food, it is important to realize that we can now easily get more than a whole day's worth of calories in a single restaurant or take-out meal. Ninety-two percent of restaurants surveyed in a recent Tufts University study served entrées that exceed the recommended calories for a single meal. A typical restaurant meal starts at about 1,500 calories for the entrée alone (not including the appetizers, bread basket, wine, and dessert). To be successful at losing weight and keeping it off, think seriously about making time in your schedule to shop, prepare, and eat at home most of the time. Many people now spend more money on food away from home than they do on groceries. Preparing food at home is better for both your waistline and your wallet.

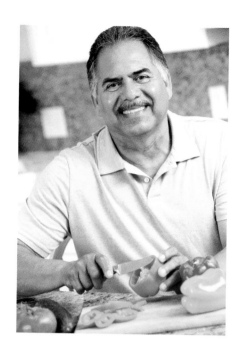

While juggling careers, family, and personal obligations, it can be easy to tell yourself that you don't have any other choice but to grab another quick take-out meal. However, developing a pattern of shopping, preparing, and storing your own "convenience" meals and snacks doesn't have to be as time-consuming as you might think. Healthier easy-to-prepare options are becoming more widely available in the grocery store. With practice and planning, making tasty, healthy food choices at home can become second nature. Read on for ideas that will help you shop, store, and prepare food that can be key in losing or maintaining your goal weight with the least amount of effort.

Planning Ahead

Next time you visit the grocery store, spend five extra minutes in each section. Focus on only one food group each time. Search for attractive low-calorie, easy prep ideas that will help you incorporate the recommended number of food group servings each day. Look for interesting options among the fresh produce. In the frozen section, explore frozen veggies as well as frozen single servings of fish and shellfish. Look for lean meats in the butcher section. If available, check out the salad bar. In the center aisle, explore, ready-to-use whole grains

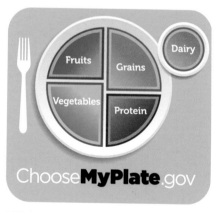

USDA My Plate. Recall the discussion of food groups from the previous chapter.

and canned legumes. You get the idea. You will see that you have a wide variety of options to build a delicious and diverse diet so you can make healthy choices without feeling deprived. With this newfound appreciation for the variety available to you, you are in a good position to begin to implement the first step in preparing healthy meals at home: making a list.

Your Personal Plan of Action will be easier to follow if you stock your pantry with food groups and Choose My Plate guidelines in mind. In fact, many of your impulsive food choices at home are really made in the grocery store. Spend 15 minutes once a week to draft a meal plan for the upcoming week. Or do this twice a week to plan out just the next three to four days. You don't need to plan every detail, but at least identify which days or nights will be the busiest and which nights or weekends you will have more time for meal prep. Make a written list of three to four complete meal options, and be sure you shop for the key ingredients and side dishes. If you typically need a snack some time during the day, plan healthy food group–based selections to keep on hand. Keep your list posted so you can refer back to it during the week.

Food Shopping Dos and Don'ts

Keep in mind that grocery stores are a lot like advertisements: they're designed to encourage you to spend your money impulsively by appealing to your senses and your desire for convenience. The following lists of dos and don'ts will help you avoid temptation and make smart grocery store purchases.

1 **Don't shop haphazardly.** Poor planning results in disorganization and may even propel you to the fast food window. Follow a routine; set aside a specific day and time that is meant for an intentional grocery run.

2 **Don't shop when you are hungry.** Shop only when you are relaxed and have had a satisfying, healthful meal. You'll be more likely to remain organized and focused, and leave the store with sensible choices.

3 **Don't be shortsighted.** Coupons are great, but only for items from the five basic USDA food groups. Clip coupons only for items that you would have purchased anyway. Avoid using coupons for versions of the five main groups with high fat or high added sugar. It's nice to save money, but most coupons are meant to encourage you to purchase foods you don't need.

4 **Do make a list.** Without a list you'll waste time, forget necessary items, and indulge in impulse buying. Making a list will encourage you to get organized. Planning at least some of your meals and snacks ahead of time will help you identify exactly what you need to shop for. Shop only for the foods on your list.

Avoid buying foods that will "call your name" once you are at home. When your cupboard is well stocked with the ingredients for preparing wholesome meals and snacks, you're more likely to make good choices.

5 **Do focus on food groups while shopping, but be selective.** Though the produce section, deli, meat counter, and bakery are where you'll find most of the USDA food group basics, such as whole grain breads, fruits, vegetables, milk, cheese, poultry, and fish, these areas nevertheless also offer many appealing, expensive, high-fat foods. For instance, the deli is great for freshly sliced lean sandwich ham, but it's also the home of six varieties of potato salad or macaroni salad drenched in oil or mayonnaise. So, be careful to stick to your list of appropriate food group selections while shopping these hot spots.

6 **Do save yourself some time.** As you focus on food groups, you'll also find that several aisles in the grocery store are almost completely unnecessary (you might call these the "empty-calorie aisles": cookies, candy, soda, chips, snacks, and frozen desserts). You'll save lots of time by simply skipping these aisles altogether while you shop.

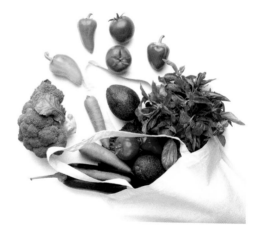

7 **Do spend much of your shopping trip in the produce department.** Choose as many richly colored items (dark green, orange, yellow, red) as possible. Most people do not eat the recommended number of servings of fruits and vegetables and cite price or time as barriers. Knowing what's in season and taking a little time to comparison shop will help you pick out excellent nutrition for the best price. For convenience (if price isn't your most pressing consideration), choose prewashed, peeled, chopped, ready-to-eat or preassembled options like baby carrots, bagged tossed salads, slaw mixtures, and cut-up, prepackaged fresh fruit. If you can't find an item on your list, or it doesn't appear fresh, or the price is outrageous, look for a reasonable alternative. Consider that many people forgo a $1.49 cantaloupe but never blink an eye at a $2.99 bag of potato chips. Don't be dissuaded from making the more nutritious purchase.

Buying Produce

Tip: If one is available in your area, consider purchasing produce from a farmer's market. Doing so will help you learn when different fruits and vegetables are in season. Since the produce for sale is locally grown, it will likely be at peak flavor. Finally, if making organic selections is important to you, you can talk to the growers directly about their practices.

8 Do consider using frozen or canned vegetables and fruits, when needed. Remember, though, that fruits, vegetables, and whole grains come in a variety of forms found in interior aisles (canned or frozen vegetables, rice, juice, etc.). These may be just as nutritious as their fresh counterparts—and, sometimes, depending on the time of year, less expensive. As always, take the time to review the food label carefully to ensure that you are not choosing options that contain added fats or sugars.

9 Don't skip calcium-rich foods, particularly if you're a woman. With low-fat milk products in abundance, there is no reason to snub these important foods, which help prevent osteoporosis. There are many varieties of low-fat cheese, yogurt, and other skim or fat-free milk products, and their taste and texture have been steadily improving. If you are lactose intolerant, choose fermented or lactase-treated milk products. Sometimes small amounts of lactose-rich foods are well tolerated even when large amounts are not. If you do not eat dairy products for personal or cultural reasons, look carefully for calcium-rich substitutes. Many soy products and some cereals and fruit juices are fortified with calcium.

10 Do beware of prominent displays and advertising gimmicks. Don't get trapped by enticing displays for inappropriate foods inside or at the ends of the aisles. Marketing strategies are meant to entice you to make impulse purchases of foods that supply very little high-quality nutrition. Remember, if it isn't on your grocery list, don't buy it.

11 Don't be tempted to buy fresh meat, poultry, and fish indiscriminately. These foods are expensive, and many are not yet mandated to have a nutrition facts panel on the package. When information is unavailable, use these rules to help:

- *White meat poultry is leaner than dark*; skinless is leaner than skin-on (you can remove the skin yourself).
- *Red meats closely trimmed of outer-layer fat are preferable;* red meats are leanest if flecks of white between red muscle (known as marbling) are

minimal; prime cuts are fattiest, round and loin are leanest; intact cuts of meat or poultry tend to be leaner than ground; and pre-breaded chops, chicken, and fish can often be high in both fat and sodium.

- **Choose white meat poultry, lean pork, and fish** much more often than beef. Keep in mind that 4 ounces (0.25 lb.) of raw lean meat will yield 3 ounces cooked, which is a reasonable serving for one meal. Even if the meat is lean, try not to eat meats at every lunch and dinner meal.

- **Substituting plant-based proteins** can increase variety and enjoyment while improving the overall nutrition profile of your sensible food plan. Don't worry about getting enough protein. Most Americans eat more protein than they need. Meals based on vegetables and whole grains can supply you with plenty of protein while increasing fiber and minimizing cholesterol and saturated fat.

Staple Foods to Consider

To help you get started, below is a list of basic supplies to keep on hand at all times. Even if you don't have all your menu details planned ahead of time, or if your schedule ends up busier than you had expected, having these types of solutions on

BOX 7-2

Go-To Grocery Items

Shop so that you always have these types of options on hand:

- precut/sliced, prewashed veggies;

- steamable bags of vegetables (limit sauces);

- ready-to-use brown rice, quinoa, ancient grains, canned beans;

- fruit cups/small cans of fruit in own juice (not syrup);

- low-fat or fat-free (skim) milk, Greek yogurt, cottage or ricotta cheese;

- reduced fat or light cheese and cheese sticks;

- single pack carrot sticks, cherry tomatoes, celery, and hummus;

- single-serve tuna/chicken; and

- containers to pack leftovers for quick/frozen lunches.

hand can encourage you to still prepare a Choose My Plate–style meal in a rush. Avoid convenience items that are also high in fat, such as rotisserie chicken, hot dogs, processed sandwich meats or packaged mixes, or saucy frozen dinners or vegetables.

Food Prep

When you come home from the grocery store, keep convenience in mind. It is worth taking the time to prepackage single servings of your favorite grab-and-go items (raw veggies, nuts, crackers, and snacks, for example) before you need them.

Keep convenient dinner options in mind: Ground meat can be formed into patties before it is frozen so they are ready to defrost and cook on a busy weeknight. Slice large chicken breasts into three- to four-ounce portions and freeze them in packs that will feed your family a single meal.

When you do have time to cook, think ahead. Every time you make a meal, make double or triple servings of everything. Pack leftovers for lunch options later in the week, or freeze for a quick single or family meal on a busy weeknight. *The trick is to pack and store leftovers in the serving sizes you will want to have on hand later.* As you get skilled in this technique, you can easily find yourself with two or three options at your fingertips or in the freezer for grab-and-go lunches or quick defrostable meals for a busy weeknight.

BOX 7-3

Freezer Ideas

- BBQ chicken
- Chili
- Stew
- Lean beef
- Shrimp
- Salmon in smaller bags
- Chicken breast (precut into 3-ounce portions)

Quick-Fix Meal Ideas

1 **Whole grain pasta is a quick and easy meal** to fix and can be finished in the time it takes to boil the water and cook the noodles (no salt or oil in the water, please!). Top with a low-fat bottled marinara sauce, sprinkle with parmesan cheese, and serve with a pre-mixed, bagged salad tossed with a low-fat salad dressing. If desired, simultaneously bake (covered) or gently boil a skinless chicken breast, chop it up, and add it to the sauce for a pseudo-chicken

parmesan. Or add a scoop of fat-free cottage or ricotta cheese for a lasagna-type effect. This freezes well.

2 **Whip up a batch of vegetarian chili**—several boxed mixes are now available and easy to prepare. Serve with quick-cooking brown rice, or ear of corn. This freezes well.

3 **Make your own pizza.** Use premade pizza crusts and canned pizza sauce. Top with pre-shredded low-fat mozzarella and parmesan cheese and any vegetables you desire. Or use a whole grain tortilla and toast in the oven or toaster oven for a quick meal for one.

4 **Make an omelet**—or fake it and scramble all your ingredients in the pan. Use two whole eggs, egg substitute, or two egg whites with one egg yolk. Use olive oil cooking spray to lightly coat the pan if needed to prevent sticking. Fill with your choice of vegetables (peppers, onions, broccoli, spinach, etc.). Lightly sprinkle with shredded reduced-fat cheese. Serve with whole grain toast or a baked sweet potato and enjoy.

5 **Use small whole grain flour tortillas,** canned black beans (rinse before use), canned chopped green chilies, reduced-fat cheese, low-fat plain Greek yogurt, and salsa. You'll have the fixings for a good, spicy meatless burrito. Roll up leftovers in singe tortillas and freeze individually. For a quick family meal on another night, defrost, add enchilada sauce, cover and bake.

6 **Soup's on!** Use up whatever leftovers are in your refrigerator—leftover turkey, chicken, vegetables, rice, pasta, etc. Add them to a can of ready-made soup (preferably clear broth and mostly vegetable), *or* to condensed tomato soup diluted with skim milk, *or* buy low-sodium chicken broth. Warm thoroughly, and serve with whole grain crackers or bread.

7 **Stir-fry in a nonstick skillet** coated with cooking spray: quickly brown lightly floured chicken breast pieces or shrimp. Add soy sauce, low-sodium chicken broth, ginger, and garlic to taste. Add a bag of frozen stir-fry veggies, or your choice of fresh vegetables (peppers, onions, broccoli, carrots, cauliflower, etc.) and bring to a boil. Cover and simmer until vegetables are tender-crisp. Serve over quick-cooking brown rice. This freezes well.

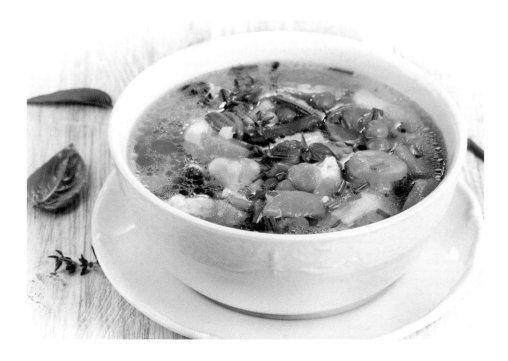

8 **Pop and top—a sweet potato,** that is. Medium sweet potatoes microwave in 4 to 8 minutes (scrub, and pierce several times with a fork first). Top with leftover stir-fry, vegetarian chili, or BBQ chicken for a one-dish meal.

9 **Mash hardboiled egg whites** with plain Greek yogurt, mustard, and relish for egg salad.

10 **Brown bag creatively.** Make extra of any of the above to take to work. Just package it up the night before while you're cleaning up dinner—then it's just a matter of remembering to grab the container as you leave the house the next day.

Eating Out

While you're actively losing weight, it's best that you prepare your own meals as much as possible. Eating away from home is generally incompatible with weight loss, and can sabotage maintenance. Here's why:

1 **You can't monitor the fat and calorie content of restaurant food.** There is often high-fat prep that you can't see, such as liberal basting of meats and veggies with fats.

2   **In restaurants, portions are almost always larger** than you would serve yourself at home. Restaurant portions have been getting even larger in recent years (even single item foods like bagels and muffins are getting bigger and bigger). The temptation to eat the whole thing can be overwhelming.

3   **Even though people are eating out more** than ever before, they still tend to regard the occasion as a reward, celebration, or opportunity to relax, often exercising less than their usual restraint in what they order and consume.

4   **The more recent appearance of things like** fast-casual restaurants and food halls has made eating out nearly a daily event for a vast number of Americans. While clever marketing (order half-items, but combine two of them for a discount) makes you think there are lower-calorie options, most people still generally select more calories than they need in a single meal.

5   **Although many restaurants are beginning to offer** a wider variety of healthier food choices, the serving sizes and the volume of high-fat "healthy fat" ingredients still tend to offer more calories than easily fit in your weight loss calorie plan.

6   **It's possible to make good choices,** but easier to say "oh forget it." The temptation of contending with the wide assortment of unhealthy choices makes for a challenging eating environment.

BEFORE, DURING, AND AFTER EATING OUT

After you have lost weight and are working on maintaining your new weight, you may be able to eat away from home more frequently, as long as control strategies are in place. Dietary control strategies for eating out can be divided into three phases: before, during, and after the event.

Before going out, follow these tips:

- **Eat regular meals.** Do not skip meals prior to eating out, or you may be tempted to "celebrate" your earlier restraint. If you plan to overindulge, eat lightly beforehand, but do eat something at the usual mealtime prior to the one eaten out. Have a low-fat snack or a glass of skim milk to help control unexpected, intense hunger between leaving home and ordering and receiving the meal.

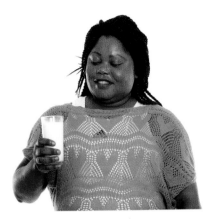

A glass of skim milk before a restaurant meal can curb hunger and help you make smarter menu choices

- **Look up the menu online.** Read carefully, looking for word clues about ingredients and food groups. Scan the menu for the signature indicator of lighter (or lower-calorie) meal selections (although even these may need to be downsized to an appropriate calorie level for your weight loss budget). Review your food groups meal plan as you browse the menu. Look for ways to select the appropriate number of servings from each food group that is planned for your Personal Plan of Action. Also utilize the posted calorie content of all your possible influences (the bread basket, appetizers, entrée, and desserts). Be aware of the calorie decisions you will need to make while you are there.

- **Know the lingo.** Menu descriptions are meant to sound enticing. But the preparation method can often make a huge difference in total calories of a single food. Words like *stuffed, breaded, fried, crispy, creamed, battered, smothered,* and *scalloped* are all indications that a food has most likely been prepared with added fat or additional indulgent ingredients, sauces, or cooking styles. Sauces like béarnaise, hollandaise, and alfredo are high in fat and calories. Look instead for words like *roasted, baked, broiled, poached, stir-fried, grilled,* and *steamed.*

- **Ask for what you want.** Most restaurants accommodate requests for fat-free or low-fat items and methods of preparation. If you want to skip the fries and get a double portion of steamed veggies instead, just say so when you order. You can even ask to create a "custom" meal using specific items that are on the menu. Start with the fresh house salad (dressing on the side, no bacon) and ask to add the grilled salmon or chicken from another menu page if that combo is not already offered. If you are going to someone's home, ask if you can bring a dish (something you know you can eat).

- **Plan ahead** whether there will be a "splurge item" in your meal. Decide on the spurge food you'll choose, then decide how many bites you'll need to be satisfied (many people find they only need two or three bites). Decide what less important choices you can avoid in order to make room for the splurge selection. For example, you may not want to "waste" calories on a glass of wine when you go to the restaurant that makes the very best french fries in the world. And you could share that one serving of fries with your friends so you can have a few without feeling like you need to eat the whole plate.

While you are out, try the following:

- **Avoid the "freebies" on the table** before your food order arrives. You can ask for these items to be eliminated or removed. If you do decide to eat the bread, however, eat it without the butter. Avoid fried tortilla chips. If it's a cracker basket, choose saltines or melba toast; the other crackers tend to be higher in fat and calories. Again, being mindful of the food groups and number of servings for this meal identified in your personal meal plan can put things into perspective while you are out.

- **Resist ordering an appetizer** unless it's a low-fat soup or salad, or a shrimp or seafood cocktail. Most other appetizers are fried or loaded with high-fat cheese.

- **Set limits for alcohol consumption.** If you do indulge in an alcoholic beverage, be sure to place your food order before you drink. Alcohol is high in calories, lowers your inhibitions (so that you may order and eat more than you intended), and temporarily shuts down the burning of fat.

- **When choosing what to order, avoid** fried foods, cream sauces and gravies, large servings of red meat, sour cream, and butter or margarine.

- **In many restaurants, liquid fat is poured over food** before it is "broiled." To avoid this, ask that it be broiled or grilled without fat (chicken, fish, crab cakes, and other foods can be broiled with water, lemon juice, or broth).

- **Order foods that are lower in fat**—for example, fish and chicken rather than pork or beef (keep preparation in mind), baked or boiled potatoes rather than french fries, tossed salad instead of coleslaw, and fresh fruit instead of cheesecake.

- **Look for nutrient-dense options.** Many restaurants are now making an effort to offer more nutritious selections. Look for whole grains such as quinoa, a variety of colorful vegetables, avocado, and salmon.

- **Ask that all dressings, condiments, gravies, and sauces** be served on the side so you can control how much you use. If a fat-free, low-calorie salad dressing is unavailable, order the regular on the side, dip your fork in the dressing first, and then spear a bite of salad. This cuts down dramatically on the amount of dressing used. Fresh lemon juice and red wine vinegar are also tasty on a salad. They can be used alone or to stretch a high-fat dressing.

- **Order à la carte** to avoid a full-course meal that may be too much for you.

- **Consider ordering** an appetizer-size portion of a favorite entrée.

- **Tell your dining companions ahead of time** that you will need help finishing your meal. When your meal is delivered, treat your plate as the serving dish by placing it near the center of the table. Use your bread plate to serve yourself only the amount you would like to eat. Then offer the serving dish to anyone else who would like some. Pack up any leftovers for another meal the next day.

- **Take your time.** Pay attention to both hunger and satiety (fullness) signals.

- **Don't try to match your dining partner(s)** bite for bite. They may be able to eat more than you can. You may feel that this is unfair, but your health is what you should be concentrating on.

- **To avoid "picking" and overeating,** be mindful to leave at least enough food on your plate to make a reasonable lunch for tomorrow. Order a "to go" box when you order your meal. Pack up leftovers right away to help avoid picking while you wait for others to finish.

- **If opting for dessert is a must,** consider selecting fruit or sorbet. If only something more indulgent will do, then share.

After eating out, particularly if you ate more than you planned, do the following:

- **Eat lightly for the next 24 hours** if the meal out was higher in calories than normal. You may wish to review your food groups meal plan for the next day and highlight a serving or two from several different food groups across the day to omit for one day to help balance out the extra calories.

- **Consider building in extra physical activity** to help compensate for any extra calories eaten.

BOX 7-4

Not All Salads Are Created Equal

When eating away from home, the word salad or vegetables isn't a guarantee that the menu item is a lower-calorie selection. Within the USDA food groups, foods in the vegetables group (dark green leafy veggies, carrots, tomatoes, broccoli, etc.) deliver taste, crunch, nutrient density, high fiber, high volume, color, and texture with very low calories. However, when finding these selections on a restaurant menu, in a salad bar, or even in the grocery store, it is wise to be on the lookout for other ingredients. What we put on those veggies can make a significant difference in calorie content. Beware that a 15-calorie cup of fresh broccoli florets could pack an additional 100-calorie wallop if topped with olive oil, cheese sauce, or similar high-fat add-on. In contrast, foods like chicken salad, potato salad, and Jell-O salad do not contain vegetables at all but are smothered in creamy mayonnaise-type dressings.

In restaurants, a salad often contains greens, carrots, and maybe a sliver of tomato but may also be loaded with bacon, cheese, nuts, berries, croutons, and high-fat salad dressing. Look for the calorie content of that salad listed on the menu. Generously assume that 3–4 cups of plain vegetables will contribute a maximum of 200 calories. All additional calories most likely come from nonvegetable (and potentially high-fat) sources. If a salad like this is an accompaniment to a main course, you do not need one that rings in at more than 500 calories. However, if you are eating a salad as your main course, it can be somewhat higher in calories, ideally if those extra calories come in the form of the addition of lean protein sources like poultry or fish.

- **Review any unplanned eating** you did and identify why it happened. Plan ways to avoid these problems in the future.

CHOOSING HEALTHFUL FOODS IN A VARIETY OF RESTAURANTS

Italian

- **Pasta is low in fat but high in refined white flour.** It is often smothered in cream, butter, and meat sauces. Order marinara, clam, or marsala sauces on whole grain pasta whenever possible. Better yet, spiralized squash is a great pasta alternative.

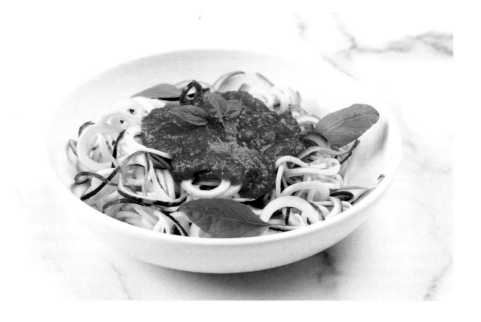

- **Try pasta primavera,** chicken cacciatore, or shrimp sautéed in white wine over linguini.

- **Avoid meat and cheese lasagna,** and dishes made with sausage.

- **Limit high-fat garlic bread.** Select one slice of plain Italian bread instead. You can use it to sop up your low-calorie marinara sauce.

- **Enjoy your pizza, but avoid meat toppings,** olives, and extra cheese. Try vegetable toppings instead (broccoli, green peppers, onions, carrots, and cauliflower) or fruit toppings like pineapple. If there are pools of oil visible on top of the pizza, soak them up with a folded paper napkin or a piece of bread (and place it to the side).

- **Choose thin crust pizza,** which has fewer calories than thick crust pizza.

- **Add a big garden salad** with low-fat or fat-free dressing to maximize volume of the meal.

Mexican
- **Stick to chicken fajitas,** black beans, vegetable tacos, soft tacos, or corn tortillas.

- **Sour cream, chips, nachos,** refried beans, guacamole, and all deep-fried foods such as chimichangas are high in fat and calories and should be eaten only in limited quantities. Salsa, on the other hand, can be poured over anything to add lots of flavor and very few calories.

French

- **Poached or steamed dishes** can be flavored with wine, as wine's calories largely evaporate with the alcohol when cooked. Oven-baked herbed chicken or poached salmon with capers are excellent choices.

- **Think twice about sauces** such as white sauce, hollandaise, béarnaise, or butter sauce. Order sauces on the side. Try dipping your fork into the rich sauce, then put the fork in your mouth so you get just a taste on your tongue, and follow with a forkful of the entrée without sauce. As with salad dressings, this trick cuts down dramatically on the amount of sauce you will consume while preserving a surprising amount of the taste.

Chinese

- **You have a lot to choose from** because a wide variety of vegetables are used in Chinese foods, and you can order entrées that are composed primarily of vegetables. If you wish to have meat, choose chicken or fish.

- **Avoid fried wontons,** egg rolls, twice-fried meat entrées like sweet and sour chicken, and any other fried foods.

- **Order clear soups** like rice broth.

- **Avoid fried rice.** Choose steamed white or brown rice instead, being mindful of portion size.

- **Ask that all dishes** be prepared with as little oil as possible.

American

- **Select small, lean cuts** of beef from the round or the loin.

- **Skip gravy and sauces,** including "au jus."

- **Have plain sweet potatoes.** Use no, or very little, sour cream, butter, or bacon.

- **Avoid fried and cheesy appetizers** like zucchini sticks, fried mozzarella sticks, and potato skins. Select clear broth soups, garden salads, or shrimp cocktail instead.

Fast Food/Fast-Casual Dining

- **Eat fast food only at mealtimes,** not as snacks. Do not supersize anything. Choose regular or small-size portions.

- **Order small burgers,** roast beef, grilled chicken, or broiled chicken with lettuce, onion, ketchup, and mustard. In most cases half the sandwich is enough for an entire meal.

- **Avoid mayonnaise-based sauces** and ask to be served an unbuttered bun.

- **Skip the french fries,** or perhaps split a small order with someone else. Blot off excess cooking oil by squeezing the fries gently with a paper napkin.

- **Most fast food restaurants offer salads.** Take advantage of this, but don't forget to focus on colorful vegetables. In some restaurants, low-fat beans or grilled chicken or fish can be added to make a complete meal. Avoid high-fat toppings such as bacon, cheese, croutons, sour cream, and so on. Use low-fat dressing or regular dressing (on the side); dip fork as described above.

- **Order diet soda, water,** unsweetened tea, or skim milk. Avoid milkshakes, sweet tea, flavored coffees, and regular soda.

- **For breakfast: avoid egg sandwiches with sausage or bacon.** Instead of big breakfast platters, have pancakes and juice or scrambled eggs with an English muffin. Request unbuttered ("dry") breakfast breads.

- **Chain restaurants are now required to post** nutrition information on the menu. Most info is also available online, so you can make your choices based on total calories and fat grams as well as personal preference.

Airline Foods

- **Preorder low-fat or diet meals** when possible.

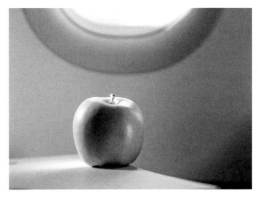

- **Try to stay on your regular eating schedule.** Plan for the time you are waiting in the airport, as well as the time you are actually in the air.

- **Bring low-fat, low-calorie foods from home.** Plan for bagged lunches and snacks just like you would on any other day.

- **Bring something to do** so you don't get bored when it is not your typical time to eat.

- **Avoid alcoholic beverages;** order tomato juice or diet soda instead. Drink lots of water to prevent dehydration and feeling empty. Treat yourself to the complementary hot tea or black coffee.

- **Refuse complementary peanuts** or other empty-calorie snack foods (such as stroopwafel or biscotti).

- **Remember, you don't have to eat it all** or eat it at all. Skip dessert.

Monitoring Strategies

Your personal strategy for selecting foods wisely and carefully should be based on your level of comfort with details and the amount of time you can devote to the task. You can be a "super analyst," a "partial analyst," or a "nonanalyst." Any of these strategies can help you succeed in losing weight. The one that is best for you depends on your personal style of dealing with tasks and problems. Which of these three styles most closely matches your preferred approach?

Strategy 1. *The Super Analyst:* "I feel most secure and in control of a situation when I know all the facts. I don't like making decisions with incomplete information. I sometimes delay making decisions I know I should make, not because

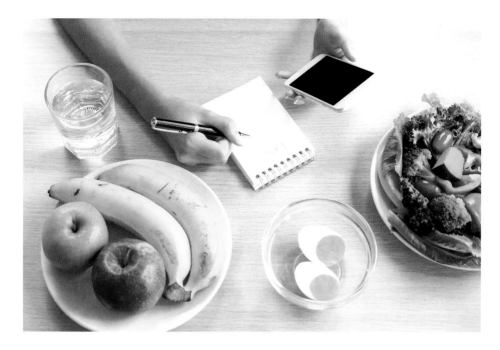

I'm really undecided, but because I don't want to take a chance that I'll make the wrong decision. I am good at detail work. I sometimes notice things other people don't. I tend to be a perfectionist."

Strategy 2. *The Partial Analyst:* "I like to understand the 'why' of things I'm doing and some of the facts, but I don't need all of the facts. I am comfortable with some gray areas but not with completely seat-of-the-pants decision-making. I am pretty good at detail work, but I'm not a real perfectionist."

Strategy 3. *The Nonanalyst:* "I make decisions mostly based on how I feel—on gut instinct. I'm comfortable if I don't have every bit of information relevant to the decision. In fact, I dislike having to hear all the so-called facts. If there's something I need to do that I don't have a choice about doing, just tell me what it is and don't bore me with the details. I tend to take things as they come, go with the flow, look at the big picture, and not sweat the details."

Which description applied most closely to you? Read on for a description of the three basic strategies. As you read, consider how you can utilize your preferred strategy in your Personal Plan of Action.

THE SUPER ANALYST

If you identified most closely with the first description, you will probably do best with the "super analyst" approach to weight loss—assuming that you're ready and willing to devote the hour or so a day that this strategy requires.

As a "super analyst," here are some steps you can follow to lose weight in a way that best suits your personal style:

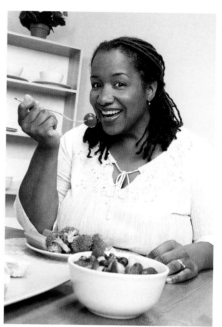

- **First, plan on eating no more than** three or four times each day.

- **Eat your first meal within** two hours of waking.

- **Try to eat only when you're hungry,** and practice stopping when you are *no longer hungry, or even well before you feel full.*

- **Choose and record your foods every day** using the food and activity log in the resources section or on a mobile phone app. Measure and record all foods as you eat them.

- **Instead of waiting until the end of the day** to see if you stayed within your food group budgets, tally the number of servings from each food group after each meal. By tracking as you go along, you can make sure that you meet your high-nutrient food group needs without going over your calorie budget. In other words, you'll know the number of servings from each food group that are left in the day *before* you eat your last meal. This will dictate the size and content of this meal.

In this way, you can maintain very tight control on a daily basis. If you are like most people, you'll probably eat more on some days than on others. It's really what happens *over time* that counts. If you find that indulgences creep in, don't despair. Each week you can total your daily caloric intake and average your weekly intake. You may find that you're meeting your budgets just fine, on average. In other words, if you overeat on one day, you can compensate on another day.

We suggest that you weigh yourself only one day per week, to avoid frustration. Try to weigh in on the same day each week, at approximately the same time.

Weigh yourself without clothing. Record your weekly weight using the weekly weigh-in log in your Personal Plan of Action. If, after two weeks, you are not meeting your weight loss goal, you will need to do one or more of these three things:

1 **Readjust your expectations**, particularly if you feel that you are doing all you can or wish to do.

2 **Adjust your personal eating plan.** Choose a lower calorie level with a corresponding food group pattern, but only if you won't feel desperately deprived. Don't dip below 1,200 calories if you are a woman or 1,500 calories if you are a man.

3 **Increase your physical activity.** This will burn more calories and create a bigger caloric deficit. You may do this either without further dietary modifications or in conjunction with additional dietary changes. In the next chapter, we will talk further about how to increase your daily movement and weekly exercise.

THE PARTIAL ANALYST, OR "ONE STEP AT A TIME, PLEASE"

If you identified most closely with the second description, you are best suited to the "partial analyst" approach.

In the role of partial analyst for weight loss, you will be making gradual changes in the degree of control and monitoring you use to achieve effective weight management. The first and simplest step is to limit your food choices using the distribution of servings from the food groups according to your daily calorie goal.

In the previous chapter, we looked at suggested daily food group menus. Each menu corresponds to a particular calorie range: 1,200–1,400, 1,400–1,600, 1,600–1,800, and 2,000–2,200. Begin your Personal Plan of Action by deciding to eat according to your personal food group pattern based on your targeted caloric intake:

- **Plan on eating no more than** three or four times per day.

- **Try to eat your first meal within** two hours of waking.

- **Practice eating only when you're hungry** and stop when you are *no longer hungry, not when you're full.*

- **Each day, use one daily food record.** Record foods as you eat them in the same way you did for your three-day evaluation. Assign your foods to the

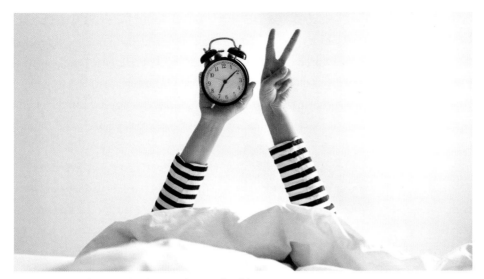
Try to eat your first meal within two hours of waking

appropriate category on the food groups part of the form. When it's time to eat your last meal of the day, refer to your food group totals and determine how many servings from each category you have left. Plan your last meal based on what and how much is left from each category.

Each day, continue recording all food intake on the food record and tallying total food group servings after each meal. At the end of one week, you will be able to average your results and compare them with your goals. Record your weight. If you are unsuccessful at meeting your weight loss goals despite your best efforts and compliance, then refer back to Strategy 1, "The Super Analyst," for instructions, since you are now in that category.

If after one or two weeks you are meeting your weight loss goals, then continue monitoring your intake according to your food group pattern only. If after two weeks you are not meeting your weight loss goal, proceed to the next decision step—you many need to refer back to Strategy 1 or increase your physical activity as described in chapter 8.

THE NONANALYST, OR "SHOW ME THE WAY"

If you identified most closely with the third description, you will probably do best with the nonanalyst, defined-diet approach. Refer back to the suggested menus from the previous chapter. For simplicity and convenience, choose and follow a menu as closely as possible based on your personal calorie budget. The daily pattern of food options corresponds to the correct food group pattern for that calorie range. Most foods within a menu food category are roughly equivalent to one another in fat and calories and were chosen based on familiarity, bulk, preference, and convenience. The idea on any given day is to glance down the appropriate meal or snack column and choose the recommended number of servings from each food group in that column. Be careful to follow the portion size as precisely as possible and follow the "key points" at the bottom of the page to ensure a *weekly average* of caloric intake necessary to achieve your weight loss goals. Each food category has five to seven options, so if you vary your choices each day, you will have a satisfying array of daily combinations. Be creative by combining and preparing your food allowances together with a variety of herbs, spices, and low-fat cooking techniques.

Weigh yourself only one day per week. Stay with the same day each week, weighing in at approximately the same time, without clothing. Record your weight on the weekly weigh-in log. If after one to two weeks you are not losing the desired amount of weight despite your best efforts, then you can either step down to the next-lower calorie level and its associated menu, increase physical activity, or both.

Action Items

- Take the time to draft a meal plan for at least the next three to four days and make a shopping list for any ingredients you need.

- While at the grocery store, shop according to food group, using the strategies discussed in this chapter, including the "shopping cart analysis."

- Review food labels when shopping for packaged foods, and choose low-fat and low-sugar options.

- Select a monitoring strategy that best fits you and update your Personal Plan of Action according to this strategy.

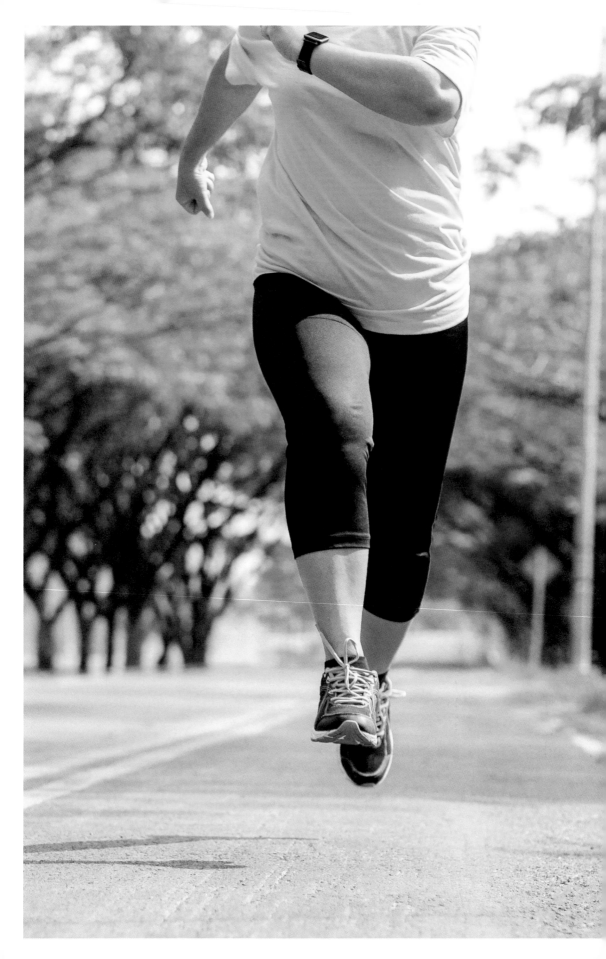

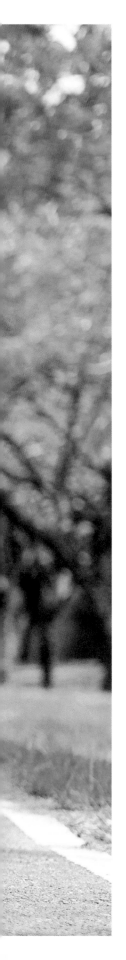

CHAPTER 8

Designing Your Daily Movement and Weekly Exercise Plan

IN THIS CHAPTER, WE WILL:

- **explain** why physical activity can make or break your weight loss and health goals,

- **describe** four ways you can assess your current levels of physical activity and fitness,

- **outline** how you can design your activity plan (with daily movement and exercise), and

- **offer** you our top ten helpful hints for sustaining your commitment to physical activity.

BY NOW YOU HAVE COMPLETED the behavior and dietary portions of your Personal Plan of Action. You've learned that what you eat and how much you eat both matter for your overall health and weight loss efforts. These considerations are in what we call the "intake" part of your weight loss program. But as we alluded to previously, your complete plan for long-term weight loss and weight maintenance does not stop there. The *energy expenditure* side of the equation also matters for your weight loss (or gain). This is where physical activity—both daily functional movement and weekly exercise—matters.

In this chapter, we will explain how you can make a physical activity plan that is truly right for you—and include it in your Personal Plan of Action. You'll discover that the latest science shows us that daily movement and weekly exercise *both* matter for your weight loss and weight management efforts, as well as your overall quality of life. You'll learn how you can create a physical activity plan that is right for you, and how our helpful hints can support you in committing to your plan over time.

BOX 8-1

The most effective way to lose weight is to reduce the intake of calories and increase caloric expenditure through physical activity—daily movement and weekly exercise.

FIGURE 8-1

Physical activity and your health

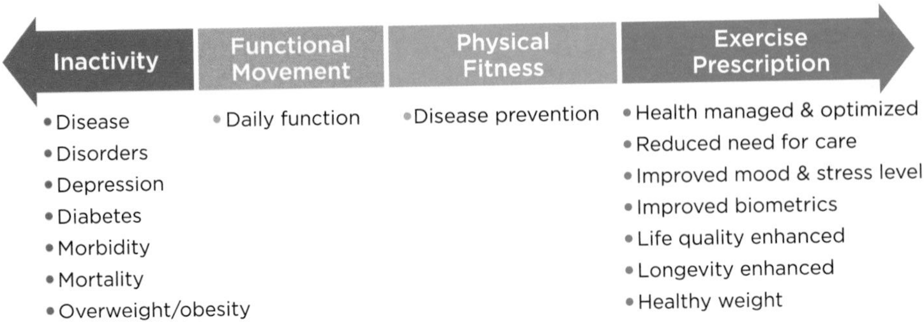

Inactivity	Functional Movement	Physical Fitness	Exercise Prescription
• Disease	• Daily function	• Disease prevention	• Health managed & optimized
• Disorders			• Reduced need for care
• Depression			• Improved mood & stress level
• Diabetes			• Improved biometrics
• Morbidity			• Life quality enhanced
• Mortality			• Longevity enhanced
• Overweight/obesity			• Healthy weight

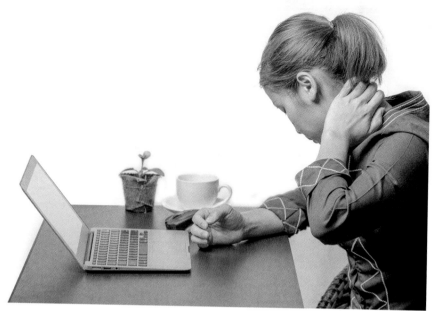

Sitting too much can be detrimental to your health

Many people focus their physical activity planning on exercise (cardiovascular training, strength training, and flexibility work) and forget the importance of daily movement. Both are key to weight management and weight loss, as well as overall health—because movement and exercise have their own risks for your health and well-being. As shown in figure 8.1, being inactive (and sitting too much) can cause or worsen up to 23 different mental and physical health outcomes. Exercising too little (being sedentary or underactive due to our busy modern lifestyles) can cause muscles to atrophy and bones to become weaker (more porous) over time.

On the other hand, moving more throughout the day, and getting the weekly recommendation of exercise, offers enormous benefits to the mind and body, your health, and your well-being. Physical activity has been shown to reduce anxiety and depression, improve mood, decrease cravings for sweets (sugar), and improve sleep—which can in turn improve the body's ability to metabolize food as fuel. For this reason, we have chosen to guide you in the creation of both movement and exercise plans in this chapter on physical activity—to support you in creating daily goals for both (in keeping with modern exercise guidelines and the latest research on the benefits of physical activity and the hazards of physical inactivity).

FIGURE 8-2

Physical activity outcomes

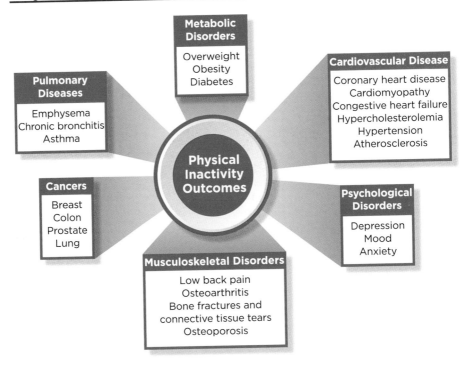

What Does "Physical Activity" Really Mean?

Although many people think of physical activity as being just another phrase referring to exercise, there is actually a large range of options on the physical activity spectrum. *Physical activity is any movement that requires your body to expend energy.* Exercise is a physical activity that is planned and intentional, such as running on a treadmill or playing a game of tennis. Functional (daily) activity includes the basic movements you do throughout your day and can vary in intensity (just like exercise). Functional activity can be as light as standing (instead of sitting) during your workday or emptying the dishwasher, or can increase with intensity and caloric expenditure. When you take a break at your desk to stretch your legs and arms, walk from your car to your workplace, take the stairs instead of the elevator, or dance at a wedding, you are engaging in different forms and intensities of functional movement (sometimes called activities of daily living, because they are so much a part of our daily routine).

Our modern lifestyle has created a world in which we all move less. And yet, recent research has shown that all forms of physical activity—light functional movement and challenging exercise—are important to maintaining the quality and length of our lives. For example, research has shown that sedentary jobs (that require long bouts of sitting) can cause as much as a 16-pound weight gain (on average) in the first year of employment. Other research examined people who were sedentary (inactive) during the day and found that participants who exercised regularly but sat more than six hours per day had a higher risk of premature death. These are just a few of many reasons why sitting has been called "the new smoking," and why both exercise and daily movement are recommended for the physical activity portion of your Personal Plan of Action.

Although it can be difficult to increase the amount of time you are moving throughout the day and are exercising weekly, we also know that it really is worth it. Both forms of physical activity will help you reduce weight gain, and improve your health and quality of life. Recent research has shown that both daily movement and weekly exercise help us to manage stress, sleep better, improve mood, and think more clearly and creatively. So, let's get moving on your physical activity plan.

Physical Activity Planning Step 1: Assessment

In order to know where you are going, it is important to know where you are. That is where the self-assessment process comes in—it helps us to determine where you are today with regard to physical activity (both weekly exercise and daily movement) and fitness level so that you'll be able to set goals that are right for you in both categories. Let's now go through a physical activity self-assessment to discover what your current level of physical activity is today. With this foundation, we can set appropriate goals for you in your Personal Plan of Action.

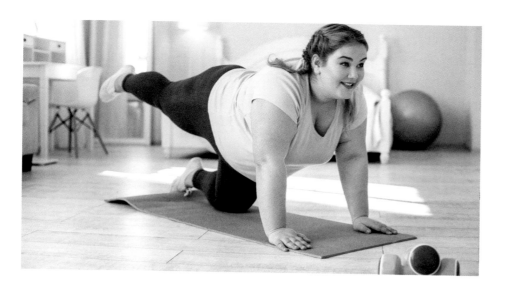

PHYSICAL ACTIVITY PLANNING ASSESSMENT 1: MEDICAL CLEARANCE FOR EXERCISE

First, meet with your health care provider to receive clearance to begin your physical activity plan. It's important to do this before you begin any exercise program, to make sure that any exercise or movement in your plan is also medically advised (and not dangerous for your unique medical situation). That's because physical activity can be much like medication—one size does not fit all, and the right "dose" for one person may not be right for another person. Many people, who would never dream of sharing a prescription medication, think it is perfectly normal to copy someone else's fitness or physical activity routine—when in fact that can be just as dangerous. In addition, certain medical conditions (like heart disease) bring with them medical concerns for exercise. For example, people with cardiovascular disease should only begin their exercise plan with medical permission, and when they do so, they must start at a light intensity level to avoid undue harm. When you ask for physical activity clearance from your medical provider, be sure to ask him or her for their guidance on your unique restrictions for both daily movement and physical activity.

PHYSICAL ACTIVITY PLANNING ASSESSMENT 2: YOUR CURRENT FITNESS LEVEL AND ADAPTATION

When you meet with your medical provider, he or she may measure your current level of fitness precisely and scientifically using special equipment not available to most individuals. This assessment will help you to know more about how your body will respond to exercise and physical activity. Knowing your current fitness level will help you to determine how light, moderate, or vigorous your exercise planning should be, and how much (or little) you will need to increase the amount of movement you are engaged in throughout your day.

In addition to learning more about your fitness level through your medical assessment, you can also assess your fitness level using cardiovascular assessment equipment found in your local gym or fitness facility. There are also fitness assessment tools that you can purchase independently, but these are not required for the success of your physical activity plan.

PHYSICAL ACTIVITY ASSESSMENT 3: YOUR PHYSICAL ACTIVITY LEVEL = MOVEMENT + EXERCISE

Equipped with an understanding of how your medical condition(s) and fitness level may impact your physical activity planning, you can now complete the third step of

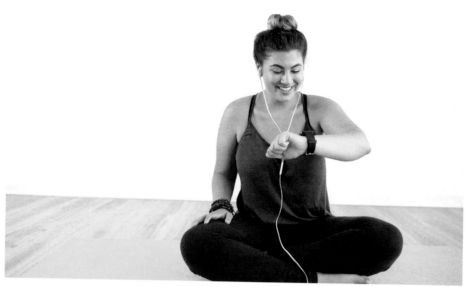
Many people find wearable fitness trackers helpful

the assessment: determining your physical activity level. In this phase, you will take an honest appraisal of how much you are (or aren't) moving daily and exercising weekly.

If you happen to own a personal activity tracker, like a Fitbit, this step is relatively easy. Simply record your standing versus sitting behavior (as a measure of your daily movement) and your step count and activity intensity level (as measures of your exercise patterns). Some mobile devices can also track these patterns. Using these technology tools can help you assess your current activity level to inform your physical activity plan in your Personal Plan of Action, and they can also help you record and track your activity patterns over time.

Although these technology tools are accurate ways to assess your physical activity today and track your progress over time, they do not tell your whole physical activity story. That is because they do not (usually) determine how you are or aren't meeting current guidelines for the three types of recommended exercise: cardiovascular activity, strength, and flexibility. Current guidelines recommend that people who are beginning or restarting their exercise program should start with slow and moderate intensity activity, and work toward a total of 150 minutes (2.5 hours) of moderate activity per week. They also recommend one to two strength training and five flexibility training sessions per week. Most fitness trackers cannot distinguish between the types of exercise or movement you are engaged in—but some do offer you the ability to manually enter your activity.

We therefore recommend that in addition to using a wearable pedometer to track your activity, you also complete the Rapid Assessment of Physical Activity designed by researchers from the University of Washington. This series of seven simple questions can easily help you determine if you are meeting current physical activity guidelines. As you can see in table 8.1, the assessment shows you how you can distinguish between functional daily movement and activities of daily living (which they describe as light activity), and exercise (which they describe as moderate and vigorous activity).

After you have taken a moment to learn the distinctions between light activity (daily movement) and moderate and vigorous activity (exercise), you can then reflect on your current activity level and complete the chart (in table 8.2).

TABLE 8-1

Rapid assessment of physical activity (RAPA)

Physical activities are activities where you move and increase your heart rate above its resting rate. You can do these activities for pleasure, work, or transportation.

The following questions address the amount and intensity of physical activity you usually do. The intensity of the activity is related to the amount of energy you use to do these activities.

Examples of physical activity intensity levels:

Light Activities
- Your heart beats slightly faster than normal
- You can talk and sing

Walking leisurely

Stretching

Vacuuming or light yard work

Moderate Activities
- Your heart beats faster than normal
- You can talk but not sing

Fast walking

Aerobics class

Strength training

Gentle swimming

Vigorous Activities
- Your heart rate increases a lot
- You can't talk or your talking is broken up by large breaths

Stair machine

Jogging or running

Tennis, racquetball, pickleball, or badminton

SOURCE: *University of Washington Health Promotion Research Center, © 2006. Funded in part by the Centers for Disease Control and Prevention.*

As you can see, the RAPA 1 focuses on your daily movement and cardiovascular activity, with scores ranging from 1 to 7. RAPA 2 focuses on your strength and flexibility activity—the two remaining components of your exercise regimen (beyond cardiovascular activity, or cardio).

Using the score sheet found below, you can assess your current level of activity—accounting for movement and exercise (cardio, strength, and flexibility) goals. You can then use this assessment to inform your physical activity plan in your Personal Plan of Action.

TABLE 8-2

How physically active are you?

(Check one answer on each line)

Does this accurately describe you?

RAPA 1	1	I rarely or never do any physical activities.	Yes ☐	No ☐
	2	I do some *light* or *moderate* physical activities, but not every week.	Yes ☐	No ☐
	3	I do some *light* physical activity every week.	Yes ☐	No ☐
	4	I do *moderate* physical activities every week, but less than 30 minutes a day or 5 days a week.	Yes ☐	No ☐
	5	I do *vigorous* physical activities every week, but less than 20 minutes a day or 3 days a week.	Yes ☐	No ☐
	6	I do 30 minutes or more a day of *moderate* physical activities, 5 or more days a week.	Yes ☐	No ☐
	7	I do 20 minutes or more a day of *vigorous* physical activities, 3 or more days a week.	Yes ☐	No ☐
RAPA 2 3=both 1 and 2	1	I do activities to increase muscle *strength*, such as lifting weights or calisthenics, once a week or more.	Yes ☐	No ☐
	2	I do activities to improve *flexibility,* such as stretching or yoga, once a week or more.	Yes ☐	No ☐

ID #:   **Today's date:**

SOURCE: *University of Washington Health Promotion Research Center, © 2006. Funded in part by the Centers for Disease Control and Prevention.*

Scoring Instructions

RAPA 1: Aerobic

To score, choose the question with the highest score with an affirmative response. Any number less than 6 is suboptimal.

For scoring or summarizing categorically:

Score as sedentary:

1   I rarely or never do any physical activities.

Score as underactive:

2   I do some light or moderate physical activities but not every week.

Score as underactive regular—light activities:

3   I do some light physical activity every week.

Score as underactive regular:

4   I do moderate physical activities every week but less than 30 minutes a day or 5 days a week.

5   I do vigorous physical activities every week but less than 20 minutes a day or 3 days a week.

Score as active:

6   I do 30 minutes or more a day of moderate physical activities, 5 or more days a week.

7   I do 20 minutes or more a day of vigorous physical activities, 3 or more days a week.

RAPA 2: Strength and Flexibility

I do activities to increase muscle strength, such as lifting weights or calisthenics, once a week or more. (1)

I do activities to improve flexibility, such as stretching or yoga, once a week or more. (2)

Both (3)

None (0)

SOURCE: *University of Washington Health Promotion Research Center, © 2006. Funded in part by the Centers for Disease Control.*

PHYSICAL ACTIVITY ASSESSMENT 4: THE TALK TEST OF EXERTION LEVEL DURING PHYSICAL ACTIVITY

In addition to completing the medical clearance, fitness level, and activity level assessments *before* you exercise, we also recommend that you conduct an additional assessment *during* exercise. It is called the Talk Test—and you can use it during exercise to determine whether you are meeting or exceeding your exertion (intensity level) goals so you can adjust your intensity of effort accordingly. Although the Talk Test is simple and easy, it has been scientifically shown to be consistent with technology-based assessments and procedures.

Here is how you can perform the Talk Test to track your exertion (effort) level: when you move or exercise, try to talk. How well you can or cannot talk determines your intensity level:

- If you can talk easily (in paragraphs), you are exercising *lightly*.

- If you can talk with some difficulty (in sentences), you are exercising *moderately*.

- If you can only talk in bullet points (not full sentences), you are exercising *vigorously*.

- If you cannot talk, you are exercising at an *extreme rate of exertion and you should cease immediately* (and call 911 if breathing does not return swiftly).

BOX 8-2

Four Key Factors

In this section, we have learned how to assess four key factors that will influence and inspire your physical activity plan:

1 **medical needs** for exercise: your provider's guidance for what to avoid

2 **fitness level** (readiness): how ready your body is to adapt to or increase activity

3 **frequency of activity** (standing and steps): your current movement and exercise patterns

4 **type of activity** (RAPA 1 and 2): how you are (or aren't) meeting movement and exercise guidelines (that is, distinguishing types of activity: cardiovascular, strength, and flexibility)

We recommend you track these four key factors, and any other factors you find relevant, in your Personal Plan of Action. You can then use this data (information) to track your progress over time.

Physical Activity Planning Step 2: Planning Daily Movement

With your assessments complete, you can now start your physical activity planning. This process begins with a reflection on the findings from your assessments, as well as goal setting aimed at meeting current guidelines for physical activity. If your assessment indicated that you are deconditioned (have a low fitness level) or are sedentary or underactive, it will be important for you to focus on the important "win" of getting started by setting small, measurable, achievable, realistic, and time-bound (SMART) goals so that you do not become overwhelmed with an "all or nothing" approach. If your assessment indicated that you are currently conditioned and active, your goal setting might focus on the "win" of sustaining your commitment to activity to increase your caloric expenditure to coincide with your weight loss or weight management goals. Whatever your win, the most important part is that you commit to creating a plan that takes you from where you are today (as found in the assessment) to where you want to be. This way, you can meet your weight loss and weight management goals, work toward meeting exercise guidelines, and improve your overall quality of life.

Let's begin by designing your daily movement plan. What do we mean by daily movement? Just as there are many ways that you can exercise, there are many ways that you can move more and sit less throughout your day. When you choose to not sit still, stand more, sit on an activity ball, sit in an active (not slouched) posture, complete daily activities and chores, and otherwise "sneak" movement into your day, you get "credit" for daily movement. In our work with patients we have found that many inactive people find it easier to begin and stick with daily movement than it is for formal exercise. We encourage you to plan for both types of physical activities in your Personal Plan of Action for weight management.

If your assessment findings found that you are sedentary or underactive, take a moment to reflect on how you could get more movement into your day through activities of daily living. For example, you could set a timer to help you remember to get up from your desk regularly and walk around or start taking the stairs instead of the elevator. The more you can sneak movement into your day like a "healthy snack," the more calories you will be spending. Here are a few ways to snack on movement:

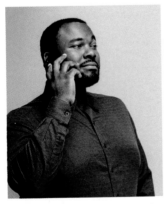

Increase your daily movement by standing during phone calls

- **stand while talking** on the phone (instead of sitting),

- **get up and change the channel** instead of using the remote control,

- **use a push mower** instead of a self-propelled or riding mower,

- **grow your own vegetables** or plant a flower garden, and

- **take out the garbage.**

What are some other activities that you can think of to increase your daily movement—and your daily calorie burning? Select the activities from the list above, and add your own as they occur to you, to your Personal Plan of Action.

Many people find it fun to brainstorm ways to increase these types of activities of daily living throughout the day. This is because they do not require setting aside a large block of time—eliminating the excuse of "busyness" that we often hear when people explain their lack of exercise. If you can take a break to grab a snack, you can take a break to move more and sit less. The good news is that the more you sneak these types of movement snacks into your day, the more calories you will burn (not keep)!

In addition to increasing these activities of daily living, another strategy for bringing movement into your day is to find "good excuses" to walk more. A substantial contributor to the increase in obesity in this country is a decrease in walking. We are much less physically active than previous generations of Americans were. Can you help counteract this trend? Perhaps you could use public transportation to get to work—helping the environment as you burn more calories walking to and from the bus stop or train station. Side benefits include reduced

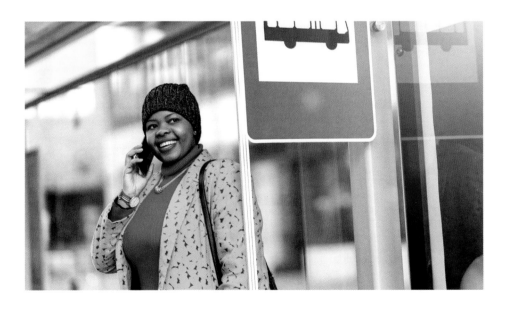

stress (no driving in traffic) and the ability to catch up on reading or work while being transported. You can also get off one stop early to work some extra walking into your day. If you must drive to work, you can choose to park farther away from your destination instead of searching for the closest parking spot. You'll be doing a kind deed for those who have mobility challenges (allowing them to park closer) as you meet your own daily activity goals.

Once you have decided what types of activities you would like to commit to in your Personal Plan of Action, you can then review them to see if they are giving you "credit" for daily movement, and also for what is called the three planes of motion. These three planes are used to describe the ways our bodies were built to move. We are healthier when we do not limit our movements to only one plane (as our modern lifestyles often do) but instead make a point to move regularly in all three planes (see figure 8.3).

FIGURE 8-3

The three planes of motion

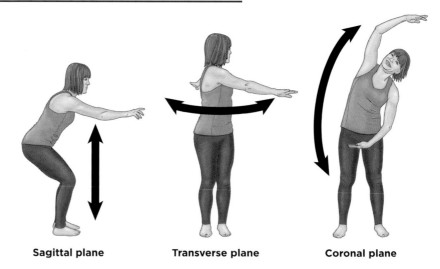

| Sagittal plane | Transverse plane | Coronal plane |

MINDFUL MOVEMENTS

Many people need a simple way to make sure they are getting all three planes of motion into their day. Using a mindful movement checklist can help ensure that you are moving all of your major joints, which in turn ensures that you are engaging all of your major muscle groups daily and that you move in all three planes of motion. The checklist, as designed by Dr. Carmack, is purposely simple so that you can easily use it to plan and manage the movement you bring into your workday or school day. You can use it to ensure that you are getting enough movement into the physical activity plan in your Personal Plan of Action. To help you carry out this plan, remember the numeric "2/4/6/8/10"—that is your checklist to remember your major joints and the ways they were built to move (in all three planes of motion):

2 (Elbows and Knees)

Your elbows and knees are hinge joints. That means that they move in two directions: (1) flexion (folding or bending) and (2) extension (opening or lengthening). Examples of moving your elbows and knees in two directions would be a squat (knees) or a bicep curl or pushup (elbows), as shown in figure 8.4.

FIGURE 8-4

Squat (a) and pushup (b)

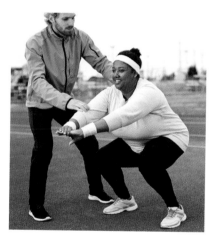 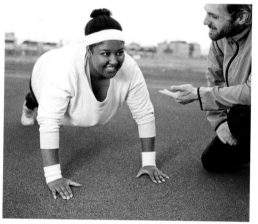

4 (Spine)

Your spine moves in four (primary) directions and also can lengthen (like a bendy straw that you stretch and turn). It is important to lengthen first, before moving in the four directions of the spine, to give yourself the most efficient movement possible:

1 forward in flexion (like a cat or ab crunch),
2 backward in extension (like a backbend or superman lift),
3 rotating (turning to hear someone behind you), and
4 sideways in lateral flexion (curling the side of your body to pick up a suitcase to your side).

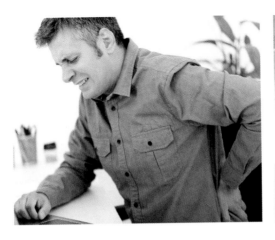
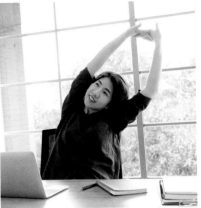

Most of our days are spent only in the cat (curl or slouched) position of spinal flexion.

This can cause back pain, muscle atrophy, and other health problems over

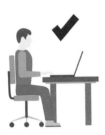

✔

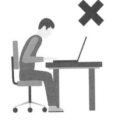

✖

Correct Position   Incorrect Position

time—because we aren't moving backward, sideways, or turning enough as our bodies were meant to do. In addition, slouching and sitting passively all day long without taking breaks diminishes the number of calories you burn per hour and per day. So, enjoy being "active" when you sit by moving the spine throughout the day and standing and moving whenever you can.

6 (Hips)

Your hips move in six directions and can also draw a circle (which is called circumduction). You can think of the six major directions of movement for the hip as:

1 flexion (folding at the hip, such as sitting in a chair or raising your leg to march),
2 extension (opening the hip, such as standing up),
3 external rotation (turning out the hip like a number 4 stretch or tree pose in yoga, as shown in figure 8.5a),
4 internal rotation (like snow plow in skiing, as shown in figure 8.5b),
5 abduction (lifting the leg sideways to the left or right; like a jumping jack out), or

6 adduction (returning the legs back to your center; like a jumping jack back into place with feet coming together, as shown in figure 8.5c).

When we sit too much and don't move enough, we are again stuck in the sagittal plane. Our hip muscles get tight and weak, which in turn starts to pull our torso forward and cause back pain and other health challenges over time, as well as hip muscle atrophy. We also have less ability to react to sudden slips and have a higher risk of falling. This is why it's important to take time to move the hips daily in six directions.

FIGURE 8-5

Hip movements

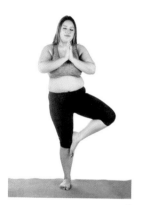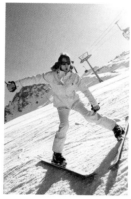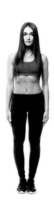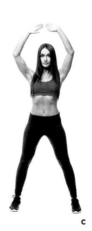

a   b   c

8 (Shoulders)
Your shoulders (specifically, where the arm meets the torso) move in eight directions:

1 forward into flexion (like you would when you put your arm up to stop someone from coming close to you),

2 backward into extension (like you would when you reach behind you to get something out of your back pocket),

3 turning out into external rotation (when you spin your biceps to face away from the middle of your body, toward the sides of the room),

4 turning into internal rotation (when you roll your biceps and thumbs inward to face toward your body),

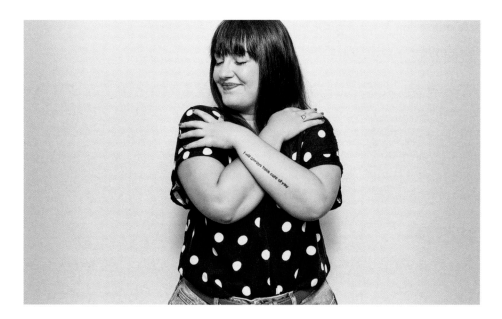

5   moving sideways into abduction out left or right (like the first part of a jumping jack),

6   moving sideways into adduction (like the return part of a jumping jack),

7   opening out to the sides of you from your chest (like you would open up for
a hug), and

8   folding in to cross your torso (like you would give yourself a hug).

Our arms are often stuck in the sagittal plane (flexion) and in internal rotation (as we type, eat, and drive). This means that the shoulders get overstretched in the back (the muscles that open us up) and we may lose our range of motion (needed when we reach for an item on a high shelf). Moving your arms throughout the day in all eight planes of motion can help to prevent this reduction in flexibility (range of motion)—and improve your ability to engage in other activities of daily living.

10 (Fingers and Toes)

The ten reminds us to move all ten fingers and all ten toes regularly—as these can get tighter as we age or spend less time out of shoes and more time typing at computers. The ten also reminds us to move at least ten minutes per day, as studies have shown this could add up to ten years to our lives.

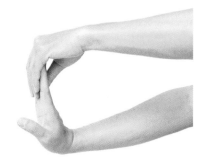

FIGURE 8-6

Warrior pose

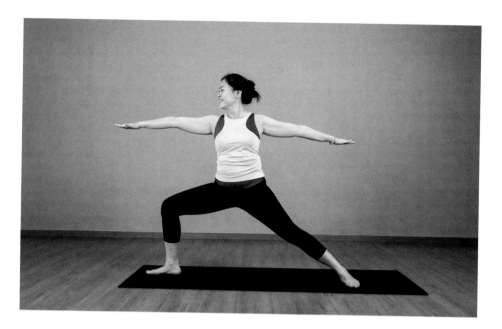

Applying Mindful Movements

To better understand just how we can actually use mindful movements, let's apply them. One way to do so is to take a look at a movement and see how it tracks against the "2/4/6/8/10" checklist (to see which joints you get "credit" for moving). In fact, you can even make a game with yourself to see how few movements or poses it takes you to complete your 2/4/6/8/10 (three planes of motion requirements), although this is less desired if you are trying to burn more calories by moving more and sitting less.

For example, figure 8.6 shows a woman performing Warrior 2 pose—a common movement (pose) in yoga classes. It is a great pose because it gets us out of our chair, and gets all of our joints moving (that is, we get credit for 2's, 6's, *and* 8's).

When we look at this pose from a mindful movement checklist (2/4/6/8/10) standpoint, we find that she gets credit for moving some joints but not all, as follows:

2's. She gets credit for the 2's for the knee because one leg is bent and the other is straight. She does not get credit for moving the arm, so later in the day she'll need to do some pushups or bicep curls to complete her 2's daily requirement for the mindful movement checklist.

4's. She does *not* get credit for moving the spine, because she is in a long yet neutral position. That means that it is not curled, bent backward, turned, or slanted to the side. (This also means that she'll have to keep practicing later in the day to get in her daily dose of the 4's—the movement of the spine.)

6's. She gets credit for *all* six hip actions! The bent leg is folded at the hip (flexion), while the long leg is extended (extension). The bent knee leg is turned out (external rotation), while the long leg is internally rotated (internal rotation). Both legs had to step out (away from midline, abduction) to get into the pose, and both legs will need to return to center (adduction).

8's. She gets credit for two of the eight shoulder actions: abduction (raising the arms out to the side) and adduction (bringing the arms back to the body—after the pose, not pictured). This means that she may want to do another pose after this that helps her get more range of motion in her shoulders, like "the butterfly stroke" from swimming.

What this 2/4/6/8/10 mindful movement review tells us is that in order to get our requirement for all three planes of motion (by completing the 2/4/6/8/10 mindful movement checklist requirements), we need to move a bit more. Specifically, we'll need to move in ways that turn the hip out and in and take it side to side (to meet the 6's) and move the shoulder out and in, side to side, and open and closed (like a hug).

In this section, we have learned many ways that you can bring more movement into your everyday life—both to increase your caloric expenditure (to lose or manage weight) and to improve your health (by reducing the risks of physical inactivity). We learned that there are three primary ways to ensure that you are moving well throughout the day, which you can build into the physical activity portion of your *Personal Plan of Action*. They are as follows:

1 sneak more activities of daily living into your day—like movement "snacks";

2 find ways to increase the amount you walk—parking far away or taking public transit; and

3 move in all three planes of motion—making sure you are moving all of your major joints (and muscle groups) by using the mindful movement "2/4/6/8/10" checklist.

Now that you have a plan in place for your daily movement, it's time to plan out your weekly exercise. Let's go there next.

Physical Activity Planning Step 3: Planning Exercise

Some people enjoy exercising. Whether it's bicycling, swimming, running, or lifting weights, they enjoy doing things that keep them moving. But there are also many people who do not find physical activity enjoyable. Since they don't like to exercise, they naturally wonder whether they really need to bother with it, or think of it as "just another thing they should be doing but they're not." Other people who want to start or restart an exercise program worry that they're too out of shape to begin or get back to it. Still others genuinely want to exercise but find it difficult to fit exercise into their daily routine. If you can relate to any of these sentiments, this chapter is here to guide you. We want to help you get past these concerns so you become more physically active and, as a result, meet and manage your weight loss goals.

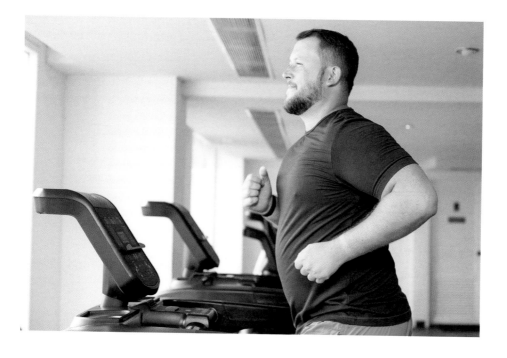

There are three important elements in any physical activity planning effort:

1 regularity: establishing a routine for exercising daily and weekly,

2 duration: being realistic about how much time you can weave activity into your day, and

3 persistence: sustaining your commitment over time (planning ahead for change).

We recommend that you weave these three elements into your plan for exercise.

Current exercise guidance recommends that you commit to 150 minutes of moderate exercise per week if you are getting started—evolving to 300 minutes over time (as you become more physically active). It may seem daunting to think about how you'll go about getting to those goals (especially if you are not exercising today and scored as either sedentary or underactive in your assessment). But do not be discouraged. Fortunately, there is a very easy-to-remember framework (checklist) that you can use to determine "how" you will work up to these goals of meeting weekly exercise requirements. It is called the FITT principle, and it refers to the components of your exercise plan listed in box 8-3.

BOX 8-3

Keeping "FITT"

F: Frequency per week
I: Intensity
T: Type
T: Time

Personal trainers are taught to use this framework when they create exercise plans for patients, but you can use it in your own exercise planning as part of your Personal Plan of Action. Let's take a moment to work through each element so you can see how they work together—like a team—to make sure you have a strong exercise plan that is truly right for you.

FREQUENCY (F): HOW OFTEN ARE YOU EXERCISING WEEKLY (NUMBER OF TIMES PER WEEK)?

- **If you aren't exercising now:**
  - set a goal for exercise two times per week at moderate intensity and
  - choose an activity that you enjoy or ask someone to join you to make it fun.

- **If you are exercising now:**
  - ◆ either increase the frequency (work up to five times per week) or
  - ◆ proceed to intensity, type, and time considerations below.

INTENSITY (I): WHEN YOU EXERCISE, WHAT IS YOUR AVERAGE INTENSITY?

- **If you are exercising at a light level,** try moderate activity for part of your session (unless medically advised not to do so) and also proceed to type.

- **If you are exercising at a moderate level,** try vigorous activity for part of your session (unless medically advised not to do so) and also proceed to type.

- **If you are exercising at a vigorous level,** proceed to the next item (time).

Please note: In order to achieve a high level of fitness, you need to exercise in your target zone for at least 20 to 30 minutes at least every other day. To burn calories, however, *any* extra physical activity will benefit you. While you may not lose very much weight by taking a leisurely stroll each day after dinner, you will at least be improving your lifestyle, and maybe the next time you can stroll a bit farther or a bit faster.

TYPE (T): WHAT TYPE OF EXERCISE ARE YOU ENGAGING IN?

Ideally, your plan should include your "macro movements":

- **cardiovascular activity** (two to five times per week)—challenge your heart rate (moderate or vigorous);

- **strength training** (one to two times per week)—build muscle and bone density and increase metabolism. You can use free weights, equipment, or "body weight" activity such as yoga; and

- **flexibility training** (one to five times per week)—increase your flexibility (range of motion) and improve your overall sense of well-being (since stretching releases "feel good" and stress-reducing hormones).

If you are relatively sedentary, it is probably best to begin with a progressive walking program, since this will provide you with a safe intensity of physical activity and still provide fitness and calorie-burning benefits. A walking program can grow with your growing level of fitness. Walking can lead to jogging or running, and can be done indoors (on a treadmill), in an enclosed public space (like a mall or an office complex), or outdoors. Walking can be a social activity, done with friends or family, or enjoyed alone as a time to think and relax. We'll use walking as an example in later sections to discuss how to schedule your formal exercise periods, how to use warm-up and cool-down exercises, and how to progressively increase the frequency, duration, and intensity of your exercise sessions.

Even if you have already been exercising regularly and are at least moderately fit, a progressive walking program can provide a structured aerobic workout and can be a part of your fitness plan. If you are in this already-fit category and have no medical problems that limit your activities, your choice of sports and exercises can be much broader right from the start.

TIME (T): HOW LONG ARE YOU EXERCISING FOR EACH SESSION?

If you are a beginner or are returning to exercise after being inactive, we recommend that you start your plan aiming for sessions lasting approximately 10 minutes. While this may not seem like much time, for those who have not exercised this can increase caloric expenditure—and therefore support weight loss efforts. Plus, studies show that moving for 10 minutes improves mood—and that the mood-boosting benefits of exercise do not increase with more activity (they are the same no matter how much longer we move, so when it comes to exercise a little really can mean a lot). As you continue to follow and refine your plan, you can aim for sessions in the 15-to-30-minute range, progressing to 45 to 60 minutes.

HOW MANY CALORIES ARE USED IN TYPICAL ACTIVITIES?

The following table shows calories used in common physical activities at both moderate and vigorous levels. This list of activities provides just some examples of the many options available. You can assess other activities, too, and determine whether they are appropriate for you. Be sure to consider whether the activity is high or low impact—and what seems best for you and your body. We also recommend that you consider whether the intensity level is right for you, whether it is competitive or noncompetitive, individual or team or group, and whether you are likely to enjoy it and be willing to employ the activity as a regular part of your fitness program throughout the year. It is best to avoid the latest fad exercises or sports, especially if they require a substantial investment in equipment or training.

TABLE 8-3

Calories used per hour in common physical activities

Moderate physical activity	Approximate calories used per 30 minutes for a 154-lb person	Approximate calories used per hour for a 154-lb person
Hiking	185	370
Light gardening/yard work	165	330
Dancing	165	330
Golf (walking and carrying clubs)	165	330
Bicycling (< 10 mph)	145	290
Walking (3.5 mph)	140	280
Weight lifting (general light workout)	110	220
Stretching	90	180
Vigorous physical activity		
Running/jogging (5 mph)	295	590
Bicycling (> 10 mph)	295	590
Swimming (slow freestyle laps)	255	510
Aerobics	240	480
Walking (4.5 mph)	230	460
Heavy yard work (chopping wood)	220	440
Weight lifting (vigorous effort)		440
Basketball (vigorous)	220	440

SOURCE: *https://www.cdc.gov/healthyweight/physical_activity/.*

SCHEDULING YOUR PHYSICAL ACTIVITY PLAN FOR EXERCISE

As you reflect on the FITT principle, what goals does it inspire you to set for yourself this coming week? To help you, we offer two examples of what a weekly exercise plan might look like for a beginner (who isn't currently exercising) and for an intermediate (someone who is aiming to meet the guidelines fully). Remember

---

BOX 8-4

Sample Beginners' Weekly Exercise Plan

Sun	10-minute family walk + 10 minutes of light stretching
Mon	10-minute bike ride (cardio) + 10 minutes of light stretching
Tues	10-minute light strength training + 10 minutes of light stretching
Wed	10-minute walk (cardio) + 10 minutes of light stretching
Thurs	Off
Fri	10-minute walk alone (cardio) + 10 minutes of light stretching
Sat	Next week: try increasing to 15 minutes of cardio, stretching, and strength

Note: You may designate Saturday or Sunday as a rest day.

BOX 8-5

Sample Intermediate Weekly Exercise Plan

Sun	30-minute family walk + 10 minutes of light stretching
Mon	30-minute bike ride + 10 minutes of light stretching
Tues	15-minute walk + 20 minutes of strength training (arms) + 10 minutes of light stretching
Wed	15-minute walk + 20 minutes of strength training (legs) + 10 minutes of light stretching
Thurs	15-minute walk + 20 minutes of strength training (arms) + 10 minutes of light stretching
Fri	15-minute walk + 20 minutes of strength training (legs) + 10 minutes of light stretching
Sat	45 minutes of yoga (30 minutes of movement at moderate level + 15 minutes meditation)

Note: You may designate Saturday or Sunday as a rest day.

---

that these examples are offered to help you brainstorm your unique plan, which should be customized to adapt to your medical and weight loss needs, your physical capabilities, your current activity level, and the type of exercise you enjoy (or would like to try).

Physical Activity Planning Step 4: Get Cleared for Takeoff

After you have created the physical activity component of your Personal Plan of Action, we recommend that you double-check with your medical provider that the plan that you created is truly right and safe for you. If your provider determines that you need additional support for your plan, they may recommend that you see an exercise physiologist (trained to customize your exercise plan) or an occupational therapist or kinesiologist (trained to customize your daily movement plan). Any of these referrals are nothing to be concerned or ashamed about and can be quite helpful. Much like how registered dietitians can help you create a customized nutrition plan based on your unique medical needs, these providers can help you create a customized and medically safe physical activity plan based on your medical needs, too.

Additionally, as you prepare to get moving, remember to pay attention to how your body feels. If you have a heart, lung, or vascular disease, you will need to start at a light intensity and use extra caution when starting any physical activity regimen (as per your medical provider's direction). And remember, regardless of how fit you are or how vigorous your exercise program becomes over time, you should *always* stop immediately if the exercise or movement causes pain, shortness of breath, or chest, jaw, or arm discomfort.

Ten Helpful Hints for Your Physical Activity Success

Although we are happy you are committed to creating your own unique Personal Plan of Action for physical activity—including weekly exercise and daily movement—we know that even the best of plans can be hard to turn into a reality. That's why we created this list of helpful hints that have helped others. We are hopeful they can help you, too.

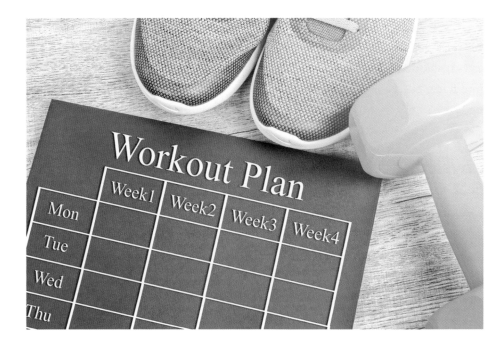

HELPFUL HINT 1. CREATE A SCHEDULE
YOU CAN LIVE WITH AND LOVE

Because sticking to a regular program of physical activities is crucial to your long-term success at weight management, it is crucial that you schedule the time to make it happen. Our experience with patients as well as in our own lives has shown us that one of the hardest parts of losing weight—and keeping it off—is making sure that you can fit your plan into your daily life.

To consistently sustain a level of physical activity above your current level, it is helpful to devise a schedule you can live with. Just as things get done more reliably at work when a time is set aside for them, your fitness plan will become a reality only if you set aside the needed time.

How much time is needed? To achieve a higher level of physical fitness and burn a significant number of calories, plan to spend 20 to 30 minutes at your target heart rate at least every other day. If you throw in 5 minutes to stretch and warm up, and 5 minutes to cool down, this is a minimum of 30 minutes per session. If the activity is done at home or at work, no travel time will need to be added. If you must travel—to a health club, for example—figure in travel time and time for changing clothes.

Regardless of how busy you are, it should be possible to schedule this amount of time if you make the commitment to do so. Many people have successfully utilized part of their lunchtime at work. Others are freshest at the start of the day and prefer scheduling activities early in the morning. Still others prefer to exercise in the early evenings during the week. On weekends, it is often best to choose a time early in the day so as not to interfere with other activities, or have other activities interfere with your exercise.

One problem many people have with scheduled fitness activities is that during the preparation and action stages of their Personal Plan of Action, they may be overly ambitious in their scheduling of physical activities, perhaps in number of sessions, intensity of exercise, or duration of each session. It may seem as if more should be better, and if that's the case, why not take advantage of your peak motivational state?

If you keep the long-term goal of weight maintenance in mind, you can see how an overly aggressive exercise schedule can have a negative rather than a positive effect. You may indeed stick to a grueling, time-consuming schedule initially, but after a while you probably won't be able to keep it up. Then, the level you are able to maintain will likely lead to weight regain rather than maintenance. Also, once you have accomplished your weight goal, the grueling schedule will seem excessive and unnecessary. There is a tendency to stop doing these activities almost entirely, yet we know that regular exercise at a moderate level is necessary for giving you the best chance at keeping your weight stable.

To avoid this problem, it is best to pick a moderate and sustainable amount of time to commit to fitness activities from the start. It will be much easier to continue a level of activity that fits comfortably into your schedule than a more aggressive level that requires putting other commitments aside. If you have worked up to exercising several times per week, schedule in one or two rest days at any point during the week to allow your body a period of recovery.

HELPFUL HINT 2. MAKE A PLAN A AND A PLAN B

Let's say that your "Plan A" for the day is to complete your day's cardio and strength exercise goals at the gym by taking a fitness class, and to build a walking meeting into your day for your daily dose of functional movement. You wake up full of optimism that you can make this plan a reality, but then your child tells you that they are not feeling well. You realize that you'll need to stay home to take care of your child, which you are glad to do for your child's sake, but you also realize that you won't be able to get your exercise or daily movement in after all. In this very common scenario, someone who only had a Plan A would give up on their exercise and movement plan for the day, and may even feel discouraged because they weren't able to follow through on their plan.

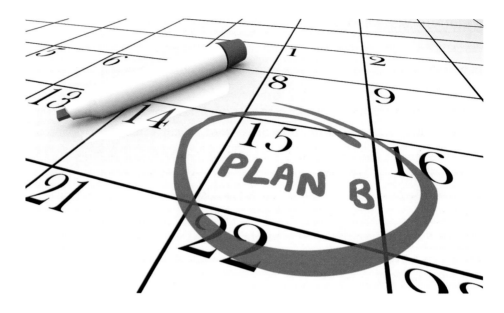

This is why we suggest you also have a Plan B for each day. Your Plan B is what you'll do if Plan A doesn't work out. It may not give you the same experience as Plan A but is "better than doing nothing." For example, your Plan B for going to the gym might be to practice a workout with your favorite app or online personal training subscription—that you have bookmarked so you can start quickly (while your child rests). And your Plan B for a walking meeting is to take a 30-minute stretch break with a colleague or a family member during your lunch hour so that you won't get bored, you'll stay accountable, and you'll have more fun.

In addition to having a daily Plan B, you might also make a Plan B for times when you are not feeling well. Plan ahead for difficulties. We do not recommend that you exercise vigorously during illness; however, we also know that most people stop exercising during an illness, and this may disrupt their commitment to their physical activity plan. While you are ill, focus on getting well, and take time to plan for getting back to moving again. Be patient with yourself by starting small—knowing that a little movement is better than no movement (unless you have been medically advised otherwise).

We also recommend the same "Plan B" approach to holidays and vacations. Create your Plan A *and* Plan B for how you will stick to your Personal Plan of Action during these periods, and decide how you will resume your exercise program *before* you begin the celebration or leave town to visit friends or relatives. Then give yourself the gift of following through!

HELPFUL HINT 3. PLAN FOR YOUR EXPERIENCE

If you desire to join a gym, fitness center, or studio, consider the facility's hours of operation, rates, location, childcare options, equipment, staffing, group exercise classes, and culture before committing. It is better to shop around and find a fitness center that meets your needs than to opt for the least expensive or most popular option for others. This is why many gyms, fitness centers, and studios offer you a trial period. Take advantage of this offer and experience multiple classes and instructors so you'll know if it feels like home to you.

Don't just decide you need to take an exercise class and then join the most convenient one. Find out about the music, the instructor, the setting, and so on. Observe the class and talk to the instructor *before* you take the class. That way the instructor knows you and has a vested interest in your enjoyment of the class. Many classes will offer a free first-timer trial.

If you prefer outdoor activities, consider gear and clothing that is appropriate for the weather and establish an indoor alternative for days when the weather is especially bad to help you stay on track. If you are exercising in extreme heat or cold, proceed with caution and hydrate often.

HELPFUL HINT 4. KEEP A JOURNAL

Much like we recommended that you document your food intake and practices in your weight loss journal, we also recommend that you track your exercise regimen in your journal. Many people find it easier to keep up their exercise regimen if they

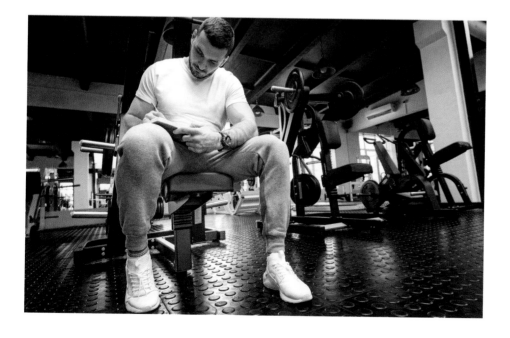

keep a written record, or use an app designed for this purpose. We have provided you with a workout planner in the resources section so you can record what days and times you have set aside for exercise to serve as a reminder of your commitment. Consider how you will schedule this time for physical activity with yourself and put it on your daily calendar, in the same way that you would any other commitment, like a meeting, medical appointment, or lunch date. If you should feel tempted to break this commitment when you are busy or tired, the idea that this is an appointment with yourself will help you stay on track and keep this important commitment to yourself.

Remember that your journal (or record) is not just about tracking whether you exercised—you can also track how it went and how you are feeling. This will give you a diary of preferences over time that you can use to inform future planning. If you have a medical challenge, this data can also be helpful for you and your provider to ensure that your wellness and health care plans are woven well together.

HELPFUL HINT 5. SET THE STAGE FOR YOUR SUCCESS

To avoid rushing around at the last minute gathering your things, set equipment or clothing for exercising out the night before, by the door, or in your car so you will see them on your way to work or upon arriving home. Nothing will deter you from exercising more than if you are always late for work because you can't find your walking shoes.

HELPFUL HINT 6. TAKE THE TIME
TO WARM UP AND COOL DOWN

Injuries are more likely to occur when you fail to get your body gradually ready for exercise, and exercise-related injuries provide a surefire excuse for abandoning your Personal Plan of Action. Once you have lost your initial momentum, it can be extremely difficult to get going again. To avoid these interruptions, stretching, warm-ups, and cool-downs are essential.

However you stretch, do not push to the point of pain. (The "no pain no gain" mindset is actually a myth and potentially harmful to many people.) When you find a point of challenge—the place between easy and ouch—hold each position for 10–15 seconds. You can rotate through the same routine if you wish, at which point you may notice a bit more flexibility the second time around. For a walking program, an appropriate warm-up is to walk more slowly than your usual exercise pace for a few minutes, then gradually pick up the pace.

At the end of your exercise session, it is best to cool down slowly, giving your body a chance to adjust gradually to less activity. You should not be exercising so vigorously that you need to lie down, panting at the end of the session. To cool down, perform the same activity you were doing at a slow pace for a few minutes. For instance, if you were jogging, begin to walk. If you were cycling at 10 miles per hour, reduce your speed to 5 miles per hour for the last five minutes. If you were playing tennis, walk instead of sitting down right away. Perform the same stretching exercises at the end of your cool-down period.

HELPFUL HINT 7. FIGHT PLATEAUS BY CHALLENGING YOURSELF MENTALLY AND PHYSICALLY

If you start an exercise program and are doing it the same way for half an hour every other day, you will soon notice that it seems to take less and less effort as the weeks go on. That's because your strength and stamina are increasing and your body is becoming more fit—which was our goal all along.

But with this win comes a new challenge to your weight management. As your body becomes more fit, you'll need to keep challenging yourself so you don't plateau. That's because as your body becomes more efficient at exercising, you'll burn fewer calories when you complete the same effort. Since our aim is to increase fitness and burn calories, and not plateau, you'll need to keep challenging yourself by using the FITT principle—increasing the frequency, intensity, time, and/or

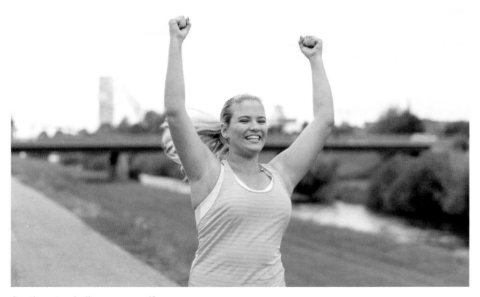

Continue to challenge yourself

type of your activity as time goes on. The good news is that as you keep changing up your routine—while sticking to it—you'll also be preventing boredom (which has derailed many physical activity plans).

As part of your efforts to challenge yourself mentally and physically, you might want to develop an intellectual interest in fitness and different sports and activities to help you maintain your enthusiasm. Subscribe to fitness magazines, join local teams or interest groups, and see your fitness program become a very satisfying and integral part of your life.

HELPFUL HINT 8. SPICE UP YOUR DAILY COMMITMENT BY EXERCISING YOUR OPTIONS

While a progressive walking program is an excellent way to burn calories and increase fitness, you may get bored with only a single activity. This does not mean that you should stop walking and replace walking with another form of exercise. It is better to continue walking, perhaps at a slightly reduced duration if you have time constraints, and add something new. Athletes call this *cross-training*. Cross-training can reduce the risk of injuries as well as add variety to your exercise routine.

We also recommend that you select activities that you enjoy. You may have to work up to these activities gradually if you have not been physically active for a while. Remember the payoff. Don't think of your fitness plan as a dreaded chore. Focus on the activities you can see yourself enjoying, and give yourself a chance to appreciate that you are indeed accomplishing something. If you're unable to enjoy physical activity or exercise, notice how you feel more fit, don't get tired as easily, and gain all of the other benefits of those physical activities, and focus on how you feel afterward, which is generally good.

You can also spice up your routine by making it interesting. For example, you can change the scenery (walk a different route); utilize your mobile apps for encouragement, music, podcasts, and audiobooks; or exercise while reading or watching TV if you can safely do so (for example, while on a reclined stationary bike).

HELPFUL HINT 9. FIND A BUDDY TO HOLD EACH OTHER ACCOUNTABLE

Find a fitness buddy—a friend or relative who is also interested in becoming more fit or losing weight—and enlist his or her support and participation. You are far less likely to skip an exercise session when you have someone you exercise with or someone who is waiting to exercise with you.

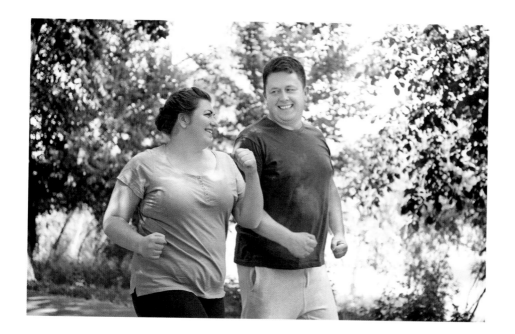

When working with a fitness buddy, remember that they may have times when they cannot make it to your exercise session. Don't let this discourage you or derail you. Make a plan for what you both will do on days you cannot exercise together—such as send a motivating text or email to each other. Be creative in how you support each other to stick to your own respective plans.

HELPFUL HINT 10. BE YOURSELF

Earlier in this chapter, we emphasized the importance of creating a physical activity component of your Personal Plan of Action that is right for you and tailored to your needs—comparing it to a medical prescription. You wouldn't go into some else's medicine cabinet and borrow their medications, so it's best not to do the same with exercise by assuming that what they do is something you should do.

Instead, enjoy creating your plan for yourself—and your own unique individuality. Set small, realistic goals, and celebrate your own successes along the way. As part of these efforts, celebrate what brings you joy and excitement, and try to link this feeling of having fun to exercise so it feels more like play and like less like a chore.

Also, enjoy "getting real" with yourself by recognizing the two or three most common excuses you give yourself for not exercising, and then develop an appropriate response. Talk back to yourself the way a good friend would talk to you. Write these responses down in your Personal Plan of Action and keep them handy. Review them regularly.

As you can see, there are many ways for you to plan for and commit to physical activity—both daily activity and weekly exercise—so you can meet your weight loss and weight management goals. Enjoy bringing these new possibilities into your life.

Action Items

- Complete the assessment in this chapter for daily movement and physical activity.

- Complete the movement and exercise assessments located in the resources section of this book.

- Use these insights to inform the creation of your Personal Plan of Action.

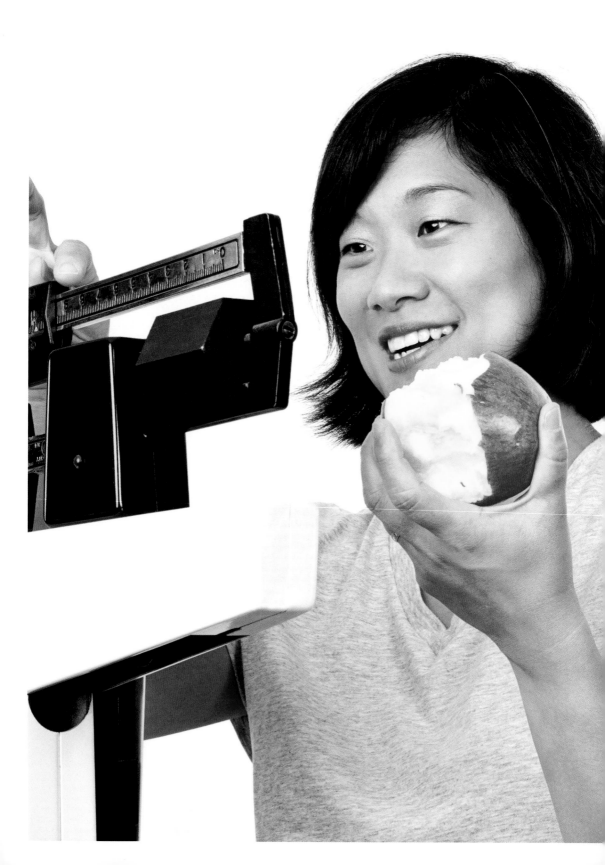

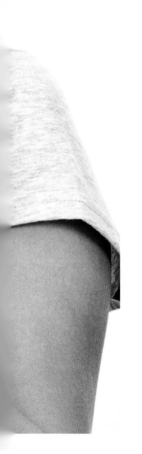

CHAPTER 9

Keeping It Off

IN THIS CHAPTER, WE WILL:

- **review** characteristics of people who have maintained long-term weight loss,

- **discuss** strategies for maintaining long-term weight loss,

- **identify** potential maintenance pitfalls to avoid,

- **offer** strategies for overcoming maintenance challenges, and

- **remind** you to believe in your ability to successfully maintain a healthy weight.

HAVING READ THIS BOOK SO FAR, *you* have designed a Personal Plan of Action for weight management after careful assessment of your individual strengths and needs. It contains not just a "diet" but also a plan for healthful eating after the weight loss, a plan for behavior change, and a fitness plan. You have looked closely at your reasons for wanting to lose weight and maintain a healthful weight. You know what motivates you best and longest. You know the stages of change, and you are ready.

The fact is that, throughout this book, you have been methodically building the foundation for maintaining your weight loss. In each chapter you learned a specific technique for maintaining the progress you make during the action stage of your Personal Plan of Action. You know what lifestyle changes are necessary for you to succeed.

The purpose of this chapter is to reinforce some of the important ingredients of long-term weight management. We will study the characteristics of people who are most successful at losing weight and keeping it off, and compare them with people who are less successful. We will then summarize how you can put yourself squarely into the "most successful" group. Let's begin by looking at the results of some recent research studies.

Successful Maintainers: What Do We Know?

First, the bad news. Most research studies have shown relatively poor long-term maintenance of lost weight a few years or more after a weight loss program. This includes programs that emphasize behavior modification as well as programs that emphasize aggressive dieting such as very-low-calorie, liquid protein diets. Fewer than one out of ten people in these studies succeeded in maintaining a substantial weight loss in the long run.

Before you get discouraged, however, let us say that these studies do not tell the whole story. There have been some studies that show a considerably better result among people *not* enrolled in formal research studies. How can this be? Probably because people who lose weight on their own, perhaps with the help of friends and information they learn from personal experience and books, are different from the average research subject. Oftentimes individuals who participate in research studies may not have health conditions linked with obesity, like depression, which can interfere with successful weight management.

Research studies also suggest that having continual contact with others in the weight loss program is an important part of weight maintenance. When a program ends abruptly, the results are poor. With ongoing support, perhaps as infrequently as every two weeks or even less often than that, maintenance of weight loss is much improved. In a self-help program such as your Personal Plan of Action, there has never been any one-on-one contact between the program and the participant. Does this mean that the benefit of personal contact would not apply in this situation? We believe that it does apply, and that ongoing contact would be beneficial even to people who have developed a Personal Plan of Action.

You can secure the additional "maintenance insurance" that regular ongoing contact provides in one of two ways. You can join or form your own support group for people who have recently lost weight and are trying to maintain the loss. Or, you can develop a support system for yourself that provides some of the same benefits as a support group.

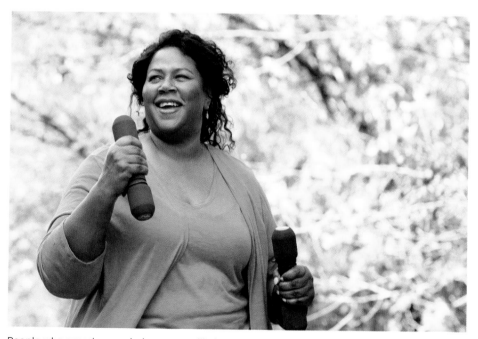

People who exercise regularly are more likely to maintain their weight loss

What do studies show about the characteristics of successful maintainers compared to regainers? There are only a handful of studies in this area, but the themes are similar to a 1990 study by Dr. Susan Kayman and others at UCLA. They compared the behaviors of a group of 30 women who had successfully lost 20% or more of their initial weight and maintained the loss for at least two years to 44 women who had regained their lost weight and 34 "control group" women who had not lost any weight. Their findings included the following useful information:

- **The successful maintainers** were much more likely (73%) than the regainers (39%) to have lost weight by devising a personal eating plan after making the decision to lose weight.

- **The maintainers** were more than twice as likely (76%) than the regainers (36%) to have exercised regularly to help lose weight.

- **The regainers** were far more likely (47%) than the maintainers (3%) to have used appetite-suppressing pills to lose weight.

- **While 72% of the regainers** attended weight loss programs and groups, only 10% of the maintainers attended such groups. Ninety percent of the maintainers achieved long-term weight loss on their own.

- **The maintainers, unlike the regainers,** were aware that they needed to continue to be conscious of their eating and physical activity behaviors.

- **Ninety percent of maintainers** were still exercising regularly after their weight loss (at least three times per week, 30 minutes per session), while only 34% of the regainers did so. Even those regainers who did exercise regularly did so less frequently and less vigorously than the maintainers.

- **Regainers ate** 4.6 snacks per day, while maintainers ate only 1.5 snacks on a typical day. Regainers also ate more candies and chocolate and were more likely to skip breakfast than maintainers and controls.

- **While women in all the groups reported** having stress or troubling issues in their lives, they coped in different ways. Few of the regainers (10%) used problem-solving or confrontational ways of coping, compared to 95% of the maintainers and 60% of the average-weight controls.

- **Many regainers (70%) reported** dealing with problems by "escape-avoidance," such as eating, sleeping, drinking, smoking, taking tranquilizers, or simply wishing the problem would go away. Fewer than half as many maintainers (33%) coped in these ineffective ways.

- **While 70% of maintainers reported** seeking outside support in dealing with problems, either by talking out their feelings or seeking professional help, only 38% of regainers did these things.

The results of the aforementioned study bring to light a number of lessons that will be useful to you in thinking about your strategies for maintaining weight loss. Most, if not all, of the habits of successful maintainers can be learned, even if they are not already a part of your repertoire. Does emulating the behavior pattern of successful maintainers guarantee that you, too, will be successful? Unfortunately, no. But it is likely that your chances will be vastly improved. Having a clear plan of action is just as critical to weight maintenance as it is to weight loss, and your Personal Plan of Action, with a few modifications, can serve you well after the action phase of active weight loss is complete.

Dietary Principles for Permanent Weight Loss and Weight Management

Presumably, if you've worked your way through the book to this point, you're well on your way to developing a new way of eating for weight loss based on sound, healthful eating habits. You can initially learn a lot about the quality of your food choices by focusing on food groups, portion sizes, and nutrient density. And you can be successful in weight loss by planning ahead; selecting, measuring, and preparing healthy foods; monitoring healthy serving sizes; and limiting empty calories. Does this mean you can't ever deviate from your plan? Do you have to "diet" forever in order to attain or maintain your goal weight? Of course not. Sustainability is the key to successful long-term weight management.

In the long run, we don't eat nutrients or food groups. We eat foods, snacks, and meals. So, as you develop your new, healthy eating pattern, it is important to also learn to build in your own personal preferences, as well as a somewhat flexible mindset, in order to encourage the "livability" or sustainability of your new patterns.

Whether you are in the process of losing weight or nearing your weight goal and beginning to focus on weight maintenance, occasionally some flexibility will

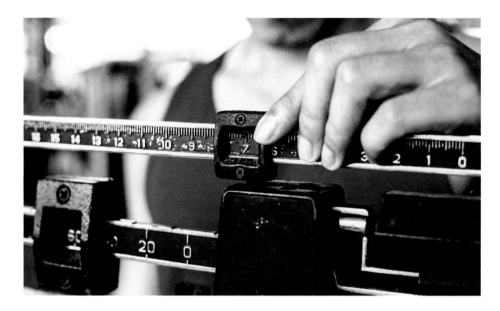

be necessary in order to navigate the eating situations that arise in everyday life. It is important to keep in mind that the *frequency* of deviating from your maintenance plan, the *size* of the deviation, and the *length of time* you allow yourself to continue deviating will affect the likelihood that you will continue to lose weight or maintain your new desired weight. If you've deviated, don't panic, and get back on track as soon as you can.

We advocate the concept of a *weight window*. This is the acceptable weight range that you'll maintain long term. Keeping an eye on it is important so that you don't "drift" back to old eating habits and food choices.

Once you have determined your "perfect" weight, then consider a three- to four-pound range that surrounds your perfect weight. If 175 is perfect, you might choose 173–176 or 174–77. Either range is fine, provided you are comfortable seeing any of those numbers on the scale at your official weigh-in. If you consider 176 on the scale to be unsatisfactory, then the top number of your weight window should be no higher than that. Give yourself permission to weigh any number inside that range. Any of the numbers within your window can be considered "weight maintenance." You can use your weight window to allow some moderate flexibility in your eating and exercise choices, but it also defines the boundary of weight regain. Sometimes selecting the ideal range takes some time and practice.

Once you have found the ideal bracket, note the bottom number as nearing the area of "trying too hard" or "unrealistic to maintain for long." And more importantly, firmly consider the top number being the *beginning of weight regain*. You

Sample Intermediate Weekly Exercise Plan

Green Safety Zone Current weight: _____ pounds Weight window: _____ to _____ pounds	Your maintenance weight, within 3 to 5 pounds. Weigh yourself at least weekly to monitor your window.
Yellow Safety Zone Weight window: _____ to _____ pounds	Sometimes you may slip beyond the 3- to 5-pound safety zone and need to take action. You may need to keep a food diary for a few days, be cognizant of your habits and attitudes, and revisit your support to get into the green zone. It's time to make a plan and take action.
Red Correction Zone	You have regained more than 5 to 8 pounds, which puts you at higher risk for continuing to regain more weight. It is vital to stop, reevaluate what happened, and avoid slipping back into your old lifestyle and behaviors. You need to reactivate your weight loss efforts with new proven methods or familiar methods you've been successful with in the past.

can use that range to allow some flexibility for "good days" and "bad days." You can use any movement within that range to gauge how much flexibility you have at your disposal (or how much has already been used). However, when you do an official weigh-in and see the top number of your weight window on the scale, then *immediately, that day, right now, no questions asked*, begin trimming back any extra calories in order to begin the gradual return to within your weight window. We don't mean engaging in a crash diet; you just need to return to the principles of careful monitoring of food groups and portion sizes and empty calories that helped you be so successful in losing weight. There is no need for self-criticism; you have simply used your flexibility, and now it's time to be a little more conservative until you return to a weight that is within your window.

For example, perhaps you have a vacation coming up. You will visit family, travel to new places, perhaps stay in a hotel for several days, and have limited choices about when and where to eat and exercise. You will be out of your normal eating routine. In addition, you might also want to enjoy an extra glass of wine,

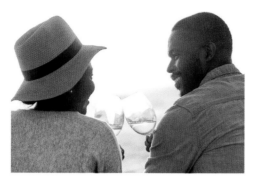

You can indulge a little on vacation as long as you make up for it before and after your trip

a fancy dessert, or the local dining scene. For several weeks *before* you leave for vacation, work to get closer to the low end of your weight window. However, even if you begin your vacation at the "bottom" of your window, you should still focus on making healthy food and exercise choices *most of the time* while you are away. But you also have the freedom to gain a pound or two on your trip and still return home *within* your window. While you're away, you may want to enjoy a few carefully selected "splurge" calories, but you will also see the importance of choosing only the very yummiest calories and avoiding the mindless over-eating and drinking that often accompanies a vacation. Once you return home and have access to your normal eating and exercise patterns, you can immediately begin trimming back extra calories in order to begin the gradual return to the middle of your window. This cycle of flexibility accompanied by self-accountability is important for building the self-trust required for enjoying flexible food choices and personal preferences without feeling that you are doomed to eventually "gain it all back."

Long-Term Eating Principles

No matter where you are on your weight loss or weight maintenance journey, it is important to make healthy eating choices most of the time. Whether you are consistently losing, maintaining, or are slightly above your weight window or square in the middle, the following healthy eating practices will always apply:

- **Eat a variety of foods in moderation** and in proportion to one another. In other words, consistently choose according to your personal food group pattern for portion control, variety, and nutrient balance.

- **Prepare foods yourself as often as possible.** Limit packaged, convenience, and processed foods as often as possible. Limit fats/oils of all kinds every day. Avoid empty calorie foods nearly all the time.

- **Practice semi-vegetarianism** by eating the combined total of vegetables and fruits, whole grains, and legumes according to your food groups meal plan. At least half should be whole grain sources.

- **Choose high-fiber options** as often as possible for low-calorie bulk and satiety.

- **Eat fewer foods with added sugars.** Avoid junk foods, including fat-free alternatives—they still have many calories and can stall your efforts if you eat too much of them.

- **Eat a minimum of three times per day.** Breakfast is essential, although you can wait up to two hours after rising to eat breakfast.

- **Avoid skipping meals** and limit grazing.

- **Eat only when you are physically hungry,** and stop eating when you are no longer hungry. Either measure specific portions according to your food groups meal plan, or start with half as much of every food as you think you need. Don't wait to stop eating until you are stuffed. Eat slowly to allow satiety to occur.

- **Plan ahead, both forward and backward.** Plan ahead for each meal or snack in relation to what you've already eaten that day and what you plan to eat later. Each meal or snack does not stand alone but rather should be viewed as part of a pattern.

- **Compensate with a little extra calorie reduction** or increased physical activity either before or after deviations from your Personal Plan of Action.

- **Prioritize weight loss over "I deserve a treat"** (instead: I deserve to feel great). It's not "too hard to pay attention" but "too hard to carry so much weight and feel so sluggish."

- **Go do something exciting.** (I have extra time when not I'm prowling around in the kitchen looking for something else to eat.)

Successful Maintenance Strategies

Even after weight loss, it is still important to pay attention to the reasons why you initially chose to lose weight, as it's a way to continue to reaffirm your commitment. It is also particularly important to remind yourself of the benefits you are enjoying since losing weight, and not to forget what your life was like before developing and following your Personal Plan of Action. And speaking of your Personal Plan of

4 M's of Maintenance

Move	Movements (physical activity) that are enjoyable and sustainable to you
Monitor	Nutrients going in, physical activity, weight, patterns, sleep
Motivation	Motivators for achieving short- and long-term goals
Make time	Prioritize and schedule healthful eating and physical activity to fit your lifestyle

Action, now is not the time to cast it aside. You should continue to refer to it regularly to help you stay on track with your successful eating and exercise strategies.

Key Ingredients of a Good Maintenance System

- Learning to talk positively to yourself. Being your own cheerleader can keep you going.

- Keeping records. Self-monitoring of food, exercise, and behavior is like discussing your progress with someone else.

- Continuing your buddy system. Keep in touch with your weight loss partner during the maintenance stage.

- Consulting your written lists of substitute activities and problem-solving actions when old eating behaviors or situations threaten.

Just as during the weight loss phase, the goal of maintenance must be reasonable. That is, you should not expect to stay within a pound of your lowest weight. Instead, recognize that weight management means managing your weight within a reasonable *range*. This may be a 5-pound or 10-pound range for some, or as much as 20 pounds for those who were obese.

Although in a Personal Plan of Action you will not have the benefit of ongoing contact through a therapist or in a group setting (unless you choose to seek one out), you can obtain much of the benefit by nurturing your own contacts, through both your support system of people and such tools as talking to yourself in a positive way, keeping written lists of useful behaviors, and self-monitoring activities.

One important strategy used by maintainers to help solve problems is having a network of friends and relatives to turn to.

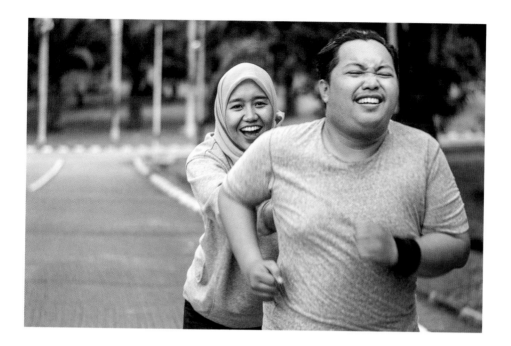

Throughout this book, we've talked about the importance of the buddy system as a key ingredient of weight loss. It is equally useful during the maintenance phase.

Being able to discuss problems with others has many advantages. Getting encouragement from others can make you feel the problem is not all that bad. Discussion will also help you crystallize the issues and create viable solutions; it will enable you to test the likely response to your solutions; and, finally, it will give you immediate positive feedback regarding the problem and your ability to solve it.

The various tools described during the development of your Personal Plan of Action were presented as assessment or weight loss devices, but they are equally useful as maintenance tools. They include:

- **stimulus-control devices,** such as keeping tempting foods out of the house or out of sight,

- **eating in only one room** of the house,

- **changing to a low-fat, higher volume diet** with increased emphasis on foods lower on the food guide pyramid, and

- **adding spices instead of fats** to improve the taste of foods.

Changes in eating habits are maintenance tools, too. They include:

- **teaching yourself to eat more slowly,** in smaller bites, on smaller plates, at regular meals, taken only when you are physically hungry; and

- **using calorie-burning devices** such as increasing incidental activities and spontaneous activities, in addition to formal exercise, to help you successfully maintain your weight loss.

To keep these tools fresh, you may find it helpful during maintenance to vary your emphasis from time to time. For example, you may engage in a different form of monitoring from month to month, setting aside February and March, for instance, for exercise monitoring, since it is a time when cold weather makes getting enough physical activity more problematic, and April and May for monitoring your fat intake as warm weather approaches. Similarly, you can vary the forms of physical activity you emphasize from season to season, or vary the kinds of foods you use to fill your pyramid boxes based on the seasonal availability of various fresh or frozen fruits and vegetables.

During maintenance, keep an eye out for adverse psychological states like depression, which might develop, and for evidence of binge eating. It is critical to deal with such problems early on. While it is important in maintenance to keep close tabs on your weight, you should recognize that your weight may vary by as much as several pounds from day to day. This is largely due to changes in the body's state of hydration—how much water you are carrying in your tissues. Increases in body water are sometimes hormonally driven. Many premenopausal women especially notice fluid retention during the days right before menstruating. For other people, eating foods high in salt may result in fluid retention. Thus, it is possible to eat the same number of calories yet gain water weight during some periods.

Within this variation, however, it is a good idea to keep close watch on your weight and on how your clothes fit. An increase above the goal range you have achieved or a snugly fitting outfit may signal a maintenance problem. Many successful maintainers weigh themselves daily (weighing yourself more than once a day yields no further information). The idea is not to focus exclusively on the number of pounds, though, since the pounds are an imperfect reflection of what is really being managed during maintenance—your behavior.

During maintenance, the best way to evaluate your behavior is through self-monitoring of as many items as you can manage. The more you monitor, the better—within limits. At a minimum you should monitor your weight, your food portions (or fat grams), and your physical activity. For those whose Personal Plan of Action reflected a need to control inappropriate eating cues, ongoing monitoring of eating situations and what you did to deal with them is critical. All this monitoring should take less than 15 minutes per day. This is a reasonable investment of time for maintaining your hard-won success. Try to stay aware of the pleasures of maintaining a healthful weight, as opposed to the pleasures of food. For instance, cancel your subscription to a food magazine and replace it with a subscription to a fitness magazine. Take pride in your fitness, positive health attitudes, and appearance.

BOX 9-4

Maintenance Check List

✓ Physical activity that I enjoy and can sustain each week

✓ Meal preparation or planning to eat healthful foods routinely and while traveling

✓ Scheduling my health in my calendar to fit with my routine and other responsibilities

✓ Updating my goals and keeping them in plain sight

✓ Monitoring my weight while living my life

Maintenance Pitfalls

Despite the best of intentions, you must recognize that there will be lapses and even relapses along the path, but we hope you will not suffer total collapse. What do these terms mean? A lapse can be described as a slip from desired behaviors. An

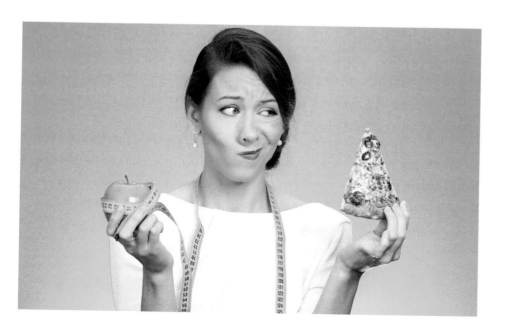

example is eating the second piece of chocolate cake when you were not hungry. Lapses are very common and no cause for alarm. We are often more concerned about people who suffer no lapses than those who have frequent lapses. Lapses are, by definition, temporary. When the cake is gone, the lapse is over. It does not spell the end of your Personal Plan of Action. You must simply move on, record the event dutifully as part of your monitoring, and learn something from it, whether it is how to avoid the situation, how to substitute another behavior, or simply how to compensate for the lapse in some other way over the next day. No lapses mean no practice in dealing with situations that need more work. No lapses may lead to or reflect all-or-nothing thinking.

A relapse, on the other hand, is when you stop adhering to your Personal Plan of Action in ongoing, major ways. Relapse may occur early, or at any time during maintenance. Often relapse happens when you stop self-monitoring. The vigilance necessary to avoid weight regain may seem too big a burden, or you may simply become confident in your ability to manage your weight with less control. Unfortunately, this doesn't usually turn out to be the case.

If rebellion or lack of interest in weight management is the problem, it can help to refocus yourself. Recall your work in chapters 1 and 2, and see whether your situation or feelings have changed. If they have not, this rethinking of your Personal Plan of Action may help reinvigorate your motivation. If overconfidence is the problem, sometimes only a trial of less vigilance was needed. Perhaps you have learned enough so that less stringent control is needed, but perhaps not—and in that case you will see that you cannot relax the requirements of your Personal Plan of Action but must learn to accept the ongoing necessity of adhering to it.

When all else fails, and it is clear that a relapse has occurred, do not lose faith in yourself. It is discouraging to relapse, but you must recognize that multiple efforts are usually required to permanently change ingrained behavior patterns, especially eating patterns that are reinforced by our environment and our culture. The average cigarette smoker trying to quit makes several attempts before success, and even then may relapse years later. Changing eating habits is, in many ways, more difficult. You can't simply quit eating. You should expect that it may take more than one try to get it right. You will learn something from each attempt, particularly if you are working from a Personal Plan of Action, which provides insights into the whys of your behavior. Positive self-talk is important in dealing with a relapse. The bottom line for relapsers is that you can pick yourself up and try again, and you'll be wiser for the effort.

When you do experience a lapse or relapse, it is helpful to apply the problem-solving approach favored by most successful maintainers—objective and specific identification of the problem. For example, "eating when X happens" is easier to solve than the nonspecific problem of "overeating." If you suspect there are inappropriate eating situations causing your relapse but are unsure of what they are, you can resurrect the "watch trick" described in chapter 5. If you think overall food quantity or dietary fat percentage is the problem, you can begin a period of "super analyst" dietary monitoring to get a better handle on where you are going wrong.

A collapse, however, is something entirely different. A collapse is a relapse accompanied by a loss of interest in change. At times the person in collapse may feel hopeless, and may be depressed. When a collapse occurs or threatens, it is often advisable to seek professional help from a physician, counselor, or therapist experienced in helping people with weight problems. The solution may be to choose a different "reasonable" goal, perhaps to stabilize at the current weight instead of trying to lose weight again.

Problem-Solving for Successful Maintenance

Whatever you do, do not allow yourself to deal with (or, rather, *not* deal with) problems by escape-avoidance behaviors such as more eating, smoking, taking pills, or engaging in wishful thinking (as in "Maybe the problem will solve itself"). This is maladaptive, self-defeating behavior that could negate everything you have accomplished.

Once you have identified one or more specific problem areas, the next step in the problem-solving approach is brainstorming to come up with a number of possible

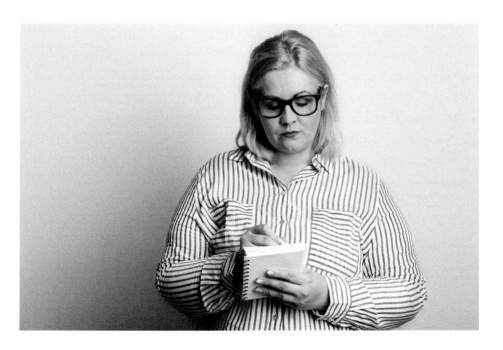

solutions. The point of brainstorming is not to arrive brilliantly at the foolproof solution, but to give yourself some ideas to try out, and the more the better. Not all the brainstormed solutions need to be good ones. It can even be helpful to think of a few ridiculous ones to give yourself a good, healthy laugh. (For example, have you considered heating all your silverware to 300° before dinner?)

Then, armed with alternative behaviors, choose one or more that you think have the best chance of working. It's not as important to be correct initially in your choice of a solution as it is just to try something. Look at this as a little experiment, knowing that the worst you are likely to do is not help the situation. You will learn something from the experiment regardless of its outcome.

The last step in the problem-solving approach, of course, is to try out your proposed solution or solutions, keeping in mind that you may need to fine-tune your solution, or try another one entirely. Even if you cannot completely resolve the problem, it is a good bet that the problem-solving approach will result in some improvement. At the same time, it will give you the confidence and pleasure that come from constructively addressing your problems instead of hiding from them.

Believe in Yourself

Perhaps the most important tool for maintenance, though, is belief in your own ability to succeed. Self-talk is important during all stages of change. There is nothing inherently different about modifying your behaviors on Day 1 of your action stage than on Day 1,000 of maintenance. Remind yourself that you have accomplished much already, and maintain your well-founded belief in your own ability to stay the course you have set for yourself. If you have followed the advice in this book, your goals are reasonable and so are the methods you have used to achieve and maintain them. They have also been carefully individualized by you to match your needs.

You have carefully assessed your motivations, diet, behaviors, and level of physical activity, and you have incorporated each in your Personal Plan of Action. Rededicate yourself to your Personal Plan of Action periodically, and watch your maintenance last and last. You deserve nothing less.

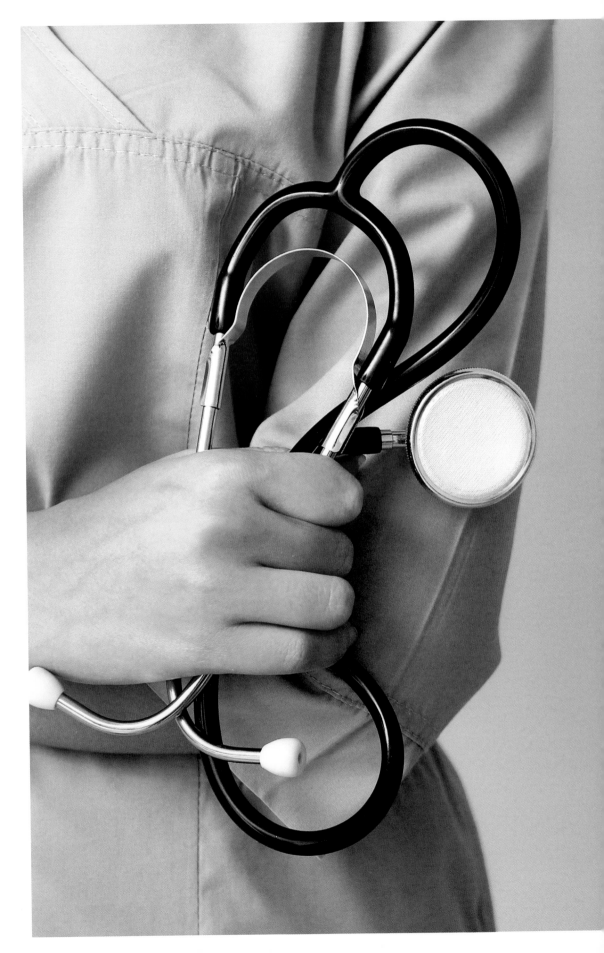

CHAPTER 10

Medical Solutions

Beyond Mindset and Behavior Change

IN THIS CHAPTER, WE WILL:

- **define** over-the-counter (OTC) weight loss supplements,

- **assess** the usefulness of OTC supplements,

- **identify** common supplement ingredients and evaluate their effectiveness,

- **discuss** MediSpas and their offerings,

- **help you decide** if prescription weight loss medications are right for you,

- **describe** the most commonly prescribed weight loss medications,

- **define** bariatric surgery,

- **help you decide** if bariatric surgery is right for you, and

- **describe** the types of bariatric surgeries.

WE STRONGLY BELIEVE THAT THE BEST WAY to take control of your weight and health is by making meaningful changes to your lifestyle, including your diet, activity level, and mindset. However, in some cases, individuals have difficulty achieving weight loss through lifestyle changes alone. At the Johns Hopkins Healthful Eating, Activity & Weight Program, we have found that these individuals may benefit from additional treatment tools in the form of prescriptions or surgery. In this chapter, we'll introduce you to additional weight loss aids. However, please note that these aids should be applied only under the guidance of a health care professional. You should discuss these options with your primary care provider or an obesity medicine specialist.

An Introduction to Over-the-Counter Supplements

Their name says it all—supplements can be a supplement to weight loss efforts. We therefore feel they should not be neglected in any discussion of weight loss, as many people have questions about this topic. *Natural, botanical, herbal, organic,* and *dietary* are terms used interchangeably when referring to supplements. In this case, we will simply use "supplements" when referring to products sold over the counter (that is, with no prescription required) for weight loss. Weight loss supplements are the most frequently purchased supplements, accounting for more than $2 billion each year in the United States. An estimated 15% of adults have tried a weight loss supplement at some point, and twice as many women have done so as men.

We do not generally recommend weight loss supplements because there are no well-designed studies supporting their efficacy and safety, so perhaps one of our first goals is to caution you against wasting money. However, that being said, if you believe you would like to try a supplement, we will equip you with the knowledge to make your decision wisely. With aisles filled with hundreds of supplements in your drug store or grocery store, you could be wandering aimlessly for hours before giving

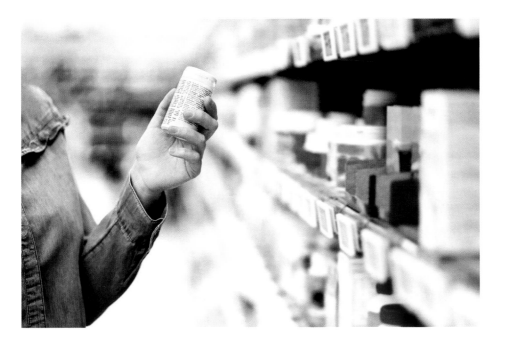

up and perhaps picking the cheapest or most heavily advertised product. As you probably know, even trying to pick out the "right" cough drops can be a challenge. So, before you enter the weight loss supplement aisle, it's important to know—for both your health and your wallet—some of the basics about what is available.

A LOOK AT THE LABELS

Just because something is labeled as a "natural" product and can be purchased over the counter does not mean there aren't risks or side effects. In fact, you will usually notice in the fine print a notification that the product has not been tested or approved by the Food and Drug Administration (FDA), meaning, among other things, that there was no official, third-party verification of what actually went into the bottle. There could be additional harmful ingredients, or not enough of the active ingredient to be effective. In fact, studies have found that the contents sometimes do not match the listed ingredients, and that there may be contaminants, at times harmful contaminants, in a substantial number of marketed products.

We recommend that you treat supplements much the same way as you do regular medications—as they have the same potential for causing allergies, side effects, and interactions with other medications you may be taking. For example, St. John's wort is well known for reducing the effect of prescription medications like blood thinners and cardiac agents. So, before taking anything, it is best to first make a list of all the ingredients on the back label of the product you want to buy. Then ask your health care provider or talk to your local pharmacist to make sure it is safe to take with your other medications or with certain health conditions you may have.

If you get the green light from your health care provider to use a supplement, choose a product that has *the* stamp of approval—the *USP Verified mark*. USP is the abbreviation for United States Pharmacopeia, and it is currently the only set of standards for supplements that we have when comparing products. No company or product is required to abide by this set of standards, but some choose to do so. Be wary of seeing just *USP*—this means they are *claiming* they meet the USP standards, but they have not actually been verified by the organization. Look for *USP Verified* or *USP-NF* (national formulary) to be certain it is legitimate. Once you've found the correct label, you can be sure the supplement (1) actually contains what it says it contains; (2) does not have harmful levels of substances like heavy metals (lead, mercury), pesticides, or bacteria; (3) will actually be broken down and released into the body instead of passing straight through; and (4) has met strict manufacturing protocols for safety and sanitation to ensure a consistently high-quality product.

COMMON INGREDIENTS

You should be aware that there is a lack of high-quality scientific evidence regarding whether many weight loss supplements work and are safe. Before considering any supplement, you should talk with your doctor to determine the benefits and risks of the supplement for patients like you. Here is a list of some of the most common ingredients in weight loss supplements and what they claim to do:

- **Psyllium:** Fiber supplement made from leafy plantain seeds
  - Reduces feelings of hunger, improves digestive regularity. Safety is well established and has potential for reducing weight by helping to reduce calories eaten.

- **Bladderwrack:** May be listed as *Fucus vesiculosis* in ingredients. A brown seaweed, you may recognize it by the air-filled pods (bladders) that help it float in the ocean.
  - It is believed the iodine levels in the seaweed stimulate the thyroid gland, which may have an effect on metabolism and weight loss.
  - Limited clinical studies testing this compound.

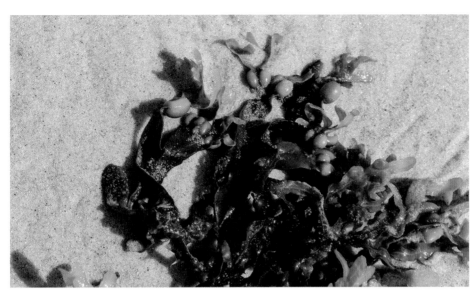

Bladderwrack is a common supplement ingredient

- **Chitosan:** Made from crab/shrimp/lobster shells and chitin, a derivative of glucose
  - ◆ Theorized to bind to fat, blocking its absorption.
  - ◆ Poor-quality studies show minimal effect, if any, on weight, and there are concerns for allergies and impaired vitamin absorption.

- **Chromium picolinate:** Mineral essential for metabolism
  - ◆ May regulate insulin and cholesterol levels
  - ◆ No high-quality data that shows an effect on body weight or appetite

- **Conjugated linoleic acid:** A chemical found naturally in foods like beef and dairy products
  - ◆ Studies have shown a reduction in body fat, but only by 0.2 pounds (0.09 kg) per week.

- **Dehydroepiandrosterone (DHEA):** Hormone produced by the kidneys that helps produce sex hormones estrogen and testosterone
  - ◆ May reduce cholesterol levels
  - ◆ No reputable evidence for reducing body weight; many safety concerns, potential interactions with medications, and side effects

- **Garcinia cambogia or brindleberry:** A green-yellow fruit that resembles a pumpkin, also called a Malabar tamarind. The rind contains a fruit acid: hydroxycitric acid, or HCA.
  - Few studies have shown little to no effects on weight loss and decreased appetite.

- **Ephedra/Ephedrine-1:** Ephedra is an herb called *ma huang* in Chinese and is often combined with caffeine or guarana. Ephedrine is an active component in ephedra.
  - Produces a stimulant effect to curb appetite and increase energy. Well-designed studies show some weight loss effects up to 2 pounds per month, although there is concern over side effects including increased blood pressure.
  - Certain ephedra species containing ephedrine alkaloids were banned in 2004 due to health risks; other types of ephedra extracts containing ephedrine are still available and legal (NIH.gov).

- **Beta-hydroxy-beta-methylbutyrate (HMB):** Substance found in the body that aids muscle growth
  - May only be beneficial for already-lean individuals; no studies available for weight loss or muscle growth in overweight individuals.

- **Teas (green, oolong, black)**
  - Potential small amount of weight loss attributed to caffeine, possible increase in metabolism and benefits from improved hydration; safety of tea concentrates is unclear.

The above list does not include all products purported to have weight loss benefits, as the number of products claiming this benefit is ever growing. When we review the available scientific evidence of such new products for efficacy and safety, we find that the studies either have not been conducted or are poorly designed. Arguably, the only currently available agents with proven efficacy are ephedra and psyllium. While ephedra may be effective, it has health risks and is not available in the United States because of these safety concerns. Psyllium-based fiber is the safest, most effective supplement for helping you lose weight because it helps you feel fuller, regulates your bowels, and may help reduce cholesterol and blood sugar levels. However, it is important to remember you can get enough fiber from eating plenty of healthful fruits, vegetables, and legumes, such as cucumbers, zucchini, squash, broccoli, lentils, black beans, chia seeds, blackberries, and many others.

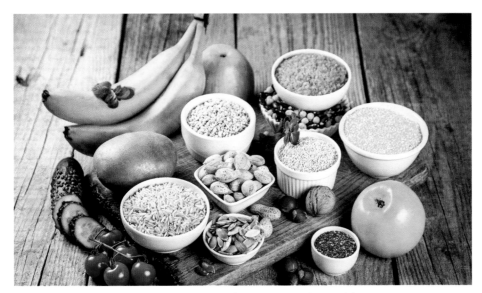
Fiber is the safest, most effective supplement for helping you lose weight

For more safety information and study results for other supplements not listed, we encourage you to visit the National Institutes of Health Office of Dietary Supplements website. Please talk to your health care provider before using any weight loss products; few have any proven efficacy, and we do not endorse their use.

hCG

Human chorionic gonadotropin (hCG) is an excellent example of a current weight loss fad. It is a naturally occurring hormone in women that increases dramatically during pregnancy and is used medically in fertility treatment. It is currently being marketed illegally by several companies, touting fast weight loss by burning upward of 3,000 calories per day of body fat without the hunger or weakness associated with the restrictive diet that is required (< 500 calories eaten per day for up to eight weeks). First of all, if it sounds too good to be true, it is too good to be true. Not to mention the FDA has officially declared the sale and use of over-the-counter hCG to be illegal, with the warning to "stop using it, throw it out, and stop following the dieting instructions" associated with its use. But let's look at the real reason it "works"—when taking or injecting hCG, you must adhere to consuming 500 calories or less per day, which is not enough to power a small rodent. Anyone would lose weight on such a restrictive diet, but he or she would also be at risk for malnutrition. This diet sounds like an introduction to an eating disorder, and there is no science to back it up, but plenty of science against it.

MediSpas

What is a MediSpa (or MedSpa)? Short for medical spa, it is a cross between a day spa and a medical treatment center. The theme is typically "wellness" or rejuvenation, emphasizing care for the whole body, at least on the outside. They offer a full variety of skin treatments, from laser hair removal to Botox injections, as well as body contouring and massages. Some MediSpas even perform liposuction. A legal MediSpa operates under a physician, often a plastic surgeon, who oversees

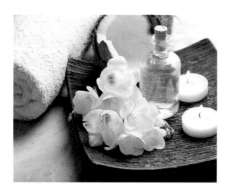

the medical aspects. Currently, it is unknown how many MediSpas are operating in the United States, but there seems to be a significant upturn, including those that may have questionable practices and legality. Be wary of MediSpas, especially those that offer easy weight loss remedies. They are not proven to be safe or effective, and you will likely have greater success working with your health care provider team.

Prescription Medications

For reasons known (environment, diet) and unknown (genetic predisposition, hormones), some people have a harder time losing a significant (more than 5%) amount of weight, even after making changes to their diet and lifestyle habits. If you

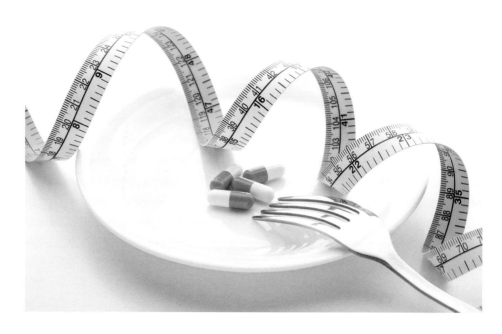

find yourself in this challenging situation, it is not unreasonable to consider adding a weight loss medication under the guidance of a health care provider with the ability to prescribe medications (such as a licensed physician, nurse practitioner, or physician's assistant). If your primary care provider is not familiar with prescribing weight loss medications, look for an obesity medicine specialist in your area at the following web address: https://obesitymedicine.org/find-obesity-treatment. Make sure to select the "ABOM Diplomate" option so that you'll know that your specialist is board-certified in obesity medicine. A comprehensive directory of all ABOM certified physicians is available at http://www.abom.org by selecting "Find a Physician/Verify Credentials."

Your decision to try a medication aid must be made with the assistance of your health care provider, but in the paragraphs that follow we will provide you with a foundation of knowledge about what medications are out there and which one might be best for you, so that you can ask the right questions and make an educated decision.

We will cover six medications that can aid in weight loss, including how they work, common side effects, average weight loss achieved in clinical trials, key points, and monthly cost without insurance. Unfortunately, weight loss medications are often not covered by insurance. It's worth a call to your insurance carrier to determine your benefits coverage and formulary options if you're interested in trying a medication.

All of the medications discussed in this chapter are approved by the FDA for weight loss, with the exception of one, metformin, that physicians sometimes prescribe "off-label" (more on that later) to patients.

WHO SHOULD CONSIDER PRESCRIPTION MEDICATIONS FOR WEIGHT LOSS?

First, it should be mentioned that no weight loss medication, including supplements, should be taken while pregnant, breastfeeding, or without first consulting your health care provider.

If you have made changes to your diet and exercise programs, and have kept them up for a reasonable length of time, you may be interested in trying weight loss medications. In addition to discussing the weight loss steps you've undertaken thus far, your health care provider will take into account whether you meet the standard guidelines

BOX 10-1

Who:

- BMI 30 kg/m2 or higher

or

- BMI 27-29.9 kg/m2 with a weight-related condition (for example, high blood pressure, high cholesterol, type 2 diabetes) and you have been unsuccessful at losing 5% of your body weight after three months of lifestyle changes

for trying medications for weight loss. If you checked either of the boxes in box 10.1, let's talk drugs.

PRESCRIPTION MEDICATIONS FOR WEIGHT LOSS

Here is a list of the most commonly prescribed weight loss medications:

- phentermine
- phentermine and topiramate combination (brand name: Qsymia)
- orlistat (brand names: Xenical, or the OTC version: Alli)
- liraglutide injection (brand name: Saxenda)
- semaglutide injection (brand name: Wegovy)
- bupropion and naltrexone combination (brand name: Contrave)
- metformin (brand name: Glucophage)

Should your health care provider prescribe any of these medications, it is important that you check in with him or her regularly to determine if it is working for you (as you would with any medication). Together with your provider, you will monitor your weight and any side effects every week for one month, and then every month for four months. You may also monitor your blood pressure and heart rate, depending on the medication used. If there has not been any significant weight loss (at least 5% of starting weight) within this time, the drug should be stopped or another medication tried. Let's take a closer look at each drug.

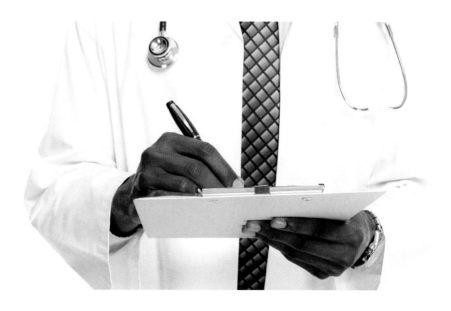

Phentermine HCl (Hydrochloride)

Let's start out with the most commonly prescribed medication nationally: phentermine. Not only is phentermine helpful for many people, but at around $10 per month, the financial risk is low, especially when used intermittently throughout the month when you need a little extra help managing your diet. In some cases, patients who take phentermine use it just on the weekends to help build a better routine for eating during this more challenging time of the week.

Say you have a solid routine during the week—you have a good breakfast early, go to work with your premade meal, get off work and hit the gym, and then come home to have a healthy dinner, some relaxation, and a good night's sleep. There is little downtime, and you get into the rhythm and habits that keep your diet and exercise on track. Work and other routines of life provide the structure for

---

BOX 10-2

Phentermine Facts

- **How does it work?**
  - Phentermine is an anti-obesity agent (technically called a noradrenergic agonist) that is taken once a day, often two hours after eating breakfast. It is unknown exactly how it causes weight loss, but it works as a stimulant (think caffeine and ADHD medications) in the central nervous system, causing appetite suppression.
  - Trade/brand name: Adipex-P, Fastin, Lomaira, others

- **Common side effects**
  - Dry mouth, insomnia, dizziness, palpitations, flushing, fatigue, and constipation (Pilitsi et al., 2018)
  - More serious side effects: increased blood pressure, increased heart rate, stroke, heart attack, psychosis (Micromedex)

- **Average amount of weight loss**
  - 12–13 kilograms (about 26–29 pounds) at nine months (Yanovski & Yanovski, 2014; site within a site, 14; up to date)

- **Key points**
  - Alcohol should be avoided
  - Cannot be taken with MAOIs (a type of antidepressant)
  - Phentermine is related to amphetamines and known to increase blood pressure and heart rate, making it potentially dangerous for those who have preexisting heart conditions

- **Cost**
  - $10–$30 for 30 tablets (one-month supply)

everything else to fall around. And then the weekend hits, and you are more likely to have social events (often that involve food) and a bit more unstructured time. Maybe your thoughts turn to food more readily, or you eat to pass the time while being with friends and family. It's easy to get off track and fall into old habits. In cases such as this, phentermine can be added to your daily routine when it is convenient for you. It is related to amphetamines (stimulants for the brain), so it reduces your feelings of needing to eat and can help you feel more motivated to get up and move. Note that there is a small risk of abuse or dependency, which your health care provider should discuss with you. However, in our experience, we have had success prescribing phentermine without seeing these effects, even when taken for up to two years or longer.

Phentermine + Topiramate Combination

Now that you have an understanding of phentermine, let's discuss combining phentermine with topiramate, a medication to treat migraines and seizures. You are probably wondering why this medication can help you lose weight, and the answer is, we're not really sure. But topiramate seems to be helpful in a variety of other conditions besides migraines and seizures, including alcohol use disorder and bipolar disorder, among others. While there are studies showing some efficacy for weight loss, topiramate alone is not FDA approved to treat obesity. However, when used in combination with phentermine, it is FDA approved specifically for weight loss and marketed as Qsymia. The combination has all the effects of phentermine but the addition of topiramate can assist in regulating appetite.

Note that the combination of phentermine and topiramate should not be mixed with alcohol. You should abstain from alcohol altogether to avoid harmful effects to the brain and respiratory system. Other medications also need to be considered by your provider before starting this combo medication. In addition, women of childbearing age should use reliable birth control, as topiramate has been linked with birth defects, specifically cleft lip and palate. The benefits are well documented in clinical trials, and it has the largest average weight loss results of any of the available drugs, but may carry a relatively high price tag at about $100 per month.

Orlistat

Next up is orlistat, which you may recognize as the product Alli, sold in pharmacies over the counter. Orlistat is a curious medication that we don't often prescribe because it does not necessarily curb appetite. It is taken as a pill when you eat fatty foods and prevents some of the fat from being absorbed, reducing excessive calories as a result. However, if the fat is not absorbed, it is expelled out the other end,

BOX 10-3

Phentermine + Topiramate Combination Facts

- **How does it work?**
  - This combination pill contains both phentermine (see above) and topiramate, an antiseizure medication. When used in combination, they are FDA approved for the treatment of obesity. Both medications suppress the appetite and cause feelings of fullness.
  - Trade/brand name: Qsymia

- **Common side effects**
  - See above for phentermine
  - Dry mouth, constipation, insomnia, anxiety, depression, numbness, and tingling (Pilitsi et al., 2018)

- **Average amount of weight loss**
  - 8.8 kilograms (about 19 pounds) at one year on highest dose (Pilitsi et al., 2018)

- **Key points**
  - Alcohol must be avoided
  - Cannot be taken with MAOIs (a type of antidepressant) and various other medications, including some OTC and herbal supplements

- **Cost**
  - $100 (one-month supply)

sometimes at unpredictable intervals. This may additionally promote avoidance of fatty foods, which is a change in diet and behavior, but it does not curb appetite directly or encourage regulation of appetite and portion control.

We typically only prescribe this medication when we can identify fried or fatty foods as the primary offender for an individual's weight gain. Purchased over the counter, the dosage is reduced to half that of the prescription, potentially reducing its effectiveness a bit. Regardless of whether it is given over the counter or comes from behind the counter, it is still quite expensive, and the amount of weight loss is typically lower than that seen with the use of phentermine or phentermine/topiramate. Be careful if buying over the counter, as it is recommended to be taken with up to three meals per day, bringing the total to 90 pills per month. A $50 box of half-strength orlistat contains only 60 pills.

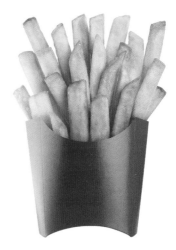

Orlistat prevents some fat in foods from being absorbed by your body

BOX 10-4

Orlistat Facts

- **How does it work?**
  - Orlistat is an anti-obesity agent that blocks some of the fat you eat from being absorbed. This means fatty foods go in and right back out without being digested and stored as excess body fat.
  - Trade/brand names: Alli, Xenical

- **Common side effects**
  - Oily discharge, oily spotting, fecal urgency, fecal incontinence, increased defecation, flatulence
  - Decreased absorption of fat-soluble vitamins (Pilitsi et al., 2018)
  - The gastrointestinal side effects may last between three and six months, and are often mild to moderate. They are the main reason for discontinuing the medication (Perrault, 2018; up to date).

- **Average amount of weight loss**
  - 10 pounds at one year (6.2% body weight; Pilitsi et al., 2018 [Xendos study])

- **Key points**
  - Orlistat can be purchased over the counter without a prescription, but only at half of the prescription dose. The full-strength must be prescribed.
  - Because essential vitamins (A, D, E, and K) require fat in order to be absorbed, these vitamins must be taken as supplements or in a multivitamin while taking orlistat to prevent malnutrition (Micromedex)

- **Cost**
  - Up to $600 for 90 tablets (taken three times per day, one-month supply) (full-strength/prescription)
  - About $70 for 120 tablets of the OTC strength

Liraglutide or Semaglutide

Before starting to read about these medications, ask yourself if you would be up for giving yourself an injection in your belly, thigh, or arm. If you're comfortable with injections, this type of medication could be an option for you. Liraglutide and semaglutide were originally designed to treat type 2 diabetes, but when used at a higher dose, their primary effect is reduced appetite and weight loss, as opposed to lowering blood sugar in diabetes patients. Interestingly, the injections are not the most common complaint with these medications. The digestive side effects of nausea, vomiting, constipation, and indigestion lead patients to stop early. Liraglutide

BOX 10-5

Liraglutide Facts

- **How does it work?**
  - Liraglutide is a daily injection that is considered an antidiabetic medication, although it is FDA approved for weight control
  - even if you do not have type 2 diabetes. Liraglutide helps control appetite, which results in fewer calories and subsequent weight loss.
  - Trade/brand name: Saxenda

- **Common side effects**
  - Nausea, vomiting, constipation, diarrhea, indigestion, headache, low blood sugar (Micromedex)

- **Average amount of weight loss**
  - 5.6 kilograms (about 12 pounds) at one year (Pilitsi et al., 2018)

- **Key points**
  - Liraglutide is not intended to treat type 2 diabetes in this case, and it can be used for weight control even if you do not have type 2 diabetes.
  - Daily injections are not difficult to perform, but it can be a deal breaker for some
  - Most likely out of all the medications to be discontinued due to side effects (Pilitsi et al., 2018)

- **Cost**
  - $300 (one-month supply), usually sold in packs of three pens for around $900

can also be particularly costly without insurance coverage—in excess of $500 per month. Semaglutide helps patients achieve a 15% total weight loss, and it has to be injected only once a week (compared with the daily injections associated with liraglutide). Given that both of these medications also improve blood sugar levels, they can be good options for patients with prediabetes/type 2 diabetes mellitus and obesity.

Bupropion + Naltrexone Combination

This combination weight loss pill is particularly beneficial for suppressing persistent food cravings. One of the two ingredients, bupropion, is a medication that increases dopamine and norepinephrine (neurotransmitters) levels in the brain, improving mood and reducing appetite. It is commonly used alone as an antidepressant, but it is also used for quitting tobacco. It is perhaps because of this that it is helpful specifically for fighting food cravings. If you are a smoker and have

Bupropion + Naltrexone Combination Facts

- **How does it work?**
  - Promotes neurotransmitters norepinephrine and dopamine, which in turn improve mood and reduce appetite
  - Trade/brand name: Contrave

- **Common side effects**
  - Nausea, vomiting, constipation, diarrhea, dry mouth, dizziness, headache, insomnia, anxiety, depression

- **Average amount of weight loss**
  - 4.9 kilograms (about 11 pounds) (5.2%) at one year (Pilitsi et al., 2018)

- **Key points**
  - Runner-up for being most commonly discontinued appetite-suppressing medication due to side effects (first place goes to liraglutide) (Pilitsi et al., 2018)

- **Cost**
  - $100 (one-month supply)

contemplated quitting during your weight loss process, this combination medication may be a particularly sensible option for you. The second ingredient, naltrexone, when used alone, can treat alcohol or opioid dependency. When combined with bupropion, they work together to reduce appetite and cravings. Consider this medication combination if you struggle at the grocery store to avoid certain foods you just can't say no to or if thoughts of these foods are disruptive and sabotage your hard work. It is taken twice a day, in the morning and evening.

Metformin

Currently, other medications have been used as weight loss aids, even if they have not been approved by the FDA specifically for weight loss. This is called using a medication "off-label," or for something other than what it was designed and tested to do. Drs. Cheskin and Gudzune sometimes prescribe metformin, a medication approved for type 2 diabetes or prediabetes, because it can be helpful in curbing appetite, even in those who do not have diabetes. Metformin can be a good option for those who have risk factors for developing diabetes or for those with high blood sugar. In fact, the American Diabetes Association now recommends treating some patients who have prediabetes with metformin. Although the weight loss results are less than those of other medications designed specifically for weight loss, it is quite inexpensive and has been a helpful aid for some of our

BOX 10-7

Metformin Facts

- **What is it and how does it work?**
  - Developed as an antidiabetic medication, metformin lowers glucose (blood sugar) levels and regulates appetite

- **Common side effects**
  - Diarrhea, nausea, vomiting, indigestion, flatulence, vitamin B12 deficiency, headache, weakness (Micromedex)

- **Average amount of weight loss**
  - Less than 5% of starting weight (Perreault, 2018; up to date)

- **Key points**
  - Metformin is recommended for people with prediabetes, making it a good option for a weight control aid if you have borderline high glucose or hemoglobin A1c levels, or if you have risk factors for developing type 2 diabetes
  - Generally very well tolerated; safety has been established in the treatment of diabetes, and it has been well studied in long-term clinical trials for type 2 diabetes
  - There is some evidence that it can have life span–prolonging properties; a clinical trial is underway to test this hypothesis

- **Cost**
  - $5 (one-month supply)

patients. It is usually taken twice a day and can be increased in dose over time. Its most common side effects are gastrointestinal upset and diarrhea.

Other Prescription Products

Recently, the FDA cleared a product called Plenity, which is available by prescription only. You take capsules of this product before lunch and dinner along with water, causing a hydrogel to form in the stomach to help you feel full. As you are able to be satisfied with smaller portions, you may lose weight. Most common side effects are gastrointestinal.

ADDITIONAL POINTS TO CONSIDER REGARDING WEIGHT LOSS MEDICATIONS

As you can see from the moderate average amount of weight loss seen with these drugs, the decision to try one of these medications should be made with the understanding that it is not a quick or easy fix. In some cases, however, these medications may be useful tools to add to your Personal Plan of Action, especially if you have been unsuccessful in your weight loss efforts. However, we recommend that medications always be used in conjunction with changes to your lifestyle, diet, physical activity, and behaviors. You may also consider the cost-benefit ratio, literally, when comparing prices with the potential weight loss results.

You should be aware that there is a frequent tendency for the effectiveness of these medications to diminish over time. Typically, the lowest weight is achieved at around six months of continuous use, with maintenance, but not much further weight loss thereafter. Stopping the medications is typically associated with weight regain, but there is some evidence that intermittent use of some of the appetite-suppressing medications, especially phentermine, may be about as effective as continuous use.

For some people, intermittent medication use may be effective. This means a cycle of use and nonuse that lasts weeks to months. The individual may begin a cycle if he or she is steadily regaining weight for some reason. The medication may begin within a week, as when patients use phentermine only on weekends, when their diets tend to be higher in calories and when eating out and social eating is most likely to occur, and then don't use it on weekdays or when they anticipate minimal food challenges. Contrave (bupropion and naltrexone) should not be

---

BOX 10-8

Additional Information on Prescription Medications

- **Liraglutide** is the most likely to be discontinued due to side effects, followed by the naltrexone + bupropion combination.

- **Orlistat** has the most data and is considered the safest weight loss medication but yields only modest weight loss on average and does not control appetite.

- **Phentermine and the phentermine/topiramate combination** are more effective but must be used more cautiously. Phentermine can increase blood pressure and heart rate, meaning too much can cause significant side effects, and there is small risk for dependency and abuse of the medication.

- **New FDA approved medications** and products to be available soon—semaglutide, Plenity, and others. Plan to check with your primary care provider at your annual physical about any new medication options in this area.

used intermittently because it contains an antidepressant component that should be taken continuously.

Nicotine

Although nicotine is not a prescription medication for weight loss, it is considered a drug. It alters body chemistry and can play a large role in your life and in your path to permanent weight loss.

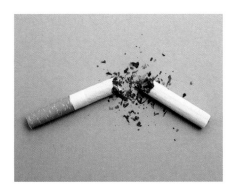

If you are a smoker or use tobacco in another form (snuff, e-cigarettes or vaping), we assume you are already well aware of the many associated health risks, so we will not burden you again with the list of reasons to quit. We will, however, acknowledge and address the reasons you may have for *not quitting*, specifically the positive effects smoking may have on your appetite and body weight. Not only does nicotine improve mood and attention, but it reduces feelings of hunger, leading to weight stabilization or weight loss in many people. In fact, dieting has been shown to actually increase smoking behavior and impede smoking cessation attempts. Nicotine was confirmed by the US surgeon general in 2010 as one of the most difficult drugs to stop, as addictive as heroin or cocaine. So it is understandable if the task of quitting feels too large to tackle, especially while trying to lose weight. It may seem counterintuitive to quit at this time. We present to you two possible options, both with the ultimate goal of helping you quit if you decide to make the attempt:

1 **Quit later.** Focus on losing that initial 5% to 10% of body weight, and then set your quit date as soon as you have reached this first weight loss goal. You may take a small step backward temporarily when you begin your attempt to quit smoking, but you've made great progress so far, and now you know you can do hard things. Reaching your first weight loss goal may provide you with the right motivation and confidence to try quitting. Talk with your health care provider about using nicotine replacements, like gum and patches, or medications like bupropion, which can additionally help curb your appetite during the process. You may also decide to keep the ball rolling with your weight loss and reach your final goal before attempting to quit, and that's okay, too. It is reasonable to reassess at each small goal you reach and decide how to proceed.

2 **Quit now.** No time like the present. Make a complete overhaul of your lifestyle, one day at a time. Clear out the cupboards, start your daily walks, and

choose a quit date with your provider. Include your friends and family in your plans to help hold you accountable. You don't have to quit cold turkey, necessarily. Studies have shown the most effective methods for quitting are nicotine replacements or medications like bupropion or varenicline. Bupropion is a daily pill that you begin taking a week before your quit date, and you can continue to take it for several months to help regulate cravings. Varenicline is another daily pill option that is started a week before your quit date, and it can be continued for three to six months. Both of these options require a prescription from your primary care provider, and he or she can help you make the best decision for you. If you decide to quit smoking during your weight loss journey, it may take you a bit longer to begin noticing changes in your weight. But keep in mind, you will be jump-starting your health by making the right changes now. Additional free quitting resources that are helpful to support this process are:

- 1-800-QUIT-NOW to get professional coaching over the phone

- BeTobaccoFree.hhs.gov to download mobile apps that will track your cravings, send motivational messages, mark milestones, and provide tips for coping with cravings and mood changes

- Text START to 47848 to receive private text message support from Smoke-Free.gov and decide on a quit date.

- Find out how much money you will save on cigarettes at SmokeFree.gov.

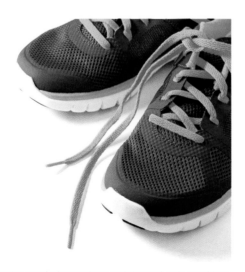

Exercise can help you lose weight and quit smoking

While you are quitting, you may find certain behaviors that help keep your mind off lighting up a cigarette or that help replace that urge. Some of these behaviors are productive to your long-term weight loss goals, such as taking a walk, hitting the gym, and staying mindful and committed to your health (remembering your "why"). It may be difficult not to replace the cigarette with a snack or meal that provides the familiar release of dopamine, a behavior that is not productive to your long-term weight loss goals. To mitigate this scenario, start with physical activity, which rapidly improves mood and reduces appetite, or choose lower-calorie foods, chew sugarless gum, and drink liquids during or after meals to help you feel fuller.

Bariatric Surgery

Thus far we have discussed an array of approaches to losing weight for good—ranging from mindset change to behavior change to the prescribed use of medications. But sometimes additional measures are needed. In the paragraphs that follow, we'll explore the option of bariatric surgery.

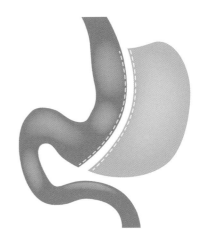

WHAT IS BARIATRIC SURGERY?

What is bariatric surgery, exactly, and why should we talk about it? The word bariatric comes from the Greek origin "baros," meaning weight, and "iatrikos," the medicine of. We use bariatric surgery interchangeably with the phrase *weight loss surgery*. In this chapter, we will use the term *bariatric*, which is the term most likely to be used by your health care provider or that you would find in your own research. It is an important topic to cover because of its growing popularity and positive results over the past decade.

The American Society for Metabolic and Bariatric Surgery estimates that 228,000 people in the United States had bariatric surgery in 2017. Of these surgeries, nearly 60% were a sleeve gastrectomy, 18% were Roux-en-Y gastric bypass, and less than 6% were gastric banding. We will take a look at these three most common procedures, with the addition of the gastric balloon, a temporary method for reducing calories and exercising portion control. All of these options work in the same way—they are just different approaches to the same result: reducing the number of calories you can ingest and absorb at one time, thereby leading to a steady, progressive weight loss.

Is bariatric surgery right for you? Maybe you've done some research already about bariatric surgery, and you think it could be your next step on your path to successful weight loss, or maybe you're not sure if you qualify yet. See if you can check two of the items below in box 10-9.

If you check a box from each category, bariatric surgery could be a good option for you. Most insurance companies require you to demonstrate a six-month trial of

Who:

☐ Unsuccessful at losing weight after trying under medical supervision for at least six months

and

☐ BMI 40 kg/m2 or higher

☐ BMI 35 kg/m2 or higher with at least one weight-related condition such as high blood pressure, high cholesterol, obstructive sleep apnea, type 2 diabetes

lifestyle modifications without significant weight loss before you are eligible to consider bariatric surgery. However, you should check with your insurance carrier (if you have one) to find out exactly how to qualify.

COSTS AND RISKS OF BARIATRIC SURGERY

Bariatric surgery can cost between $12,000 and $26,000, depending on the procedure and the medical facility. Your health care provider will help determine if you are healthy enough to undergo anesthesia and the healing process. To be a good surgical candidate, you should have a full physical exam and blood tests, and, with your health care provider, weigh the risks and benefits of the surgery.

Some of the risks of bariatric surgery are uncontrolled bleeding, infection, leaking from the incision, developing a blockage or tear in the intestine, heart and lung problems, gallstone formation (a more common side effect), nutritional deficiency, diarrhea, further surgical interventions, and, as with any surgery, death, although this outcome is extremely rare (estimated between 0.1% and 0.5%).

BENEFITS OF BARIATRIC SURGERY

It is important to understand that there are real risks involved, but it's also worthwhile to discuss the benefits of bariatric surgery. It is likely that you know most of the benefits to bariatric surgery, as they are the same benefits associated with weight loss, regardless of how it is accomplished. You may enjoy a longer and healthier life, have less risk of diseases (including stroke, heart attack, cancer), less physical stress on your joints, less fatigue, more endurance for everyday activities, improved confidence, and hopefully, achieve your own goals and expectations that you've laid out in your Personal Plan of Action.

LIFESTYLE CHANGES ASSOCIATED WITH BARIATRIC SURGERY

Bariatric surgery may help you to lose weight faster, but we caution you that this is not an easy fix. You will still need to make serious lifestyle, behavioral, and food changes, with food perhaps being the most important and also the most difficult adjustment. A registered dietitian will help you develop a meal plan for before, during, and after the surgery. You should expect to stick to foods high in protein and low in fat and sugar, and be prepared to eat four to six small meals per day. Realistic expectations and readiness to make these diet changes long term are part of the prerequisites for surgery. Weight regain in the years after is common; it is estimated that about half of bariatric surgery patients regain 5% of their initial excess weight.

TYPES OF BARIATRIC SURGERY

Sleeve Gastrectomy

Currently, a popular option in bariatric surgery is the sleeve gastrectomy. Gastrectomy is the medical term for removing part of the stomach; thus, sleeve gastrectomy means part of the stomach is permanently removed so that the remaining stomach resembles a sleeve, or a narrow tube. This modification will prevent you from eating large or even moderate amounts of food at one time. You will feel full from a small amount of food because your stomach is significantly smaller. One of the benefits of this surgery is that everything else (namely, the intestines) is left intact, and only the stomach is modified. The surgery is performed using laparoscopy, a technique that uses long, thin surgical tools inserted into two small openings in the abdomen instead of one large incision. This reduces recovery time, risk of infection, and amount of scar tissue.

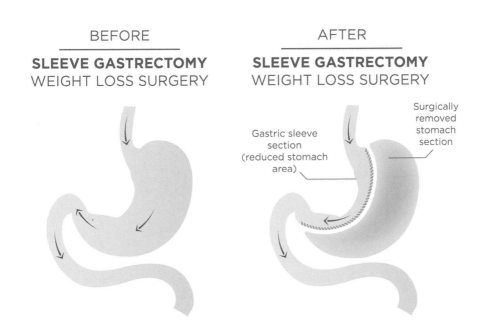

BEFORE

SLEEVE GASTRECTOMY
WEIGHT LOSS SURGERY

AFTER

SLEEVE GASTRECTOMY
WEIGHT LOSS SURGERY

Gastric sleeve section (reduced stomach area)

Surgically removed stomach section

- **Average weight loss:** 25% to 35% body weight, or *60% of excess weight.* The amount of weight you can expect to lose after gastric bypass may vary depending on your *percentage of excess weight*, a figure that is calculated by subtracting your ideal weight from your current weight.
- **Complication rate after 1 month:** < 1%
- **Complication rate total:** 13%

Roux-en-Y Gastric Bypass

The other common bariatric surgery is the Roux-en-Y gastric bypass, named for the surgeon César Roux and the Y shape that is created out of the new stomach and adjoining intestine. In this surgery, sometimes simply called gastric bypass, most of the stomach is removed, and a small pouch is formed in its place. This small pouch is then connected to the lower small intestine, thereby preventing many calories from being absorbed. As an added effect, if certain foods like sweets and fat are eaten, the lower small intestine will produce symptoms of nausea and diarrhea known as "dumping syndrome," although this can be quite dangerous. This surgery is the most invasive, requiring an open incision to be made in the abdomen and more time under anesthesia and in recovery.

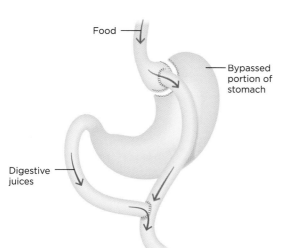

Food

Bypassed
portion of
stomach

Digestive
juices

- **Average weight loss:** 30% to 40% body weight, or *70% of excess weight.* The amount of weight you can expect to lose after gastric bypass may vary depending on your *percentage of excess weight,* a figure that is calculated by subtracting your ideal weight from your current weight.
- **Complication rate after 1 month:** 1.25%
- **Complication rate total:** 21%
- **Reoperation rate:** 3% to 20%

Gastric Banding

Gastric banding, sometimes referred to as a lap band, is third in line for the most common bariatric surgery, perhaps due to the slower rate of weight loss when compared to sleeve gastrectomy and Roux-en-Y gastric bypass. An inflatable band is placed around the stomach, acting as a kind of girdle. The band causes a small pouch to form above it, where only a small amount of food can collect, causing a feeling of fullness after only a small amount of food has been eaten. The rest of the stomach is still intact, pushed down below the band, and functions as usual after the food passes through the narrowed, banded area. The idea is the same: to limit the amount of food consumed at one time, without the feelings of hunger. Gastric banding is performed by laparoscopy, as is

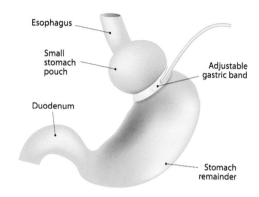

done in the sleeve gastrectomy, and is therefore a less invasive surgery than open gastric bypass. The gastric band can be removed if desired, and there are no permanent modifications to the stomach or intestines.

- **Average weight loss:** 5 to 10 pounds per month, or *50% of excess weight*
- **Complication rate after 1 month:** 0.25%
- **Complication rate total:** 13%
- **Reoperation rate:** 10% to 50%

Gastric Balloon

The gastric balloon is not technically a surgery because it is done by endoscopy and does not require an incision, but you will be slightly sedated. Endoscopy is a nonsurgical procedure involving an endoscope: a small, flexible tube with a camera on the tip. The endoscope enters through the mouth and travels down the throat into the stomach, into which it places a small fluid-filled balloon. This balloon takes up space in the stomach, preventing large amounts of food from entering

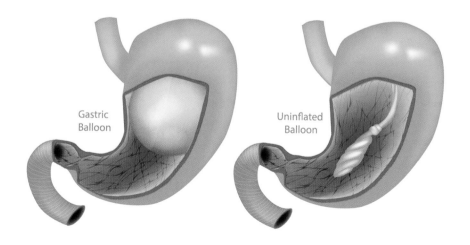

while reducing feelings of hunger. The procedure takes about 15 minutes in all. The balloon is typically removed after several months, during which the patient has been able to regulate his or her appetite and portion sizes. Over half of people who undergo this procedure are able to lose 10% of their body weight. Almost all are able to lose at least 5% after removal.

- **Average weight loss:** 5% to 10% total body weight, or *20% to 30% of excess weight*
- **Complication rate:** early removal required in 4% to 9% of patients

A LOOK INTO THE FUTURE: BARIATRIC EMBOLIZATION

We are now finding that not only do weight loss surgeries and procedures reduce hunger and the volume of the stomach, but they also trigger changes in the digestive hormones and body chemistry that have a profound influence on weight loss, perhaps even more so than do the physical changes. New evidence of these metabolic changes has prompted studies to investigate how we can achieve these changes in a patient without performing surgery.

One promising noninvasive method is called bariatric embolization, performed by an interventional radiologist and bariatric team. An embolus refers to something that causes a blockage. In embolization, one or more of the arteries leading to the stomach is blocked with tiny, gelatin beads that cut off the blood supply. A small catheter is guided from the femoral artery up to these arteries near the stomach, and the gelatin beads are deposited. One study showed striking improvements in hunger and reduced appetite, low complication rates, and a 6% to 9% loss of excess weight.

Resources

Personal Plan of Action Template

This Personalized Plan of Action is your "road map" for *Weight Loss for Life*. The plan includes the following sections, which together will help you get to your desired destination of weight management. We recommend that you start this plan **after** you have received medical clearance (required). You can complete your plan as you read this book or after you finish the book (recommended).

Weight Loss Goals

Note: *An average rate of safe, achievable, and sustainable weight loss is 1 to 2 lbs per week.*

Initial weight: _____

Goal weight in 2 weeks: _____
Goal weight in 1 month: _____
Goal weight in 3 months: _____
Goal weight in 6 months: _____
Goal weight in 12 months: _____

My goal is to lose _____ pounds in _____ weeks by losing _____ pounds per week.

Medical Conditions

Current Medical Conditions: _____

_____

_____

What guidance has my medical provider given me for weight management? _____

_____

_____

Weekly Weight Tracker

Date	Week	Weight	Amount Lost or Gained
	1		
	2		
	3		
	4		
	5		
	6		

Motivation and Support System

My main motivations to lose weight are: _____

_____

_____

_____

I will hold myself accountable by

_____ *keeping a daily journal*

_____ *using an app to track my* _____ *behavior*

_____ *other* _____

I will ask for support from (name here): _____, who is

a ____ friend ____ family member ____ coach ____ counselor ____ group, so that I can celebrate

my successes along the way and not feel like I have to go it alone.

Positive Self-Talk

When I feel discouraged, I will say the following to myself: _____

_____

_____

Stress Management and Behavioral Change Plans

STRESS

What changes will I make in how I manage stress?

_____

In order to make this change, I will commit to _____

_____

Common Reasons for Overeating	Flexible Solution
Stress	
Anxiety, nervousness	
Weekends	
Fatigue, tiredness	
Watching TV	
Feeling down or depressed	
Social settings (parties)	
Anger, irritation	
Pressure from others	

Common Barriers to Physical Activity	Flexible Solution
Too hot, too cold, too rainy, too windy	
Too busy	
Too tired	
Too sad, angry, stressed, depressed	
Too painful	
Too boring	
Too unenjoyable	

SLEEP

In order to ensure I meet my daily sleep requirement of seven hours per night, I will commit to _____

HEALTHY REWARDS/MOTIVATION TECHNIQUES:

I will celebrate my successes with the following healthy, nonfood rewards:

Eating for Weight Loss Plans

DAILY CALORIE INTAKE

I have chosen my weight loss caloric intake goal to be _____ calories per day.

My monitoring strategy: _____

_____

CALORIC INTAKE BEHAVIOR GOALS

_____ Eat more of these healthy and nutritious foods: _____

_____ Eat less of these sweet and "empty calorie" foods: _____

_____ Eat more carbohydrates with the following choices: _____

_____ Eat more vegetables with the following choices: _____

_____ Eat more protein with the following choices: _____

_____ Drink more water

_____ Drink _____ less or _____ no alcohol

_____ Drink less sweet and high-calorie drinks

_____ Other _____

_____

Foods to Reduce (that is, empty-calorie / high-fat foods)	Alternatives

MEAL PLANNING

Busiest days: _____

Strategies for staying on track on busy days: _____

_____

Healthful, low-calorie, low-fat snacks:

Snacks	Food Groups/Ingredients

Healthful, low-calorie, low-fat meals:

Meals	Food Groups/Ingredients
Meal 1	
Meal 2	
Meal 3	

EXCEPTIONS

If I want to indulge by eating a favorite/craved food (_____), I will increase my physical activity by _____ moving more throughout the day or _____ adding additional physical activity by _____.

Physical Activity for Weight Loss Plans

Current fitness level (beginner, intermediate, advanced)

Current physical activity amount: _____

Physical Activity (Caloric Output) Behavior Goals

_____ Increase amount of time sitting actively (with stability ball or other item)

_____ Increase amount of time standing throughout the day

_____ Increase amount of time moving throughout the day

_____ Move in all three planes of motion, using the mindful movement checklist

_____ Increase exercise activity (check all that apply)

_____ cardiovascular activity _____ times per week (start with 2x; aim for 4–5x)

_____ strength training _____ times per week (start with 1x; aim for 2x)

_____ flexibility training _____ times per week (aim for 5x week, 5–20 minutes)

Exercise Plan

My goal is to _____ for _____ minutes on _____ days of the week. I will start

by _____ .

Then, I will increase duration or intensity by _____ .

Month	Physical Activity Goals
Month 1	
Month 2	
Month 3	
Month 4	
Month 5	
Month 6	

Weekly Exercise Planner

Monday	**Plan A: Best Plan**
Tuesday	
Wednesday	**Plan B: Backup Plan**
Thursday	
Friday	**Notes:**
Saturday	

Preferred Exercises

Type	Location	Physical Activity Goals

Exceptions

If I want or need to skip an exercise session (_____), I will commit to

_____ in order to meet my physical activity requirements.

If I want or need to ____sit more or ____move less throughout the day, I will commit to

_____ in order to meet my physical activity mindful movement checklist

requirements.

Maintenance Plan

Zones

Green Safety Zone Current weight: _____ lbs Weight window: _____ to _____ lbs	My maintenance weight, within 3 to 5 pounds. I will weigh myself at least weekly to monitor my window.
Yellow Caution Zone Weight window: _____ to _____ lbs	If I slip beyond the 3 to 5 pound safety zone, I need to make a plan and take action (e.g.: keep a food diary for a few days, be cognizant of my habits and attitudes, and/or revisit my support to get into the Green zone).
Red Correction Zone	Regaining more than 5 to 8 pounds puts me at higher risk for continuing to regain more weight. It is vital to stop, reevaluate what happened, and avoid slipping back into my old lifestyle and behaviors. I will reactivate my weight loss efforts with new or familiar proven methods that have worked for me in the past.

Maintenance Goals

Maintenance goal physical activity: _____ for ____ minutes on ____ days of the week

Maintenance calorie intake goal:_____per day

Maintenance Check List

☐ Engage in physical activity that I enjoy and can sustain each week
☐ Prepare/plan to eat healthful foods routinely and while traveling
☐ Schedule my health in my calendar to fit with my routine and other responsibilities
☐ Update my goals and keep them in plain sight
☐ Monitor my weight while living my life
☐ In short, follow the 4 M's of Maintenance

Move	Movements (physical activity) that are enjoyable and sustainable to you
Monitor	Nutrients going in, physical activity, weight, patterns, sleep
Motivation	Motivators for achieving short- and long-term goals
Make time	Prioritize and schedule healthful eating and physical activity to fit your life

Food and Activity Log

Instructions: Use this log for your initial three-day food evaluation as well as continued trackir

Date:

Place	Time	Food/Beverages	Food Group
Home	2:00 p.m.	Crackers	Grains

Water (check one box for each 8-ounce glass)				Total Servings:
				Grains ____
				Fruits ____
				Vegetables ____
				Protein ____
				Dairy ____

SOURCE: *Adapted from the American Dietetic Association, copyright 2009.*

Amount	Calories (optional)	Hunger (0–4)	Triggers?
2 handfuls	300	1	Boredom, TV

Total Calories	

Physical Activity (type and duration)	Comments

Movement and Activity Assessment

Date: _____

Age: _____

Sex: _____

Weight (lbs): _____

Height (inches): _____

BMI: _____

Goal weight: _____

Fat (%): _____

Physical limitations: _____

Medications taken: _____
_____

Exercise/physical activity history: _____
_____

Barriers to exercise: _____
_____

Occupation/location: _____
_____

Describe current activity:

☐ Frequency: _____

☐ Intensity: _____

☐ Time: _____

☐ Type: _____

What types of exercise/physical activity do you enjoy/would you be interested in? _____
_____

Close proximity to exercise facility/interest in joining a facility? _____
_____

Do you prefer to exercise at home, in a gym, or outside? _____

What, if any, exercise equipment do you own? _____

If not currently active, when was the last time you were consistent with physical activity?

_____

_____

Readiness

Time (days/hours) per week? _____

Solo / partner / groups / classes / trainer

Goals:

1 _____
2 _____
3 _____
4 _____
5 _____

Comments:

_____
_____
_____
_____
_____
_____
_____
_____
_____
_____

The Energy Balance Equation Assessment

This optional assessment can help you understand what your caloric intake versus expenditure (energy balance equation) looks like today.

Please note: In order to determine your daily caloric needs, you can use the Mifflin–St. Jeor equation:

- **Men:** calories/day = 10 × weight (kg) + 6.25 × height (cm) − 5 × age (y) + 5
- **Women:** calories/day = 10 × weight (kg) + 6.25 × height (cm) − 5 × age (y) − 161

Multiply your result by an activity factor—a number that represents different levels of activity:

- **Sedentary:** × 1.2 (limited exercise)
- **Lightly active:** × 1.375 (light exercise less than three days per week)
- **Moderately active:** × 1.55 (moderate exercise most days of the week)
- **Very active:** × 1.725 (hard exercise every day)
- **Extra active:** × 1.9 (strenuous exercise two or more times per day)

The end result gives you your total daily energy expenditure, or TDEE—the total number of calories you burn on a given day. The formula helps you determine your TDEE, which is a combination of your resting energy expenditure (REE, the number of calories a person burns at rest) and your nonresting energy expenditure (NREE, the number of calories burned during activity and digestion).

After you have computed your TDEE, you can then determine what your daily caloric intake goal can be.

- **If you are trying to manage your weight,** you can aim to consume the same number of calories as your TDEE, while maintaining your activity level.
- **If you are trying to lose weight,** you can aim to consume fewer calories than your

TDEE and/or to increase your activity level so that you have a caloric deficit.

Tip: Since a pound is 3,500 calories, you might aim for a 500-calorie deficit daily. This can be achieved by eating less, moving more, or both. Doing so would yield you a pound of weight loss per week. Studies show that losing 1 to 2 pounds per week is a healthy goal, and has a higher likelihood to be sustained (not gained back) over time.

Remember: If you consume more calories than your TDEE, over time you will gain weight. If you consume fewer calories than your TDEE, you will lose weight.

What is your TDEE based on your current activity level: _____

How many pounds do you want to lose per week?
- If 1 pound per week, deduct 500 calorie deficit per day: _____
- If 2 pounds per week, deduct 1,000 calorie deficit per day: _____
- Your daily caloric goal for weight loss: _____

Please note:
1 You can increase your TDEE by increasing your activity level.
2 You can accomplish your calorie deficit by reducing food intake, increasing exercise, or both (recommended).

SMART Framework

What is the SMARTest way to get to success?

This optional exercise will help you get "SMART" about how you plan for success. SMART is a framework for planning that helps you ensure your goal setting is "specific, measurable, achievable, realistic, and time-bound." Creating a SMARTer plan will make sure you are working smarter, not harder, at losing weight for good.

Specific: How will you define weight loss and management success? (Check all that apply.)

____Improved health status (disease management)

____Improved wellness (ability to perform and "do" life well)

____Improved well-being (overall experience and quality of life)

____Other: _____

Measurable: How will you measure success in your body, mind, and life beyond the scale?

Improvement in body (physical function)

____Improved (or managed) medical status

____Improved physical health

____Improved strength and muscle tone

____Improved core strength and balance

____Improved cardiovascular function

____Improved flexibility

____Improved sleep ____ quality (deep) or ____ quantity (length of time)

____Other: _____

Improved mind (mental health function)

____Improved mood (experience of emotional well-being)

____Improved focus (reduction of brain fog)

____Management of mental health conditions (anxiety, depression, illness)

____Other: _____

Improved life (daily function, including social support and stress management)

_____ Improved stress management (emotional regulation)

_____ Improved social experience (relationship engagement)

_____ Improved communication (expression of voice)

_____ Other: _____

Achievable: What weight loss goals do you want to set for yourself for the next year?

_____

_____

_____

_____

_____

_____

Weight Loss Journal

References

Chapter 6. Designing Your Dietary Plan

Young, K. "Artificially Sweetened Drinks Linked to Stroke, Heart Disease." *New England Journal of Medicine: Journal Watch*, February 14, 2019, https://www.jwatch.org/fw115067/2019/02/14/artificially-sweetened-drinks-linked-stroke-heart-disease.

Chapter 7. Food Shopping, Meal Planning, and Monitoring Principles

Anderson, B., A. P. Rafferty, S. Lyon-Callo, C. Fussman, and G. Imes. "Fast Food Consumption and Obesity among Michigan Adults." *Preventing Chronic Disease* 8, no. 4 (July 2011): A71.

Bowman, S. A., and B. T. Vinyard. "Fast Food Consumption of US Adults: Impact on Energy and Nutrient Intakes and Overweight Status." *Journal of the American College of Nutrition* 23, no. 2 (April 2004): 163–68.

Rosenheck, R. "Fast Food Consumption and Increased Caloric Intake: A Systematic Review of a Trajectory Towards Weight Gain and Obesity Risk." *Obesity Reviews* 9, no. 6 (November 2008): 535–47.

Tandon, P. S., C. Zhou, N. L. Chan, P. Lozano, S. C. Couch, K. Glanz, J. Krieger, and B. E. Saelens. "The Impact of Menu Labeling on Fast-Food Purchases for Children and Parents." *American Journal of Preventive Medicine* 41, no. 4 (October 2011): 434–38.

Urban, L. E., J. L. Weber, M. B. Heyman, R. L. Schichtl, S. Verstraete, N. S. Lowery, S. K. Das, M. M. Schleicher, G. Rogers, C. Economos, W. A. Masters, and S. B. Roberts. "Energy Contents of Frequently Ordered Restaurant Meals and Comparison with Human Energy Requirements and US Department of Agriculture Database Information: A Multisite Randomized Study." *Journal of the Academy of Nutrition and Dietetics* 116, no. 4 (May 2016): 590–98.

Chapter 10. Medical Solutions: Beyond Mindset and Behavior Change

National Center for Complementary and Integrative Health. https://nccih.nih.gov/health/ephedra.

National Institutes of Health. https://ods.od.nih.gov/factsheets/WeightLoss-HealthProfessional/.

Perreault, L., and C. Apovian. "Obesity in Adults: Overview of Management."
UptoDate, 2020. Retrieved February 6, 2021, from https://www.uptodate.com/
contents/obesity-in-adults-overview-of-management.

Pilitsi, E., O. M. Farr, S. A. Polyzos, N. Perakakis, E. Nolen-Doerr, A.-E. Papatha-
nasiou, and C. S. Mantzoros. "Pharmacotherapy of Obesity: Available
Medications and Drugs under Investigation." *Metabolism* 92 (2019): 170–92.

US Pharmacopeia. http://www.usp.org/verification-services/verified-mark.

Whigham, L. D., A. C. Watras, and D. A. Schoeller. "Efficacy of Conjugated
Linoleic Acid for Reducing Fat Mass: A Meta-analysis in Humans." *American
Journal of Clinical Nutrition* 85, no. 5 (2007): 1203–1211.

Yanovski, S. Z., and J. A. Yanovski. "Long-Term Drug Treatment for Obesity: A
Systematic and Clinical Review." *Journal of the American Medical Association*
311, no. 1 (2014): 74–86.

From Micromedex

American Society for Metabolic and Bariatric Surgery. "Metabolic and
Bariatric Surgery." October 2018, https://asmbs.org/resources/metabolic-
and-bariatric-surgery.

———"Studies Weigh in on Safety and Effectiveness of Newer Bariatric and
Metabolic Surgery Procedure." June 20, 2012, https://asmbs.org/resources/
studies-weigh-in-on-safety-and-effectiveness-of-newer-bariatric-and-metabolic-
surgery-procedure.

Falk, V., J. K. Eccles, S. Karmali, and R. Sultanian. "A313 Intragastric Balloon
Removal: Puncture, Dilate, Deflate." *Journal of the Canadian Association of
Gastroenterology* 1, no. S2 (March 2018): 449–50.

Hollander, P. A., S. C. Elbein, I. B. Hirsch, et al. "Role of Orlistat in the Treatment of Obese Patients with Type 2 Diabetes." *Diabetes Care* 21, no. 8 (1998):
1288–1294.

Imaz-Iglesia, I., E. E. Garcia-Alvarez, J. Gonzales-Enriquez, C. Martínez-Cervell,
and J. M. Sendra Gutlérrez. "Safety and Effectiveness of the Intragastric Balloon
for Obesity." *Obesity Surgery* 18, no. 7 (August 2008): 841–46.

Ma, I. T., and J. A Madura. "Gastrointestinal Complications after Bariatric
Surgery." *Journal of Gastroenterology and Hepatology* 11, no. 8 (2015): 526–35.
Retrieved from https://www.ncbi.nlm.nih.gov/pmc/articles/PMC4843041/.

Obesity Coverage. "Expected Weight Loss from Gastric Bypass—Calculator."
June 4, 2020, https://www.obesitycoverage.com/weight-loss-surgeries/
gastric-bypass/how-much-can-i-expect-to-lose.

Richelsen, B., S. Tonstad, S. Rossner, et al. "Effect of Orlistat on Weight Regain and Cardiovascular Risk Factors Following a Very-Low-Energy Diet in Abdominally Obese Patients: A 3-Year Randomized, Placebo-Controlled Study." *Diabetes Care* 30, no. 1 (2007): 27–32.

UC San Diego Health. "Gastric Banding." Accessed February 6, 2021, from https://health.ucsd.edu/specialties/surgery/bariatric/weight-loss-surgery/gastric-band/pages/default.aspx.

Resources

Mifflin, M. D., S. T. St. Jeor, L. A. Hill, B. J. Scott, S. A. Daugherty, and Y. O. Koh. "A New Predictive Equation for Resting Energy Expenditure in Healthy Individuals." *American Journal of Clinical Nutrition* 51, no. 2 (1990): 241–47.

Index

Boxes are indicated by b, figures by f, and tables by t following the page number.

daily activity. *See* functional activity

daily energy audit: daily weight loss calorie budget, 205–6; estimated caloric intake chart, 203f; level of daily activity, 202–3; weight loss by caloric reduction, 204–5

dairy products, 187–88, 220

dehydroepiandrosterone (DHEA), 313

depression and anxiety: depression questionnaire, 162–63b; diagnosis and management, 37b; finding professional help, 80; identifying, 162–63; weight changes and, 36–37; weight maintenance and, 302

DiClemente, Carlo, 29

diet and nutrition: caloric overload in U.S., 172; calorie consumption outside home, 174; dietary assessment, 80–82; dietary intake, declining quality of, 173; environmental influences, 172; fad diets, 175–76, 175b; foods to limit or avoid, 197–98, 198b; good diet, 176–79; lifestyle changes and sustainable weight loss, 176–79; low-calorie diet, 69–70; nutrition density, 179b, 185b; nutrition fact label, 173f; obesogenic diet, 173, 174; permanent weight loss/management, principles for, 295–98; portion sizes, increase in, 198–200; unconscious calorie consumption, 197b, 198; USDA Primary Dietary Guidelines, 179–97. *See also* calories and caloric intake; eating; foods

dietary evaluation, three-day (action item), 216–24; combination foods, 221; dairy and proteins, 220; diet modification tips, 222–23; eating events, 221; fats and oils, 219; food and activity log (resource), 348–49; food record (example), 217f; fruits and vegetables, 220; grains, 220; miscellaneous foods, 221; steps in, 218–19

dietary plan, designing, 172–224
choosing foods to match caloric needs, 206–7, 216
foods to limit or avoid, 197–98
healthy portion sizes, 198–200
low-calorie free foods, 224b
recommended servings by daily calorie goal: 1,600 calories, 208t; 1,800 calories, 209t; 2,000 calories, 210t; 2,400 calories, 212t; 2,600 calories, 213t; 2,800 calories, 214t; 3,000 calories, 215t
sample diet, 1,800 calories, 207t
three-day dietary evaluation (action item), 216–24
See also calories and caloric intake; USDA Primary Dietary Guidelines

dietitians, 70b, 80

diseases of despair, 9

dopamine, 115

drugs, weight loss. *See* over-the-counter supplements; prescription medications

dumping syndrome, 332

foods (*continued*)
high-sodium, 192, 192b; high-volume, 185b; intake, scheduling and tracking, 61–62; portion sizes, 198–200; as reward, avoiding, 123–25; as stress reliever, 116; water content, 196. *See also* diet and nutrition; USDA Primary Dietary Guidelines

food shopping: calcium-rich foods, 232; do's and don'ts, 230–33; food groups, 229, 231; frozen/canned fruits and vegetables, 232; go-to grocery items, 233b; meat, poultry, and fish, 232–33; planning ahead, 229–30; produce, 231, 232b; staple foods, 233–34, 233b; using list, 230–31

Ford, Henry, 65

forgiveness, and stress reduction, 107b

French food: caloric intake, 228; dangers for weight loss and maintenance, 236–37; healthful choices, 236–37, 243

frequency (exercise), 274–75

friends. *See* buddy system; social support

fruits, 184, 220

Frutchey, Robin A., 10–11

fullness cues (eating behavior), 150

functional activity: adding movement to daily activities, 264–66; level of, 202–3; types of, 256, 264–65. *See also* daily energy audit

Garcinia cambogia (brindleberry), 314

gastrectomy, sleeve, 329, 331–32

gastric balloon, 333–34

gastric banding., 329, 332–33

gastric bypass, Roux-en-Y, 329, 332

genetics and healthy weight, 14

ghrelin, 137

Glascoe, Shavise, 11

gradual change, 96–97

grains, 183–84; dietary evaluation, 220; whole grains, 184b

grazing (eating behavior), 219

Gudzune, Kimberly, 10

habits: as triggers for overeating, 143, 148; weight gain and, 69

happiness, food as, 123

hCG (human chorionic gonadotropin), 315

health improvement, as weight loss motivator, 40

heart disease: obesity and risk of, 17, 18f

hips: mindful movements, 268–69, 269f

history of present illness (HPI), 73

HMB (beta-hydroxy-beta-methylbutyrate), 314

home environment: preparation for weight loss program, 59–60

hormones: overeating and, 136

hot-button topics, avoiding, 106b

human chorionic gonadotropin (hCG), 315

hunger: continuum of, 112; as physical trigger for overeating, 136

medications: causing weight gain, 38; over-the-counter supplements, 310–16. *See also* prescription medications

MediSpas, 316

menopause, 136

menstrual cycle: overeating and, 136

mental health: body weight and, 36–37

mental triggers for overeating, 142–43

metformin, 324–25, 325b

Mexican food, healthful choices, 242–43

milk, 188, 189

mindful movements: application, 271–73; checklist, 266–70; elbow and knee, 267; fingers and toes, 271; hips, 268–69, 269f; readiness for weight loss, expert assessment, 70b; shoulders, 269–70; spine, 267–68; three planes of motion, 266f

mindfulness: definition, 62; mindful eating, 62–64; mindful movement and exercise, 64–65

mindset barriers to weight loss: expecting better treatment by world following weight loss, 8; lack of personal commitment, 7–8; weight loss as personal choice, 6b

mindset mastery: action items, 101; as key to weight loss success, 93–96, 156–58; lifestyle change and sustainable weight loss, 179; self-talk, 93–94, 158; statements of, 95b, 96

monitoring strategies, weight loss:

nonanalyst, 246, 249–50; partial analyst, 246, 248–49; super analyst, 245, 247–48; types of, defined, 245–46

motivation: lack of, in weight loss failure, 54; weight loss readiness and, 27f, 39–45

naltrexone, bupropion with, 323–24, 324b

National Weight Control Registry, 6, 34

Neff, Kirsten, 144–45b

neurotransmitters, 115

nicotine, 140, 327. *See also* smoking cessation

nutrition density: definition, 179b; empty calories, 192–93, 193b; energy-dense high-volume foods, 185b. *See also* diet and nutrition

obesity: diet and fitness industries exploiting, 5; global rates, 9f; overweight vs., 18, 19t; portion size and, 199; risk factors, 17–18, 18f

obesity medicine specialists, 317

obesogenic diet, 173, 174

occupational therapists, 279

orlistat (Alli), 320–21, 322b, 326b

osteoarthritis: obesity and, 17

osteoporosis: excess protein intake and, 186

Overeaters Anonymous, 59

over-the-counter supplements, 310–16; common ingredients, 312–14; hCG (human chorionic gonadotropin), 315; labels, importance of reading, 311–12

overweight: BMI interpretation, 19t; health risk, 18

past medical history, 75–76

Patient Health Questionnaire (PHQ), 163

pedometers, 259

percentage of excess weight, 332

perfectionism, avoidable stress and, 107b

personal appearance, as weight loss motivator, 39–40

Personal Plan of Action
daily movement plan, 264–66
family involvement, 135
keys to weight loss success: clear, attainable and reasonable goals, 90–91; commitment to journey vs. destination, 88–89; flexibility, 99–100; gradual changes, 96–97; journaling the journey, 100–101; making weight loss activities fun, 97–99; mastering mindset, 93–96; reliable support system, 91–92
low-calorie diet and individualized weight loss plan, 69
physical activity plan, 254, 272–73
reassessing needs to avoid burnout, 100
as road map for weight loss/ management, 7, 15, 88, 89
template (resource), 338–47
weight maintenance, 299–300

personal trainers, 83

pets: avoid sleeping with, 138b

phentermine HCl, 320–21, 326b; facts about, 319b; with topiramate, 320, 321b, 326b

physical activity: daily movement, health benefits of, 254f, 255; energy expenditure, 254, 256; exercise as full range of, 82; intensity levels, 260, 260t; mindful movement breaks, scheduling, 62; movement and activity assessment (resource), 350–51; three planes of motion, 266f; tracking daily movement and weekly exercise, 61; weight changes and, 36. *See also* exercise; inactivity (sedentary lifestyle)

physical activity planning
action items, 288
daily movement (step 2), 264–76; adding movement to daily activities, 264–66; mindful movements, 266–73; SMART goals/framework, 264, 354–55 (*see also* functional activity)
exercise planning (step 3), 273–79
helpful hints for success, 279–88; create schedule you can live with, 280–81; cross-training, 286; fighting plateaus with self-challenge, 285–86; fitness buddy, 286–87; have Plan A and Plan B, 281–82; plan exercise experience, 283; set stage for success, 284; track exercise in journal, 283–84; warm up and cool down time, 284–85